PRACTICUM AND INTERNSHIP

Completely revised and updated, the fifth edition of *Practicum and Internship* is an eminently practical resource that provides students and supervisors with thorough coverage of the theoretical and practical aspects of the practicum and internship process.

New to this edition is:

- an accompanying website with downloadable, customizable forms, contracts, and vitae;
- thoughtful discussion of the *Diagnostic and Statistical Manual of Mental Disorders* (5th ed.; *DSM-5*) and the Health Insurance Portability and Accountability Act (HIPAA) guidelines, and the most recent standards of the Council for the Accreditation of Counseling and Related Educational Programs (CACREP);
- expanded analysis of the use of technology and social media in counseling;
- expanded discussions of ethical decision making and ethical guidelines for informed consent and for supervision contracts in individual settings;
- new and updated materials on case conceptualization, assessment, goal setting, and treatment planning;
- new materials reviewing third-wave counseling theories and practices, including mindfulness-based stress reduction, mindfulness-based cognitive therapy, acceptance and commitment therapy, and dialectical behavior therapy; and
- detailed presentation of a skill-based model for counseling training, and self-assessment questionnaires and guided reflection exercises for application and orientation to the model.

Judith Scott, PhD, is professor emeritus of the Department of Psychology in Education at the University of Pittsburgh and maintains a private practice in outpatient psychotherapy in Pittsburgh, Pennsylvania.

John C. Boylan, PhD, was professor of counseling and psychology at Marywood University in Scranton, Pennsylvania.

Christin M. Jungers, PhD, LPCC, is an associate professor in the clinical mental health counseling program at Franciscan University of Steubenville in Steubenville, Ohio.

PRACTICUM AND INTERNSHIP

Textbook and Resource Guide for Counseling and Psychotherapy

Fifth Edition

Judith Scott, John C. Boylan, and Christin M. Jungers

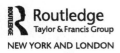

Routledge
Taylor & Francis Group

NEW YORK AND LONDON

First published 2015
by Routledge
711 Third Avenue, New York, NY 10017

and by Routledge
27 Church Road, Hove, East Sussex BN3 2FA

Routledge is an imprint of the Taylor & Francis Group, an informa business

Fourth edition published 2008 by Routledge

First edition published 1988 by Accelerated Development

Library of Congress Cataloging-in-Publication Data
  Scott, Judith, 1940–
Practicum and internship : textbook and resource guide for counseling and psychotherapy / by Judith Scott, John C. Boylan, and Christin M. Jungers. — Fifth edition.
    pages cm
Previous edition cataloged under John Charles Boylan.
  Includes bibliographical references and index.
  1. Psychotherapy—Study and teaching (Internship)—Outlines, syllabi, etc.
  2. Psychotherapy—Study and teaching—Supervision—Outlines, syllabi, etc.
  3. Psychotherapy—Study and teaching (Internship)—Forms. 4. Psychotherapy—Study and teaching—Supervision—Forms. I. Boylan, John Charles. II. Jungers, Christin M. III. Title.
  RC459.B68 2015
  616.89'140076—dc23
  2014011115

ISBN: 978-1-138-80147-9 (hbk)
ISBN: 978-1-138-79651-5 (pbk)
ISBN: 978-1-315-75489-5 (ebk)

Typeset in Stone Serif
by Apex CoVantage, LLC

Printed and bound in the United States of America by
Edwards Brothers Malloy on sustainably sourced paper

To my children and their spouses: Kristin and Bill Pardini; Troy and Kristin Scott; Megan and Adam Swift; and Neil and Shannon Scott for their loving support of my life and work.

To my grandchildren: Brenna, Katrina, and Nate Scott; Josie and Mica Swift; Riley, Aiden (AJ), and Ellie Scott; and Roman and Levi Pardini, who bring me constant joy and hope for the future.

And to the memory of my dear friend and colleague, Jack Boylan.

Judith Scott

To Jean Boylan, Jack's wife and constant support.

To his children and their spouses: John and Lisa Boylan; and Meghan and Ken Senisi, who meant the world to him.

And to his grandchildren: Luke and Emily Boylan; and Molly and Caroline Senisi, who were truly his blessings.

John C. Boylan

To my family, who have brought so much happiness to my life; and especially to my niece, Natalie, and my nephews, Nicholas and Benjamin. May you grow up to know how special each one of you is and how much you have to offer this world.

Christin M. Jungers

CONTENTS

About the Authors   xvii
Preface   xix
Acknowledgments   xxi
Overview of the Book   xxiii

SECTION I PREPRACTICUM

CHAPTER 1 Preparing for Practicum and Internship   3

Becoming a Professional Counselor   3
  Steps to Becoming a Professional Counselor   4
Accreditation Standards for Practicum and Internship   4
  CACREP Standards for Practicum and Internship   5
  CORE Standards for Practicum and Internship   6
  CACEP Standards for Initial and Final Practicum   6
  APA-CoA Standards for Practicum and Internship in Counseling Psychology   7
  AAPC Standards for Practicum and Internship for Pastoral Counselors   7
Counselor Certification   7
  National Certified Counselor (NCC)   7
  NBCC Specialty Certifications   8
  Certified Rehabilitation Counselor (CRC)   8
  Canadian Certified Counsellor (CCC): CCPA   8
  Registered Professional Counsellor (RPC): Canadian Professional
    Counsellors Association   8
  Other Specialty Counseling Certifications   9
State Licensure for Counselors and Psychologists   9
Prepracticum Considerations   10
  Checklist of Questions to Be Researched and Answered Before
    Practicum Site Selection   10

Phases of Practicum and Internship   11

    Development Reflected in the Program Structure   11

    Development Reflected in the Learning Process   12

    Development Reflected in Supervisor Interaction   12

Implications   12

Summary   12

References   13

CHAPTER 2   Securing a Practicum/Internship Site   **15**

Guidelines for Choosing a Practicum/Internship Site   15

Criteria for Site Selection   16

    Professional Staff and Supervisor   16

    Professional Affiliations of the Site   16

    Professional Practices of the Site   16

    Site Administration   17

    Training and Supervision Values   17

    Theoretical Orientation of the Site and Supervisor   17

    Client Population   17

Negotiating the Practicum/Internship Placement   19

    Typical Questions Asked at the Interview   19

Getting Oriented to Your Field Site   20

Role and Function of the Practicum/Internship Student   21

Summary   22

References   22

SECTION II   BEGINNING TO WORK WITH CLIENTS

CHAPTER 3   Starting the Practicum   **25**

Beginning the Practicum Experience   25

    Getting Started: Where Do I Begin?   25

    I've Taken the Classes, but Do I Really Know What to Do?   26

    What if I Say Something Wrong?   26

    How Do I Know When to Use the Right Techniques?   27

    But I'm Just a Rookie! (Learning to Trust Yourself and Your Inner Voice)   27

    When in Doubt, Consult! (Your Faculty and Site Supervisors Are There to Help You)   28

Preparing to Meet With Your First Client   28

    The Health Insurance Portability and Accountability Act (HIPAA)   29

    Informed Consent   30

Sample Informed Consent and Disclosure Statement   31

Establishing a Therapeutic Alliance   34

The Initial Session With the Client   35

Structured and Unstructured Interviews   35

Basic and Advanced Helping Skills   36

Procedural and Issue-Specific Skills   37

Structuring the Initial Session   38

Closing the Initial Session   39

Pretherapy Intake Information   39

Intake Summary   40

Client Record Keeping   40

Progress Notes   40

The DAP Format   41

The SOAP Notes Format   41

Record Keeping and the School Counselor   41

Documenting Practicum Hours   45

Summary   45

Note   45

References   45

CHAPTER 4   Assessment and Case Conceptualization   47

Initial Assessment   48

Gathering Family History Data   49

Gathering Personal History Data   49

Obtaining Information From Others   50

Goals of Assessment   50

Processes and Categories for Assessing Client Problems   50

Assessing the Client's Mental Status   52

Mental Status Categories of Assessment   52

Diagnosis in Counseling   53

DSM-5   54

Elimination of the Multiaxial Assessment System   55

Subtypes and Specifiers   55

Other Specified and Unspecified Designation   55

DSM-5 Codes and Classification   56

Sharing Assessment Information With the Client   56

Gathering Additional Data   57

Assessing the Client's Progress   57

Reporting Therapeutic Progress   60

Implications   60
Case Conceptualization   60
    Case Conceptualization Models   61
        The "Linchpin" Model   61
        The Inverted Pyramid Model   62
        The Integrative Model   63
Summary   63
References   64

■ **CHAPTER 5**   Goal Setting, Treatment Planning, and
                   Treatment Modalities   **67**

Goal Setting in Counseling   67
    Goals and the Stages of Change Model   67
    Types of Goals   68
Developing a Treatment Plan   69
A Review of Philosophy, Theories, and Theory-Based Techniques of Counseling   71
Identifying Your Theory and Technique Preferences   75
Extending the Counselor's Theory-Based Techniques   80
    Solution-Focused Brief Therapy   80
    Strategic Solution-Focused Therapy   82
    Cognitive Restructuring Brief Therapy   83
    Rational Emotive Brief Therapy   83
    Coping Skills Brief Therapy   83
Third-Wave Therapies   84
    Mindfulness-Based Therapy (MBT)   84
    Mindfulness-Based Stress Reduction (MBSR)   85
    Mindfulness-Based Cognitive Therapy (MBCT)   85
    Acceptance and Commitment Therapy (ACT)   86
    Dialectical Behavior Therapy (DBT)   86
Summary   87
References   87

SECTION III SUPERVISION IN PRACTICUM AND INTERNSHIP

■ **CHAPTER 6**   Group Supervision in Practicum and Internship   **93**

Identifying Counseling Skill Areas   93
    Skill Area One: Counseling Performance Skills   93
        Basic and Advanced Counseling Skills   93

Theory-Based Techniques   94
Procedural Skills   94
Professional and Issue-Specific Skills   94
Skill Area Two: Cognitive Counseling Skills   94
Skill Area Three: Self-Awareness/Multicultural Awareness Skills   94
Self-Awareness Skills   94
Multicultural Awareness Skills   95
Skill Area Four: Developmental Level   95
Self-Assessment in the Skill Areas   96
Sample Supervisee Goal Statement   96
Concepts in Group Supervision   97
Group Supervision in Practicum   99
Sample of Course Objectives and Assignments in Group Practicum   101
Activities in Group Supervision   102
Peer Consultation   102
Evaluation of Practicum in Group Supervision   104
Formative Evaluation   104
Summative Evaluation   104
Transitioning Into Internship   105
Recommended Skill Levels for Transitioning Into Internship   105
Group Supervision in Internship   105
Group Supervision Models in Internship   107
The SPGS Model   107
The Structured Group Supervision (SGS) Model   108
Evaluation in Group Supervision of Internship   108
Summary   109
References   109

CHAPTER 7 Individual Supervision in Practicum and Internship   111

Role and Function of the Supervisor in Practicum and Internship   111
Administrative and Clinical Supervision   112
The Supervisor–Supervisee Relationship   112
What Is "Lousy" Supervision?   113
Overarching Principles   114
General Spheres   114
Approaches to Individual Supervision   114
Models Grounded in Psychotherapy Theory: The Psychodynamic Model   115
Developmental Models: The Integrated Developmental Model   115
Process Models: The Discrimination Model   116

The Triadic Model of Supervision   117
The Clinical Supervision Process   119
    Informed Consent in Supervision   119
    Sample of a Supervisor Informed Consent and Disclosure Statement   119
    Forming a Supervision Contract   121
    Sample Supervision Contract   122
    The Supervision Session Format   123
    Supervising the Developing Counselor-in-Training   124
Evaluation of Individual Supervision in Practicum and Internship   126
    Summative Evaluation in Practicum   126
    Sample of a Midpoint Narrative Evaluation of a Practicum Student   126
    Summative Evaluation in Internship   128
    Documenting Internship Hours   129
Summary   129
References   129

SECTION IV PROFESSIONAL PRACTICE TOPICS

CHAPTER 8   Selected Topics on Ethical Issues in Counseling   135

Definitions: Ethics, Morality, and Law   135
Ethical Codes for Counselors   136
    Websites for Ethical Codes and Related Standards for Professional Organizations   136
Codes of Ethics: Similarities   137
Ethical Decision Making   137
    Principle-Based Ethics and Ethical Decision Making   137
    Virtue-Based Ethics and Ethical Decision Making   140
    Self-Tests After Resolving an Ethical Dilemma   142
The Use of Technology in Counseling   142
Summary   145
References   146

CHAPTER 9   Selected Topics on Legal Issues in Counseling   149

The Law   149
Classifications of the Law   149
Types of Laws   150
The Steps in a Lawsuit   150
Elements of Malpractice   151

Why Clients Sue   152

Risk Management and the Counselor   153

Liability Insurance   154

Privacy, Confidentiality, and Privileged Communication   154

Release of Information   156

When the Counselor Must Breach Confidentiality   156

    The Law and the Duty to Protect: The Suicidal Client   156

    The Law and the Duty to Warn: The Potentially Dangerous Client   157

    Mandatory Reporting: Suspected Child Abuse and Neglect   158

    Mandatory Reporting: Suspected Harm to Vulnerable Adults   159

    The Law and the Practice of Counsellor–Client Confidentiality in Canada   159

Managed Care and the Counselor   159

Client Records   161

Summary   162

References   162

CHAPTER 10 Working With Clients in Crisis and Other Special Populations — 165

Understanding Crisis and Trauma   165

    The Kanel Model of Crisis Intervention   166

    The James and Gilliland Model of Crisis Intervention   167

Crisis Intervention in Schools   169

    School Counselors as Prevention Consultants for Crises   170

    Suggestions for a School-Based Training on Crisis Response   170

    Post-Crisis: Understanding Children's Responses   172

The High-Risk Client: Understanding and Assessing Harm to Self   173

    Defining Suicide and Debunking Common Myths   173

    Warning Signs for Suicide   175

    Risk Assessment for Suicide   176

        Assessment Point 1: Desire to Die   176

        Assessment Point 2: Capacity to Commit Suicide   176

        Assessment Point 3: Suicidal Intent   177

        Assessment Point 4: Buffers Against Suicide   177

        Evaluating Suicide Risk: Putting It All Together   178

    Suicide Risk Assessment Instruments   178

    Intervention and Planning   179

    Ethical and Legal Mandates Relating to Danger to Self   180

        Professional School Counselors   180

Professional Counselors 180

Suicide Risk Assessment and Prevention in Schools 181

Basics of Suicide Prevention Programs in Schools 181

Learning About and Responding to Potentially Suicidal Students 182

Suicide Risk Assessment for Students 183

The High-Risk Client: Potential Harm to Others 184

The *Tarasoff* Case: The Events 184

Implications of the *Tarasoff* Case 185

What *Tarasoff* Did Not Require 185

Post-*Tarasoff* 185

Risk Assessment for Potentially Dangerous Clients 186

Task I: Risk Assessment 186

Task II: Selecting a Course of Action 188

Task III: Monitoring the Situation 188

Clients' Past Criminal Acts 188

The Client Who Is Being Abused: Responding, Reporting, and Intervening 189

Legal Issues Related to Reporting Child Abuse 192

Making a Report Related to Child Abuse 192

Interviewing Children Who May Have Been Sexually Abused 193

Before the Interview 193

Interviewing the Child 193

Counseling the Sexually Abused 194

The Client Who Is Dealing With Addiction 196

Understanding Addiction 196

Diagnosing Alcohol and Drug Use 196

What Is Treatment? 197

What Is Recovery? 198

Stages of Recovery 198

Counseling Recommendations for Clients With Addiction 199

Preventing Relapse 200

Summary 201

References 201

■ **CHAPTER 11** Consultation in the Schools and
Mental Health Agencies: Models and Methods 207

Definition of Consultation 207

Types of Mental Health Consultation 208

Characteristics of Mental Health Consultation   209
Dimensions of Internal and External Consultation   210
Consultation or Collaboration?   210
Assumptions of and Metaphors for Consultation   211
    The Purchase-of-Expertise Model   211
    The Doctor–Patient Model   212
    The Process Consultation Model   212
Cultural Issues in Consultation   212
School Consultation   213
    Consultation Models and Practices in Schools   215
    Sensorimotor   216
    Concrete   216
    Formal-Operational   216
    Dialectic/Systemic   217
General Guidelines for Consultation   218
    Preentry   218
    Entry Into the System   219
    Orientation to Consultation   219
    Problem Identification   220
    Consultation Intervention   220
Assessing the Impact of Consultation   221
Resistance to Consultation   222
Contracting and the Forces of Change in the Organization   223
Summary   224
References   224

CHAPTER 12 Final Evaluations   **227**

Appendix I: The Supervisee Performance Assessment Instrument   231
Appendix II: Psychiatric Medications   237

FORMS
    Form 2.1   Practicum Contract   247
    Form 2.2   Internship Contract   249
    Form 2.3   Student Profile Sheet   251
    Form 2.4   Student Practicum/Internship Agreement   252
    Form 3.1a   Parental Release Form: Secondary School Counseling   253
    Form 3.1b   Elementary School Counseling Permission Form   254
    Form 3.2   Client Permission to Record Counseling Session for Supervision Purposes 255
    Form 3.3   Initial Intake Form   256

Form 3.4   Psychosocial History   258
Form 3.5   Case Notes   262
Form 3.6   Weekly Schedule/Practicum Log   264
Form 3.7   Monthly Practicum Log   265
Form 4.1   Elementary School Counseling Referral Form   266
Form 4.2   Secondary School Counseling Referral Form   267
Form 4.3   Mental Status Checklist   269
Form 4.4   Therapeutic Progress Report   272
Form 5.1   Counseling Techniques List   273
Form 6.1   Self-Assessment of Counseling Performance Skills   277
Form 6.2   Self-Awareness/Multicultural Awareness Rating Scale   279
Form 6.3   Directed Reflection Exercise on Supervision   280
Form 6.4   Supervisee Goal Statement   281
Form 6.5   Tape Critique Form   282
Form 6.6   Peer Rating Form   283
Form 6.7   Interviewer Rating Form   284
Form 7.1   Supervision Contract   286
Form 7.2   Supervisor Notes   288
Form 7.3   Supervisee Notes on Individual Supervision   289
Form 7.4   Supervisor's Formative Evaluation of Supervisee's Counseling Practice 290
Form 7.5   Supervisor's Final Evaluation of Practicum Student   292
Form 7.6   Supervisor's Final Evaluation of Intern   293
Form 10.1   Suicide Consultation Form   295
Form 10.2   Harm to Others Form   298
Form 10.3   Child Abuse Reporting Form   301
Form 10.4   Substance Abuse Assessment Form   302
Form 12.1   Weekly Internship Log   305
Form 12.2   Summary Internship Log   306
Form 12.3   Evaluation of Intern's Practice in Site Activities   307
Form 12.4   Client's Assessment of the Counseling Experience   308
Form 12.5   Supervisee Evaluation of Supervisor   309
Form 12.6   Site Evaluation Form   311

Index   313

ABOUT THE AUTHORS

Judith Scott, PhD, is a licensed psychologist, certified school counselor, National Certified Counselor, and professor emeritus of the Department of Psychology in Education at the University of Pittsburgh. During her tenure at the University of Pittsburgh she served as director of doctoral studies and as field site coordinator in the CACREP-accredited counseling programs. She is a past president of Pennsylvania ACES and was awarded Counselor Educator of the Year by the Pennsylvania School Counselors Association. Dr. Scott maintains a private practice that specializes in outpatient individual psychotherapy in women's issues and infertility counseling. Her research focuses on counseling supervision and women's adult development.

John C. Boylan, PhD, was a licensed psychologist, certified school counselor, and certified sex therapist. Dr. Boylan was professor of counseling and psychology at Marywood University, Scranton, Pennsylvania. During his long tenure at Marywood, he served as chairperson of the Graduate Psychology and Counseling Program and director of Career Planning and Placement. In addition to his academic duties, Dr. Boylan maintained a private practice in individual, marital, and sex therapy in Clarks Summit and Scranton, Pennsylvania. After moving to South Carolina, he taught part time in the Department of Psychology and Sociology at Coastal Carolina University and in the Graduate Counseling Program at Webster University, Myrtle Beach, South Carolina.

Christin M. Jungers, PhD, LPCC, is an associate professor at Franciscan University of Steubenville in the Clinical Mental Health Counseling Program. She is a licensed professional clinical counselor who has experience working with a variety of life span issues faced by individuals and couples. Dr. Jungers has co-authored two other books and numerous articles. She is currently a member of the counselor licensure board in Ohio.

PREFACE

Since the publication of the first edition of this text in 1988, each new edition has evolved to provide materials which support the many changes and developments in the counseling profession and the preparation of professional counselors. In particular, the experiences and competencies required of counselors-in-training while involved in their practicum and internship placement have been and continue to be the focus of this book. As a counselor educator, it has been exciting and my privilege to have been a part of participating in a process that enhances the quality of those who become certified as professional counselors. For the first four editions, John C. Boylan shepherded the work through the updates, revisions, and additions. It is now my turn to carry the work forward and to bring in a counselor educator from a new generation, Christin Jungers, to continue with this gratifying and important work. This fifth edition has benefited greatly from new views and new voices. I am excited about the reorganization of this text, respectful of the maturation of our profession, and hopeful about the many contributions of the new professional counselors.

Judith Scott

ACKNOWLEDGMENTS

The authors gratefully appreciate the efforts of the following individuals, who were instrumental in the development of the fifth edition of this textbook:

The graduate counseling students at Marywood University, the University of Pittsburgh, and Franciscan University of Steubenville for all they have contributed to our professional growth and enhancement;

Anna Moore, editor at Routledge, whose understanding and editorial suggestions were invaluable in the development of the textbook;

Elizabeth Graber, editorial assistant, whose help with obtaining the needed permissions and being available for assistance was very much appreciated;

Our reviewers, especially Dawn McBride, who provided valuable recommendations about how to reorganize and streamline the text, as well as thoughtful insight into new topics that might be addressed;

Jocelyn Gregoire, PhD, for his helpful and constructive feedback on the manuscript, especially related to risk assessment and crisis intervention;

Patrick Malley, PhD, for his many contributions to the development of this text, especially the first three editions, and many conversations regarding ethics and the law in counseling;

Daria Brown and Troy Scott, for providing assistance and guidance with the much-needed computer skills for producing the manuscript for this text;

Therese Dumas, a graduate student at Franciscan University, for her careful review of the references and citations in the manuscript.

OVERVIEW OF THE BOOK

The fifth edition of this text guides students through the important preprofessional training experiences, from the selection of an appropriate practicum site to the final evaluation of the internship. The text is reorganized related to a skill-based approach to the practicum and internship experience. Separate chapters related to counseling performance, cognitive skills, group and individual supervision, and selected topics in professional practice include related professional resource materials, practical self-assessment instruments, and guidelines, formats, and forms to assist in applied counseling and supervision practices.

The first part of the text focuses on the preparation, identification, and application process to secure a field site placement. Chapter 1 provides foundational information which students must consider as they prepare to identify their practicum/internship placements. Chapter 2 guides students through the process of selecting, applying for, securing, and orienting to a site appropriate to their professional goals and specializations.

The second part of the text emphasizes counseling performance skills and cognitive counseling skills. Chapter 3 emphasizes starting the practicum and initiating contact with clients and includes a sample informed consent statement and current HIPAA (Health Insurance Portability and Accountability Act) guidelines. Chapter 4 includes assessment and case conceptualization practices, references, and models to be used in practice with clients. An overview of the new *DSM-5* (*Diagnostic and Statistical Manual of Mental Disorders*, 5th ed.) coding and classification system is included. Chapter 5 content areas include goal setting, treatment planning, and theory-related approaches to treatment. A new section which reviews the "New Wave" theories of mindfulness-based practices, acceptance and commitment therapy, and dialectical behavior therapy has been added.

The third section is focused on group and individual supervision. Chapter 6, on group supervision, begins with a full description of the skill-based model and includes self-assessment exercises for the supervision group to use to become more familiar with the model. Chapter 7, on individual supervision, describes several regularly applied models of individual supervision which students may encounter as well as an expanded section about the triadic model of supervision. A sample informed consent and disclosure statement for supervisors and a sample supervision contract consistent with the Association for Counselor Education and Supervision's best practices guidelines are included. New forms which support the application of best practices, such as supervisor notes, supervisee notes, and evaluation checklists and formats, have been added.

The fourth section of the text includes chapters on selected topics related to professional practices in ethics, law, and assessment of and response to crisis situations and substance abuse.

Current guidelines for the use of technology in counseling and the application of principle-based, virtue-based, and self-review approaches to ethical decision making are included. Information on crisis intervention and response as well as risk assessment tools and revised content related to substance abuse assessment and related forms has been updated.

Forms and samples of completed forms have been referenced throughout the text. A complete set of available forms is provided in the Forms section at the end of the text. They can now be accessed for download on the website for this edition of the text at www.routledgementalhealth.com/cw/scott.

We are very pleased with this new edition and hope that the information, materials, and resources included will provide the student, counselor, and supervisor with a useful and reader-friendly approach to the practicum and internship experience.

SECTION I

PREPRACTICUM

CHAPTER 1

PREPARING FOR PRACTICUM AND INTERNSHIP

The focus of this book is on fostering the development of qualified, competent practitioners in the helping professions. It is written for students registered in graduate programs in professional counseling and psychology. The first two chapters of the book are designed to provide the counselor-in-training with foundational information about what the professional accreditation requirements are for practicum and internship and how to identify, apply for, and secure a field placement. The emphasis in practicum and internship is on the application of basic knowledge in the practice of counseling at the field site of choice. It is possible for the professional counselor to practice in a variety of settings (i.e., schools, colleges and universities, mental health agencies, career centers). Practicum and internship experiences are required in a broad variety of preparation programs in the helping professions. Counselor education and psychology training programs, national associations, and the accrediting bodies related to these specializations continue to clarify and solidify the definitions of practicum and internship, along with their field experience requirements. They also specify activities, experiences, and knowledge base requirements that are appropriate to each component of training. Similarly, national accrediting bodies specify the qualifications and levels of experience of both field and campus-based supervisors. Practicum and internship are measured by clock hours, with the required number increasing as the profession advances.

Becoming a Professional Counselor

The new consensus definition of counseling is that "counseling is a professional relationship that empowers diverse individuals, families, and groups to accomplish mental health, wellness, education, and career goals" (American Counseling Association, 2010, para. 2). Counseling, over the last 75 years, has evolved into achieving a recognized professional status. Professionalization has been accomplished through forming associations, changing names to reduce identification with its previous occupational status, developing a code of ethics, and obtaining public sanction through the passage of licensure laws in all 50 states. Changes taking place in the last 30 years include increases in the credit hours required in training, the establishment of accreditation and certification standards, increases in the body of knowledge in counseling as distinguished from psychology, and the passage of state laws granting privilege in interactions between counselors and clients (Remley & Herlihy, 2014).

Professional counselors apply a wellness model of mental health in their work which emphasizes helping people maximize their potential rather than curing their illness. Counselors emphasize prevention and early intervention rather than remediation. In addition, the training of counselors focuses on teaching counseling skills rather than physical health care and psychopathology (Remley & Herlihy, 2014). It is important that the student identifies a field site setting that understands and respects the foundational values of the professional counselor.

Steps to Becoming a Professional Counselor

Schweiger, Henderson, McKaskill, & Collins (2012) have reviewed the steps one must take in order to become certified and recognized as a professional counselor. A summary of these steps is

1. Complete a master's degree program in counseling. The program may or may not be a nationally accredited program.
2. Complete a practicum.
3. Complete a supervised clinical internship with clients in your specialty area.
4. Graduate from a master's degree (or higher) counseling program.
5. Apply to the national certification board or the appropriate credentialing association and obtain certification. Completion of an accredited program usually allows one to sit for certification exams immediately following graduation.
6. Apply to the state board and obtain state licensure. (pp. 4–5)

Accreditation Standards for Practicum and Internship

Accreditation of counselor preparation programs in the United States and Canada is a voluntary process; the accreditation bodies are independent from federal and state and provincial governments. In most cases, the accreditation body was initially established by a professional association. For example, the American Counseling Association established the Council for the Accreditation of Counseling and Related Educational Programs (CACREP); the American Association for Marriage and Family Therapy established the Commission on Accreditation for Marriage and Family Therapy Education (COAMFTE); the American Association for Pastoral Counselors (AAPC) became the accrediting body for pastoral counselors; the Council on Rehabilitation Education (CORE) became the accrediting body for rehabilitation counselors; the American Psychological Association Commission on Accreditation (APA-CoA) became the accrediting body for psychologists; and the Canadian Counselling and Psychotherapy Association (CCPA) established the Council on Accreditation of Counsellor Education Programs (CACEP—Council on Accreditation). Each accrediting body established criteria to be met by programs before accreditation. If a department offers more than one program, each program must be evaluated separately for accreditation. Thus, a department may have some programs that are accredited and others that are not. Graduation from an accredited program has a number of significant advantages for students. For example, accredited programs

- provide assurance that the program meets high professional standards,
- provide periodic review of the program,
- offer graduates of the program advantages such as sitting for the national certification exams immediately following graduation, and
- provide a source of pride for faculty, students, and the college or university as they become involved in a nationally recognized program (Schweiger et al., 2012, pp. 7–9).

The major applied components in counselor preparation are practicum and internship. Professional practice provides for the development of counseling skills under supervision. Practicum/internship students will counsel clients in their specialty who represent the ethnic and demographic diversity of the community. Their hours of direct service will be with actual clients, which will contribute to the development of required counseling skills. The internship is begun after successful completion of the practicum. The internship should reflect the comprehensive work of a professional in the designated program specialty and include individual and group counseling.

Practicum and internship requirements have undergone four major changes in recent years: (a) the amount of time spent in practicum and internship has increased, (b) the setting in which the experience occurs has changed, (c) the specifications for the supervisor doing the clinical supervision of practicum and internship have become more stringent, and (d) the number of hours spent in supervision has increased. These four aspects could make major differences in the job opportunities, types of practice, clientele, philosophical orientation, and techniques emphasized throughout the student's professional life. For these reasons, as well as others (e.g., personalities involved, practicum and internship sites available), each student needs to give considerable attention to practicum and internship: under whose clinical supervision it occurs, and for what period of time.

If a student is attending a counselor preparation program that has not sought accreditation, it may be wise to consider standards regarding practicum and internship when fulfilling the professional practice requirements of the counselor preparation program. The student is encouraged to keep careful records of total practicum and internship hours, client contact hours, supervision hours, and supervisor credentials—both on-site and on campus. The forms in this textbook can be helpful for such record keeping. For the student who wishes to pursue state licensure and national certification, evidence of a practicum and internship equivalent to those in an accredited program may be necessary.

CACREP Standards for Practicum and Internship

CACREP accredits entry-level programs at the master's degree level in six areas:

> Addictions Counseling (60 semester hours)
> Career Counseling (48 semester hours)
> Clinical Mental Health Counseling (60 semester hours)
> Marriage, Couple, and Family Counseling (60 semester hours)
> School Counseling (48 semester hours)
> Student Affairs and College Counseling (48 semester hours)

CACREP guidelines are expected to increase the total semester hours required in each of these specialties to 60 semester hours beginning in 2020. The following summarizes information about the primary aspects of practicum and internship in each of the above specializations:

Setting: An agency, institution, or organization appropriate to the specialization in one of the above identified specialties.

Practicum: Minimum of 100 clock hours over a minimum 10-week academic term with 40 hours of direct contact with actual clients in the area of specialty; weekly average of 1 hour of individual or triadic supervision with site and/or faculty supervisor; and weekly average of 1 1/2 hours of group supervision by faculty.

Internship: Minimum of 600 clock hours with at least 240 clock hours of direct service, including leading groups; weekly average of 1 hour per week of individual or triadic supervision, usually by site supervisor; and weekly average of 1 1/2 hours per week of group supervision by a faculty supervisor.

Supervisor: Faculty supervisor must have a doctoral degree and/or appropriate counseling preparation. Site supervisor must have a minimum of a master's degree in counseling or a related profession with appropriate certification or license and two years of experience as a practicing counselor in the specialty area of the student (CACREP, 2009).

CORE Standards for Practicum and Internship

CORE is the accrediting body for master's degree programs in rehabilitation counseling. In October 2013, CACREP and its affiliate CORE announced the establishment of accreditation standards for a Clinical Rehabilitation Counseling specialization which would be jointly administered. For more information about this new specialization, access www.cacrep.org. A summary of the practicum and internship requirements follows (CORE, 2012).

Setting: An agency or facility that provides services to disabled persons from diverse populations.

Practicum: 100 hours of supervised rehabilitation counseling experience with 40 hours of direct service to persons with disabilities; an average of 1 hour per week of individual supervision or 1 1/2 hours per week of group supervision (maximum of 10 persons) by faculty or a qualified individual.

Internship: 600 hours of applied experience in a rehabilitation agency or program with 240 hours of direct service to individuals with disability; weekly on-site supervision by a certified rehabilitation counselor; and an average of 1 hour per week of individual supervision or 1 1/2 hours per week of group supervision (maximum 10 persons) by faculty or a qualified individual.

Supervisor: Certified rehabilitation counselor or rehabilitation education faculty member.

For more information regarding CORE requirements and standards, access www.core-rehab.org.

CACEP Standards for Initial and Final Practicum

The Council on Accreditation of Counsellor Education Programs (CACEP) is the accreditation body established by the Canadian Counsellors and Psychologists Association (CCPA). CACEP established standards for accrediting master's degree programs in School Counselling, Counselling in Higher Education, Community/Agency Counselling, Rehabilitation Counselling, and Family Counselling, each of which requires a minimum of 48 credit hours. A summary of the requirements for the initial and final practicum in these programs follows (CCPA, 2003).

Setting: An agency, institution, or organization appropriate to the specialization and career goals of the student.

Initial practicum: 100 hours of supervised practice with 50 hours of direct service with clients (40 hours with individual clients and 10 hours in group work); an average of 1 hour per week of individual or joint supervision and 1 1/2 hours per week of group supervision by a faculty member or a supervisor under the supervision of a faculty member.

Final practicum: 400 hours of supervised practice with 200 hours of direct client contact (160 hours with individual clients and 40 hours of group work) under the supervision of the site supervisor in collaboration with a faculty member.

Supervisor: The site supervisor must have a minimum of 4 years of experience as a counselor, recognized competence, and knowledge of program expectations, requirements, and evaluation procedures. Doctoral students in counseling may supervise under the supervision of a faculty member.

APA-CoA Standards for Practicum and Internship in Counseling Psychology

Practicum: 1500 hours of supervised professional experience; 50% in service-related activities, 25% of which are in face-to-face client/patient contact; supervision is part of the 1500 hours. Individual face-to-face supervision shall be no less than 25% of the time spent in service-related activities; 25% of supervision may be in a group setting (Association of State and Provincial Psychology Boards, 2009).

Internship: Full time for 1 academic year or part time for 2 academic years, with a minimum of 4 hours per week of scheduled supervision, at least 2 of which will be individual supervision (APA, 2007).

AAPC Standards for Practicum and Internship for Pastoral Counselors

The AAPC was founded in 1963 in response to the need for leadership and standards for the involvement of religious organizations in mental health care. Institutions can be accredited as training centers, service centers, or both. Currently 33 training programs are identified as accredited. The following requirements are applicable (AAPC, 2011).

Setting: Active relationship to a local religious community.

Practicum: Complete formal, in-depth, supervised pastoral care experience equivalent to pastoral care specialist.

Internship: 375 hours of pastoral counseling with a variety of clients with a variety of cases (i.e., individual, couples, families, therapeutic groups); a total of 125 hours of supervision—60 hours with at least 2 supervisors (30 hours with 1 supervisor), 35 hours of continuous group supervision, 30 hours in clinical case conference.

Supervisor: One-third of supervision with a supervisor who is an AAPC Diplomat, AAPC Fellow (who is under supervision of a supervisor), or in an AAPC-approved training program.

For more information on AAPC requirements, access www.aapc.org.

Counselor Certification

National Certified Counselor (NCC)

Counselor certification proves to the public that the counselor has met national standards established by the counseling profession. It is not a license to practice. In some states, national certification can help with getting a state license. The National Board of Certified Counselors (NBCC) is the certifying body that administers the National Counselors Exam and awards the designation of National Certified Counselor (NCC) to those who are approved to sit for the exam and successfully pass the exam. CACREP accredits counseling programs in six specialty areas: Addictions Counseling; Career Counseling; Clinical Mental Health Counseling; Marriage, Couple, and Family Counseling; School Counseling; and Student Affairs and College Counseling. Applicants completing a

CACREP-accredited program in any of these specialties may sit for the exam immediately upon completion of their master's degree program.

Applicants graduating from programs that are not CACREP approved must complete a master's degree in counseling or master's degree with a major focus in counseling from a regionally accredited institution. They must also complete 3000 hours of counseling experience and 100 hours of supervision by a supervisor who holds a master's degree (or higher) in a counseling field in their specialty or a related mental health field. These hours must be completed in a 2-year post-master's time frame. They may then be approved to sit for the National Counselor Exam (NCE) and will be awarded the designation of NCC upon successfully passing the exam (NBCC, 2012).

NBCC Specialty Certifications

NBCC also awards specialty counseling credentials in three areas: addictions, clinical mental health, and school. The requirements for specialty certification require additional post–master's degree coursework and supervised experience and the completion of an exam. With any NBCC specialty certification, the general counseling practice certification (NCC) is a prerequisite. For more information regarding specialty certification, access www.nbcc.org.

Certified Rehabilitation Counselor (CRC)

Rehabilitation counselors may sit for the CRC exam upon completion of a CORE-accredited master's degree program to be awarded the credential of CRC. For information regarding additional requirements if one is completing a degree in a master's degree program that is not accredited by CORE, access www.core-rehab.org.

Canadian Certified Counsellor (CCC): CCPA

The CCPA offers the credential of CCC after one has met specified training and practice standards. First, one must be a member of CCPA. Then one can apply for certification. Certification is different from membership. Certification represents a successful evaluation of a member's qualifications to practice. A member of CCPA must apply for certification and go through an evaluation process; if approved, one will be permitted to use the CCC when practicing as a counsellor. Those graduating from a CCPA-accredited program can apply for the CCC certification immediately upon graduation. Those graduating from other degree programs in counselling or a related field must meet specific course and direct practice experience requirements. For more information, access www.ccpa.ca/en/certificationrequirements.

Registered Professional Counsellor (RPC): Canadian Professional Counsellors Association

The Canadian Professional Counsellors Association, as part of its membership, offers the designation of RPC upon attaining the level of Full Member (CPCA, 2013). The levels of membership are Student Member, Intern (RPC candidate), Full Member (RPC), and Master Practitioner Practicing Counselling Psychology (MPPCP). Each level of membership specifies coursework, direct practice, and supervision requirements. To progress to the Intern level, you must complete and pass an exam package consisting of a qualifying exam and a personality exam. At the Intern level, you must complete supervision requirements in a 24-month period, whereupon you can become a Full Member (RPC).

Other Specialty Counseling Certifications

The American Association for Marriage and Family Therapy offers a specialty professional counseling credential entitled Clinical Member Status. For more information regarding this designation, access www.aamft.org/membership/levels of membership.

The National Career Development Association offers specialty professional credentials entitled Fellow, Master Career Counselor, or Master Career Development Specialist. For more information, access www.ncda.org/membership.

State Licensure for Counselors and Psychologists

Government-sanctioned credentialing is usually called licensure. Passage of a state licensure law for a given profession restricts or prohibits the practice of the profession by individuals not meeting the state-determined qualification standards (American Counseling Association, 2013). At the present time, in the United States all 50 states and Washington, D.C., and Puerto Rico have passed licensing laws for counselors. The laws, however, are not consistent from state to state, so you must go to the website of the state in which you intend to practice to become informed of the requirements for licensing in that state. Currently, school counselors are certified but not licensed by each state. In Canada, there is no licensing law, but the practice of counselling is variously regulated by the provinces. To learn about standards established by state licensure laws and provincial regulations within specified counseling or psychology professions, the following websites are recommended:

Addictions Counselor: access www.naadac.org/certification, then click on "state licensing boards."

Canadian regulation standards for counselling and school counselling: access www.ccpa-accp.ca/en/pathways.

Clinical Mental Health Counselor or Licensed Professional Counselor: access www.nbcc.org/stateLicensure.

Marriage, Couple, and Family Therapist: access www.aamfte.org/MFTLicensingBoards.

Pastoral Counselor: access www.aapc.org/membership/licensing.

Psychologist: In the United States, all states require psychologist licensure in order to practice as a psychologist, and a doctoral degree is required. About half of the states and the Canadian provinces have a category for licensure for the practice of psychology under the supervision of a doctoral-level licensed psychologist. A person practicing at this level is called a psychological associate, which usually requires a master's degree in psychology (ASPPB, 2009). For more information, access asppb.net/Licensing Board/Contact Information.

Rehabilitation Counselors: access www.crccertification.com/pages/state_licensure_boards.

School Counselors: access www.schoolcounselor.org; then click on "school counselors and members," then "Careers/Roles," then "State Certification Requirements." It should be noted that school counselors are state certified but not state licensed.

Preceipracticum Considerations

All individuals involved in the applied training components of counseling and psychology need to carefully examine the expectations they bring to the practicum and internship. The practicum professor, practicum student, site supervisor, and professional accreditation agencies all have expectations about practicum and internship, which may vary. We are providing a list of questions which counseling students should research and answer for themselves before proceeding to select a field site for a practicum and/or internship. Students should modify and adapt this list in keeping with their own training program and specific practicum situations.

Checklist of Questions to Be Researched and Answered Before Practicum Site Selection

- What are the practicum and internship (or final practicum) requirements to become credentialed in my specialty?
- What are the practicum and internship (or final practicum) requirements for securing certification and/or licensure in the state or province where I intend to be employed?
- What are the basic skills and content areas that are necessary to begin the practicum experience in my program?
- What are the prerequisites for the practicum? Where in the program is it placed?
- What number of credit hours are devoted to the practicum and internship (or final practicum)? Do practicum hours include class on campus?
- Will I be retained in practicum until minimal competencies are demonstrated?
- How will I be expected to demonstrate identified competencies, and how are they to be evaluated?
- How much time will be spent in direct service with individual clients? With groups? With other professional activities?
- What is the role of the faculty supervisor in the field site experience? Instructional leader? Liaison? Role model? Evaluator?
- What is my responsibility for site placement?
- What are the guidelines and procedures for practicum and internship placement?
- What field site placements are recommended and available? Is there a list of approved field sites? If I want to go to a previously unknown field site, how do I know if they have an approved supervisor?
- How does the site supervisor communicate with the university training program?
- Who are the other students in my practicum group? How many? Will we have the same counseling specializations?
- Who gives me a grade and recommends that I have met the expected standards to complete my practice requirements?

In some cases, you may have to do website searches to get information regarding state and provincial requirements. In other cases, you may have to check your student handbook or program procedures and syllabi for the needed information.

Phases of Practicum and Internship

The phases of practicum/internship can be described from a variety of perspectives. For example, one might describe the practicum/internship from the categories of level of skill, such as beginning, intermediate, or advanced. Another way of categorizing phases of practicum might be according to functions, such as structuring, stating goals, acquiring knowledge, and refining skills and interventions. We prefer to describe practicum/internship phases from a developmental perspective. Several principles regarding development can be identified within practicum/internship:

1. *Movement is directional and hierarchical.* Early learning in the program establishes a foundation (knowledge base) for later development in the program (applied skills).
2. *Differentiation occurs with new learning.* Learning proceeds from the more simplistic and straightforward (content) toward the more complex and subtle (process).
3. *Separation or individuation can be observed.* The learning process leads to progressively more independent and separate functioning on the part of the counselor or therapist.

These developmental principles can be identified within the specific program structure, the learning process, and the supervisory interaction encountered by the student.

Development Reflected in the Program Structure

Students in a counseling or psychology training program can expect to proceed through a well-thought-out experiential component of their programs. Generally experiences are orderly and sequentially planned. A typical sequence would be as follows:

Foundations of Counseling

   Prepracticum

      ↳ Practicum

         ↳ Internship (or final practicum)

           ↳ Full professional status

Some variations exist in counseling and psychology programs regarding the number of credit hours required in each component of training. Some variations also exist in training programs regarding the range and depth of expected skills and competencies that are necessary before a student can move to the next component in the program. Generally, programs begin with courses that orient the student to the profession. The history of the profession and its current status might well be a beginning point. Early courses tend to be more didactic and straightforward. As the student enters the prepracticum phase of the program, he/she can generally expect more interaction and active participation with the professor. In this stage, the focus is on basic skill development, role playing, peer interaction and feedback, and observation activities in a classroom or counseling laboratory. In the practicum component, the student is likely to be functioning at a field site with supervision and on campus in a practicum class with university faculty. The focus in both of these settings is on observation by functioning professionals as well as on initial interactions with clients. As time progresses, the student becomes more actively involved with a range of clients and is given increased opportunities to expand and develop the full range of professional behaviors. At the internship end of the continuum, the student is expected to be able to participate in the full range of professional counseling activities within the field site under the supervision of an approved field site supervisor.

Development Reflected in the Learning Process

As students progress in their training, they tend to progress across several stages or steps of learning. Initially, counselors often lack confidence in their skills and tend to imitate the type of supervision they receive. Counselors look to others for an indication of how they should function in the setting. Counselors tend to question their level of skill development. As time passes, they tend to fluctuate between feeling competent and professional and feeling inadequate. At this point, most counselors see the need to develop an internalized theoretical framework, to give them a sense of "grounding" and to help them to develop their own approach to counseling. Further learning helps counselors to develop confidence in their skills and an awareness of their strengths, weaknesses, and motivations. Finally, counselors internalize and integrate their personal theories with their counseling practice.

Development Reflected in Supervisor Interaction

Supervisory interaction between supervisor and student begins with a high level of dependence on the supervisor for instruction, feedback, and support. This interaction is modified as skill, personal awareness, and confidence increase for the student. The student becomes more likely to explore new modes of practice that reflect his/her own unique style. The interaction continues to move more gradually toward a higher level of independent judgment by the student and a more collegial and consultative stance on the part of the supervisor.

Implications

The implications for students in professional counselor training are becoming quite clear. In addition to requirements for practicum and internship as stipulated by the counselor preparation program, each student will need to give careful consideration to (a) the selection of sites where practicum and internship are experienced, (b) a review of required supervisory credentials, (c) a determination of the amount of supervisory time available, (d) the identification of a site that provides opportunities to work with one's chosen population, (e) an understanding of program accreditation or its equivalent, and (f) an understanding of the credentialing requirements of organizations with which the student hopes to affiliate.

Summary

In this chapter the current accreditation, certification, and licensing standards that apply to students in a variety of counseling and psychology training programs in the United States and Canada have been described. Specific attention was directed to the CACREP, CACEP, APA-CoA, CORE, and AAPC guidelines for practicum and internship. In addition, we provided students with a checklist of questions to be answered prior to selecting and procuring a field site for the applied supervised practice component of their master's degree program. We hope that the information in this chapter will help the beginning counseling student to gain a fuller understanding of the professional training and certification requirements for counseling specializations as they relate to the practicum and internship experience.

References

American Association of Pastoral Counselors (AAPC). (2011). *Membership manual.* Fairfax, VA: Author.

American Counseling Association. (2010). *20/20: Consensus definition of counseling.* Retrieved from www.counseling.org/knowledge-center/20-20-a-vision-of-the-future-of-counseling.

American Counseling Association. (2013). *Licensure and certification.* Retrieved from www.counseling.org/knowledge-center/licensure-requirements.

American Psychological Association Commission on Accreditation. (2007). *Guidelines and principles for accreditation of programs in professional psychology.* Washington, DC: Author.

Association of State and Provincial Psychology Boards (ASPPB). (2009). *Guidelines on practicum experience for licensure.* Peachtree, GA: Author.

Canadian Counselling and Psychotherapy Association (CCPA). (2003). *Accreditation manual.* Retrieved October 2013 from www.ccpa.accp.ca/en/accreditation/standards.

Canadian Professional Counsellors Association. (2013). *Membership criteria.* Retrieved October 2013 from www.cpca-rpc.ca/membership/membership-criteria.html.

Council for Accreditation of Counseling and Related Educational Programs (CACREP). (2009). *CACREP standards.* Alexandria, VA: Author.

Council on Rehabilitation Education (CORE). (2012). *CRC certification guide.* Schaumburg, IL: Author.

National Board of Certified Counselors (NBCC). (2012). *National certification and licensure.* Greensboro, NC: Author.

Remley, T. P., Jr., & Herlihy, B. (2014). *Ethical, legal and professional issues in counseling* (4th ed.). Upper Saddle River, NJ: Pearson.

Schweiger, Wendi K., Henderson, Donna A., McKaskill, Kristi, Clawson, Thomas W., & Collins, Daniel R. (2012). *Counselor preparation: Programs, faculty, trends* (13th ed.). New York: Routledge.

CHAPTER 2

SECURING A PRACTICUM/INTERNSHIP SITE

Chapter 2 has as its focus the process of selecting and negotiating a site placement. We provide you with guidelines for choosing a field site, recommendations for interviewing with the site coordinator, and specific orientation information which will allow you to make a smooth transition into the role of counselor-in-training at the site.

Guidelines for Choosing a Practicum/Internship Site

The practicum placement is often the first opportunity that a student has to gain experience working with a client population. Approval to proceed to a field site placement usually occurs after the completion of academic prerequisites and prepracticum or practicum lab situations with volunteers or with peer counseling interactions where basic counseling skills are demonstrated. Many counselor preparation programs offer the student an opportunity to have some say in determining practicum placement. For example, you may prefer to complete your initial practicum at one site and move to a different site for your internship. Or you may wish to do half of your internship hours at one site and the rest at a different site. Some school settings prefer that you split your internship between the elementary or middle school and the high school. Some mental health agencies provide both outpatient services and extended day care treatment for another patient population, and you may wish to have experience in both settings. Your career and specialization goals as well as the flexibility of the site influence how you may wish to pursue these options. Variations of your site hours and patient population are best accomplished by negotiating for different placements in one system.

Although some programs may assign students to a site which fits their career goals, it is students' responsibility to identify and get their own field placement. Students are required to contact the appropriate person at the site and go through a formal interviewing process at the field site of their choice. The field site coordinators are responsible for selecting students who they believe will benefit from the placement and who will best serve the needs of the site's client population. The student is responsible for obtaining a field site, but the training program establishes the guidelines and procedures for approval of the site. Most counselor training programs have established guidelines and procedures for procuring a field site placement which can be approved by the program, and they provide a list of possible sites where previous students have successfully completed practicum and internship. If you identify a possible practicum/internship site which meets your career and specialization goals but the site has no previous connection to your university program, check with your university coordinator about how and whether to proceed. An important consideration is always the credentials of the site and the proposed site supervisor, as well as the site supervisor's knowledge of the university's requirements.

The student can select sites of interest to him/her and then, with the university site coordinator's approval, apply for placement. A list of approved sites and the contact person may be provided by the student's training program. Identifying and applying for a field placement should take place the semester before the student begins the practicum. At this time, the student should purchase malpractice insurance. Your professional counseling organization can provide you with information regarding insurance options. The student must also obtain appropriate state or provincial clearances prior to beginning the placement. An example of these clearances would be the completion of a criminal background check and completion of a clearance to work with children or vulnerable others. These clearances are managed through state regulatory agencies in the United States and through the Royal Canadian Mounted Police in Canada. Clearances can take as long as a month to process. Be sure to obtain these clearances before applying to your practicum site.

Prior to applying to the site, the student should thoroughly research each field placement of interest. Some of this information can be obtained by reviewing the website of the school or agency. Other information can be learned from informal sources such as previous students or other professional counselors. The selection and application process for practicum/internship sites can be confusing and at times overwhelming. To alleviate some of the frustration, the student might find it helpful to have a set of criteria in mind.

Criteria for Site Selection

In the sections that follow, we list questions pertaining to important categories that may be helpful in determining the selection of a practicum site.

Professional Staff and Supervisor

- What are the professional credentials of the site personnel?
- Do their credentials meet the standards of your professional credentialing bodies?

Professional Affiliations of the Site

- In what association does the site hold membership?
- Does the site hold the approval of national certifying agencies?
- What is the reputation of the site among other organizations?
- Does the site have affiliations or working cooperations with other institutions?

Professional Practices of the Site

- Does the site follow the ethical guidelines of the appropriate profession (American Psychological Association [APA], Canadian Psychological Association [CPA], American Counseling Association [ACA], Canadian Counselling and Psychotherapy Association [CCPA], etc.)? Which code(s) of ethics is followed?
- What kinds of resources are available to personnel (e.g., a library, computer programs, ongoing research, professional consultation)?

- What are the client procedures, treatment modalities, and staffing and outreach practices? How are these practices consistent with the goals of the practicum/internship?
- What are the policies and procedures regarding taping (audio/video) and other practicum support activities?
- Do the staff members regularly update their skills and participate in continuing education?
- Are continuing education opportunities available to counselor trainees?

Site Administration

- What resources, if any, are directed toward staff development?
- Does the administration of the site provide in-house funds for staff training or reinforcement for college credit?
- How is policy developed and approved (corporate structure, board of directors, contributions)?
- How stable is the site? (Does the site receive hard money or soft money support? What is the length of service of the director and staff? What is the site's mission statement or purpose?)

Training and Supervision Values

- What values regarding training and supervision are verbalized and demonstrated?
- Will the supervisor be available for individual supervision for a minimum of 1 hour per week?
- Will practicum/internship students have opportunities for full participation?
- What kinds of counseling and professional services are offered by the site, such as individual counseling and/or therapy, group counseling and therapy, couples/family therapy, psycho-educational group guidance or workshops, consultation with professionals or families, career counseling, proposal writing, or student advising?
- Are adequate facilities available for practicum/internship students?

Theoretical Orientation of the Site and Supervisor

- What are the special counseling or therapy interests of the site supervisor(s)?

Many therapists are eclectic in their counseling practice, but many may also favor a particular therapeutic approach over others. Thus, if students are exposed to a supervisor who favors and supports the use of a particular theoretical approach, it requires the student to have grounding in the knowledge base of that theory. Naturally, the advantage of having one approach to counseling is that it affords the student the opportunity to become more proficient at it. Also, in mastering one approach, the student begins to develop a clearer, firmer professional identity regarding his/her goals in counseling practice. Conversely, the disadvantage of learning only one approach is that it limits the student's opportunity to measure other approaches that could be more in keeping with his/her own style and personality.

Client Population

- What are the client demographics in the placement site?
- Who is the client population served? For example, is it a restricted or open group? Is the age range narrow or wide? Are clients predominantly of a low, middle, or high socioeconomic level?

- Do clients require remedial, preventive, and/or developmental services?
- What opportunities exist for multicultural counseling?
- Do the site and its professional staff demonstrate high regard for human dignity and support the civil rights of clients?

Multicultural counseling skills have become increasingly important for the practicing professional counselor. The American Counseling Association's *Code of Ethics* (2014) under Section F.11.c asserts that "Counselor educators actively infuse multicultural/diversity competency in their training and supervision programs. They actively train students to gain awareness, knowledge, and skills in the competencies of multicultural practice." The American Mental Health Counselors Association's *Code of Ethics* (2008) and the American School Counselors Association's *Ethical Standards for School Counselors* (2010) similarly emphasize the importance of multicultural competency in the practice of counseling. Sections A10, B9, and D10 of the Canadian Counselling and Psychotherapy Association's *Code of Ethics* (2007) emphasize that counsellors respect and understand diversity, do not condone or engage in discrimination, and demonstrate sensitivity to diversity when assessing and evaluating clients.

The demographic composition of clients is and will be of a different nature than it was a few years ago in the United States. The projected changes from 2012 through 2060 indicate that the United States is set to become a more diverse nation (US Census Bureau, 2012). The non-Hispanic white population is expected to peak in 2024 at 199.6 million and then slowly decrease, falling nearly 20.6 million by 2060. The Hispanic population will increase from 17% in 2012 to 31.3% in 2060. By 2060 nearly one in three US residents would be Hispanic. The black population is expected to increase from 41.2 million to 61.8 million over the same period. Its share of the population would increase from 13.1% to 14.7% in 2060. The Asian population is projected to more than double, increasing from 15.9 million in 2012 to 34.4 million in 2060 (8.2% of the US population). Other remaining racial groups and those people identifying as being of two or more races will continue to grow. Minorities, now 37% of the US population, are projected to become 57% of the population by 2060 (US Census Bureau, 2012).

The demographic composition of clients is also changing in Canada. Statistics Canada projects that by 2031 approximately 28% of the population will be foreign born. The number of people belonging to "visible minority" groups will double and make up the majority of the population in Toronto and Vancouver. The Southeast Asian population is expected to double to between 3.2 and 4.1 million in the next 20 years. The Chinese population is expected to grow from 1.3 million to between 2.4 and 4 million in the next 20 years (Statistics Canada, 2010).

Constantine and Gloria (1999) noted that studies have suggested that counseling students' "exposure to multicultural issues may increase their sensitivity to and effectiveness with racially and ethnically diverse clients" (p. 21). Sue and Sue (2008) described multicultural counseling competencies as consisting of three areas:

- attitudes and beliefs—awareness of one's own values, assumptions, and biases;
- knowledge—understanding the worldview of culturally diverse clients; and
- skills—developing appropriate intervention strategies and techniques.

It is clear that the majority of counselor education and professional psychology programs have responded to multicultural imperatives by examining their curricular offerings and reacting positively to the need for multicultural training. Some training programs recommend that trainees have caseloads of at least 30% minority clients or other clients who represent diversity. Practicum and internship students must consider the client population of the field site to ensure that they will have the opportunity to increase their understanding and application of multicultural counseling skills in their practice.

Negotiating the Practicum/Internship Placement

At this point in the process, you should have determined your preferred practicum/internship structure (same site, different sites), obtained malpractice insurance and appropriate clearances, and identified two or three field sites where you will apply. In many instances, several students may be applying for the same practicum/internship site, which may have only a limited number of openings. Consequently, you must approach the application process the same as you would in applying for a job in the profession. Start by preparing a résumé which identifies your objectives and the relevant educational, work, and volunteer experiences which support your application as a counselor-in-training at that site. You may also prepare a cover letter which includes comments on what training opportunities specific to that site make you especially interested in doing your practicum/internship there. Thinking this through will prepare you for a face-to-face interview with the contact person who will be making the decision about whether your background, goals, and personal impression seem to be a good fit with their site. The cover letter, with your résumé as an attached document, can be sent to the contact person at the site. Next, call the identified contact person to follow up and set up an interview. The contact person may be a supervisor of outpatient services at an agency, a director of counseling or student services, an administrator at a school district, or a specific supervisor at the site. When you go to the interview, remember to dress as other professionals do at that site. Remember, you are the one who is to be interviewed at the site. Be prepared to answer questions about the skills, interests, and experiences which make you a good fit for the site.

Typical Questions Asked at the Interview

Be prepared to answer the following kinds of questions at your interview. You may want to work with some of your peers to brainstorm other possible questions and give thought to how you may respond.

- Tell me what you know about the students/clients we serve? What makes you want to work with them?
- What do you hope to gain from training at this site?
- What's your comfort level working with diverse clients?
- How would you describe your role as counselor to a student/client?
- Is there a theory that influences your practice as a counselor?
- Have you had any life experiences that help you relate to the concerns that students/clients may have?
- What student/client concerns are you ready to begin seeing now?
- Are there any problems that a student/client might present in counseling that would be challenging for you to work with?
- Describe your strengths as a counselor.
- How can a supervisor support your development as a counselor?

- Why did you choose our agency/school to do a practicum/internship?
- What types of professional experiences are you most interested in? Least interested in?
- What do you consider to be a rewarding practicum/internship experience?

In addition to answering questions, you may also ask questions to clarify information you have gotten from your research about the site.

- You may need more information about how audio- or videotaping of sessions is permitted and managed.
- Are there any releases to be signed or guidelines to follow, and how is confidentiality safeguarded? This can be a concern if you are required to bring taped session material to university-based supervision.
- You could ask about what population of students/clients you would begin working with and how will you make initial contact with them. In a school setting, counselors sometimes do outreach by introducing themselves through classroom guidance activities, or they shadow another counselor before seeing students one-to-one.
- In general, what kind of applied experience occurs at the beginning of the placement, and what range of practices are gradually added to the trainee's responsibilities? What kinds of groups are offered at the site?

When you are accepted as a counselor-in-training at the site, a written exchange of agreement is made so that all parties involved in the practicum/internship placement understand the roles and responsibilities involved. With regard to written contracts, most counselor or psychology training programs have developed their own contracts. Specific guidelines followed in the practicum or internship are stated as part of the agreement. Guidelines identified by national certifying agencies are often used or referenced in formalizing the practicum/internship placement.

In the guidelines of the Council on the Accreditation of Counseling and Related Educational Programs (2009) and the Canadian Counselling and Psychotherapy Association's Council on the Accreditation of Counselling Education Programs (CACEP; 2003), the development of counseling skills is emphasized. We suggest that the counselor preparation program identify the guidelines and standards that it follows and include the guidelines in the contract. An example of a formal contract between the university and the practicum/internship field sites is included in the Forms section at the end of the book for your review. The sample Practicum Contract and Internship Contract (Forms 2.1 and 2.2) can be adapted to the specific needs of your training program. The contract includes a statement concerning guidelines to be followed, conditions agreed on by the field site, conditions agreed on by the counselor or psychologist preparation program, student responsibilities, and a list of suggested practicum/internship activities. Form 2.3 is a Student Profile Sheet, which can be filled in and submitted to the field site supervisor. Form 2.4 is a Student Practicum/Internship Agreement which the student completes and submits to the university practicum/internship coordinator.

Getting Oriented to Your Field Site

Some field sites have a specific orientation for all new personnel to acquaint them with policy and procedures for working with clients/students. Other sites have no formal orientation, and you must seek out needed information. When you meet with your site supervisor, start by asking what you need to know about operations at the site in order to begin. Information about site operations is related to space (offices, study areas), support people (receptionists, secretaries), and access to resources (computer, phone, fax, forms). Site operations also specify how client records are kept (what is in the record, what notes and in what form, where and how records are kept and secured).

It would be helpful to know about the process a client/student follows when coming for counseling. How does a client/student get an appointment, how are they assigned to a particular counselor, what is the intake process, and how and with whom do they schedule a next appointment? Inquire about site policy regarding phone, e-mail, or other media-related contact with clients/ students.

You will want to know what a typical day's schedule looks like for a counselor at the site. Often, a new practicum/internship student will shadow the supervisor or another staff member as an orientation. This gives the student an opportunity to experience the range of professional practices at the site and the procedures associated with them. Finally, you will need information about policy and protocols related to managing crisis situations or dealing with client/student behaviors of concern.

Role and Function of the Practicum/Internship Student

The student who has been accepted to the field site will start as a novice in the counseling profession but at the same time will be a representative of his/her university training program and of other student counselors and psychologists. The student is working in the setting as a guest of the practicum/internship site. The site personnel have agreed to provide the student with appropriate counseling experiences with the clientele they serve.

Although the individual freedom of the student counselor is understood and respected, the overriding concern of the site personnel is to provide role-appropriate services to the client population. The role of the practicum/internship student is to obtain practice in counseling or psychotherapy in the manner in which it is provided in the field site setting. The student counselor is expected to adhere to any dress code or expected behaviors that are existent at the field site. In some instances, the student may disagree with some of the site requirements; however, the role of the student counselor is not to change the system but to develop his/her own abilities in counseling practice.

Occasionally tension or conflict may arise between the student and site personnel. Although such events are upsetting to all involved, these events can provide an opportunity for the student to develop personal insight into and understanding of the problem. After all, practicum/internship placement is real-life exposure to the realities of the counseling profession; however, should the tension or conflict persist, the student should consult with the faculty liaison, who is available to assist the student in the process of understanding his/her role within the system and to facilitate the student's ability to function in the setting.

A Student Profile Sheet (Form 2.3) and a Student Practicum/Internship Agreement (Form 2.4) have been included in the Forms section. The profile sheet guides the documentation of the student counselor's academic preparation and relevant experience prior to practicum. The agreement form demonstrates the formal agreement being entered into by the student. Form 2.3 can be a valuable resource for the site supervisor in assessing the practicum/internship student's preparation for the field site experience.

Summary

The information presented in this chapter is designed to assist the counseling student in the process of choosing and negotiating a practicum and/or an internship placement. Several aspects of the practicum/internship experience need to be carefully considered by the student prior to making this important decision, and to this end, we have provided a number of questions that warrant attention. It is recommended that the student make an effort to answer these questions to understand fully the benefits and disadvantages of a particular site. Additional information concerning the role and function of the practicum/internship student has been discussed. Finally, sample forms have been included for use in preselection planning and ongoing practicum/internship activities; the student can adapt these to fit his/her own needs.

References

American Counseling Association. (2014). *Code of ethics*. Alexandria, VA: Author.

American Mental Health Counselors Association. (2008). *Code of ethics*. Alexandria, VA: Author.

American School Counselors Association. (2010). *Ethical standards for school counselors*. Alexandria, VA: Author.

Canadian Counselling and Psychotherapy Association. (2003). *Accreditation manual*. Retrieved October 2013 from www.ccpa.accp.ca/en/accreditation/standards.

Canadian Counselling and Psychotherapy Association. (2007). *Code of ethics*. Retrieved from www.ccpa-accp.ca/_documents?CodeofEthics_en_new.pdf.

Constantine, M. G., & Gloria, A. M. (1999). Multicultural issues in predoctoral internship programs: A national survey. *Journal of Multicultural Counseling and Development, 27*, 42–53.

Council on the Accreditation of Counseling and Related Educational Programs. (2009). *CACREP standards*. Alexandria, VA: Author.

Statistics Canada. (2010). *Study: Projections of the diversity of the Canadian population*. Retrieved from www.statcan.gc.ca/daily-quotidien/100309/dq100309a-eng.htm.

Sue, D. W., & Sue, D. (2008). *Counseling the culturally diverse: Theory and practice* (5th ed.). New York: Wiley.

US Census Bureau. (2012). *U.S. Census Bureau projections show a slower growing older, more diverse nation a half century from now*. Washington, DC: Author.

SECTION II

BEGINNING TO WORK WITH CLIENTS

CHAPTER 3

STARTING THE PRACTICUM

This chapter is designed to assist the counseling student in understanding the importance of developing a therapeutic alliance with the client and how to proceed with privacy and informed consent requirements in the initial interview. The emphasis is on how the counselor-in-training develops and applies counseling performance skills with clients at the field site. A review of basic and advanced helping skills, the initial intake, and suggestions for opening and closing the initial session have been included. Formats for taking case notes in clinical and school settings will also be reviewed.

Beginning the Practicum Experience[1]

Getting Started: Where Do I Begin?

In my experience, the practicum course tends to bring out the most anxiety in students. Prior to the start, most students have not had the experience of interacting one-on-one with "real" clients, or, at the least, their exposure has been very limited. By this time, most students have completed several foundational classes including theory, techniques, and very structured applied work but have not yet begun a true ongoing counseling relationship. This can make students feel very apprehensive and anxious about their upcoming practicum experience.

It has also been my experience that once students break down the requirements and begin to work, the anxiety does begin to slowly decline. As with most things, the anticipation is often much worse than the actual event. The key is for them to take things one step at a time so they don't become overwhelmed by details. Some common tips for students to consider prior to beginning the practicum course include the following:

1. *Choose an appropriate field site.* Students tend to choose the field site that they are most familiar with, which isn't always the best option. It is better to investigate possible field sites (whether in a school or an agency) to see what best fits with their personal style and learning goals. The field site should be a place where the students feel they will gain the most valuable experience and where they will get the best support in mentoring and supervision. If your university program chooses your site for you, it is best to arm yourself with as much information as possible about the mission, objectives, and goals of the field site. Find out everything you can so you are as prepared as possible, and show your site supervisor that you are prepared to hit the ground running.

2. *Be aware of course requirements.* Practicum course requirements can vary considerably from school to school and program to program. Some requirements are based on accreditation standards and others on professional ideology. For example, some programs may require sessions to be taped and monitored by a third party. A prospective practicum site supervisor needs to be aware of this requirement in the event the field site does not permit such practices. Most programs require a specific amount of direct contact hours and one-on-one sessions. These requirements must be communicated early in the process so that the field site supervisor can make provisions for these types of tasks to be available to the counselor trainee. It is imperative that students make the site supervisor aware of all class requirements so the student can be sure that all course objectives and requirements are attainable during the field placement.

3. *Plan your time wisely.* After you have been given all the specific requirements for your practicum course, be sure to create a realistic schedule to make the most of your time. Don't try to do too much in too short a period of time. We all know that unforeseen circumstances can arise, so be sure to give yourself room for unplanned situations. For example, if your course requires 100 on-site hours, you may want to plan for 120 hours of fieldwork so you have room in your schedule to accommodate a variety of occurrences (illness, holidays, missed appointments, etc.) that may affect your scheduled time at the field site. Plan for extra time, and if you don't need it, be happy that you have completed your requirements without any difficulty.

I've Taken the Classes, but Do I Really Know What to Do?

Now that you've taken all the classes you need prior to moving on to your practicum experience, you are ready, confident, and completely sure of yourself, right? Most likely you are experiencing the exact opposite emotions as you get ready to begin your on-site hours. Most students at this stage are feeling anxious, frightened, incompetent, and unsure of their skills. You would not be alone by any means if this description fits you at this point in your academic career, but hold on—there's hope!

So how do you deal with these feelings and jitters? First of all, take a long, deep breath and relax (and feel free to repeat this as often as you deem necessary). You would not have gotten this far if you didn't *successfully* complete the critical components of your program. Remember, you chose this college or university for a reason, so have confidence in your training and in your professors' and instructors' support as you begin your field site experience.

What if I Say Something Wrong?

One of the greatest fears of many students is doing or saying the wrong thing to a client and not knowing when or how to use the appropriate techniques. One of the most frightening aspects is that this may depend to a large degree on the client's needs. In addition, there is no cookie-cutter way to perform successfully in a counseling session.

So what happens if you say something wrong? In most situations, honesty is the best policy. If it is a minor offense and you feel you may have slightly offended the client, apologize ("I'm very sorry. It appears that I may have offended you by asking that question. Please permit me to rephrase the question."). It is important that your clients know you are being authentic and are tuned into them and their needs. Remember, the counseling relationship is a two-way street. You need to be genuine with your clients if you expect them to reciprocate.

If you feel you have made an egregious error, consult with your faculty or site supervisor and have him/her assist you in coming up with a plan to deal with the situation. Remember, first and foremost, "do no harm," and if you feel that somehow you have crossed into that territory, you need to deal with the issue as quickly and thoroughly as possible. Don't be afraid to ask for help if you need it. Recognizing when this has happened and seeking appropriate help are signs of a competent counselor.

How Do I Know When to Use the Right Techniques?

Finding the appropriate techniques can be difficult for beginning counselors. It is best if you review a prospective technique or intervention before using it and consult with your supervisor to get his/her input as to its suitability for the client and your ability to execute it properly. Chances are you have the capability to implement the technique but need some extra support and feedback as to how to use it and ensure its appropriateness.

As we stated before, there is no perfect cookie-cutter way to proceed in your treatment of clients. However, one of the greatest benefits of your practicum experience is knowing that you have experienced professors and supervisors who are willing to provide you with the needed support in your efforts to implement the appropriate techniques and strategies in your counseling session.

But I'm Just a Rookie! (Learning to Trust Yourself and Your Inner Voice)

When students are first beginning to work with clients in live sessions, it is common for them to try to recall all of the knowledge and skills they have learned in the classroom. Although this can be beneficial in some ways, it may actually stifle the session and the client.

If the student counselor is distracted by attempting to recall all of the information learned in coursework, he/she may not be fully present with the client. It is critical to the counseling process that you are as completely present with the client as possible to ensure that the correct information is taken in and also to assure the client that you are listening attentively. The client should be encouraged by the fact that you are attentive and feel that what he/she is saying has value. In addition, the counseling process cannot proceed if you are not authentic to yourself. In other words, be yourself! If the client senses that you are not being genuine, he/she may reciprocate in kind. If you want the client to truly be himself/herself and to be open to you, you must be open yourself. The process becomes easier if you have the confidence in the knowledge and skills learned in your training program.

So how does one go about doing this? Of course, it does take time and experience to relax and be yourself. The goal of the practicum experience is to assist student counselors in honing their therapeutic skills and building a level of confidence and comfort in their counseling. It is important to note that the field site experience is the most appropriate setting for honing skills in a clinically supervised environment.

One of the most difficult aspects of counseling is learning to trust one's own instincts or inner voice. This does occur over time, but like many other aspects of counseling, it often needs some tweaking in the beginning stages of the counseling experience. To accomplish trust in oneself, the student must first listen to his/her inner voice and instincts, trust them, and then observe the outcome. As when you are learning techniques and interventions, there are trials and errors, but if you can learn to trust yourself and that inner voice, you will be more genuine in your counseling relationships, which will serve to greatly enhance the counseling process. It is only when you learn to listen to and use your inner voice that you can truly see the counseling process at work—and it can be really wonderful when you do.

When in Doubt, Consult! (Your Faculty and Site Supervisors Are There to Help You)

One of the most important aspects of counseling is for you to know when to seek professional or supervisory assistance. Throughout your coursework, you have been taught to recognize your strengths and weaknesses. This is vital to your success as a counselor. As mentioned in the previous section, your instinct or inner voice plays a large part in knowing when to seek assistance, because it can let you know when you are in over your head or if you are unsure of your boundaries.

If you are not certain of how to proceed with a client, if you feel your ethics may be at risk, or if you are dealing with an issue you know is a difficult one for you, it is important for you to seek consultation with another professional. Your practicum experience will help you with these issues because you are already receiving close supervision and support. When you are finished with your school requirements and are on your own, you will find it is still critical to seek consultation when you deem it necessary. This is always the best practice to be sure that you are helping your clients appropriately and professionally.

Consultation happens at all levels, not just at the novice level. Professionals who have been in the field for many years often consult with others when they feel it is necessary. It is a process that ensures that you have your client's best interest at heart. Consultation should never be seen as a sign of weakness or incompetence but rather as the hallmark of a professional working ethically and responsibly. It is a truly professional counselor who realizes and accepts his/her limitations and is not too proud or overzealous to seek assistance and consultation from another professional. If you need to consult, it is important to be sure to consult with a trusted and ethical professional.

Preparing to Meet With Your First Client

Several things must be accomplished in the first session with your client. First, and most important, from your first contact with your client you are establishing a warm and genuine helping relationship. The importance of establishing a therapeutic alliance cannot be overstated. In clinical settings, clients come to counseling with concerns, vulnerabilities, and apprehensions about what kinds of responses they are likely to receive. In school, career, or post-secondary settings, clients can come to counseling with similar dynamics, but many of their concerns can be of a developmental or life transition nature. Although they may be experiencing emotional discomfort or confusion, they are often functioning adequately in their life circumstances but require support, clarification, and assistance with their concerns. The counselor must greet each client with empathy for his/her unique situation and make every effort to reduce any discomfort. The counselor must establish himself/herself as someone who can be both approachable and helpful.

Specifics that must be accomplished in the first session are

- making certain that clients are informed of their privacy rights as required by federal law in settings where health information is managed electronically;

- providing the client with informed consent about the counseling process they are about to begin; and
- helping the client talk about the concerns and life situations that motivated them to seek counseling.

Prior to meeting with your first client, it is necessary to review required federal guidelines that mental health practitioners, and others who provide health services to clients, must review with clients about the privacy practices at the site. These requirements must be posted in a prominent place at the site. Counselors must be prepared to answer any questions a client may have regarding these guidelines. In the United States, these guidelines are referred to as HIPAA. Any site which transmits records electronically is required to comply with this law. We are including information about the law so that you will be able to answer questions clients may have regarding this process.

The Health Insurance Portability and Accountability Act (HIPAA)

HIPAA is the first federal privacy standards law in the United States intended to protect patients' health information and medical records. This first took effect in 2003. Then the standards were revised, and the revised standards were placed into effect in September 2013. HIPAA rules apply to therapists (sites) who transmit records electronically in carrying out financial transactions or administrative activity such as claims submission. This includes the internet, e-mail transmissions, and the use of electronic media such as CDs. HIPAA is a federal law that applies throughout the United States and overrides state laws unless state laws are stricter in protecting consumer health care privacy. Civil penalties for violation of HIPAA rules have been identified. Criminal penalties for providers who knowingly and improperly disclose information include fines and prison terms.

HIPAA identifies three core compliance areas:

1. *The privacy rule* restricts use and disclosure of an individual's "protected health information" (PHI). The privacy rule provides for individual rights such as a patient's rights to access their PHI, restrict disclosures, request amendments or an accounting disclosure, and complain without retaliation.
2. *The security rule* requires covered practices to implement a number of administrative, technical, and physical safeguards to ensure confidentiality, integrity, and availability of electronic PHI. "Electronic PHI" refers to all individually identifiable health information a covered entity creates, receives, maintains, or transmits in electronic form.
3. *The breach notification rule* requires covered practices to notify affected individuals, the secretary of the US Department of Health and Human Services, and, in some cases, the media when they discover a breach of a patient's PHI (American Medical Association, 2013).

The Notice of Privacy Practices (NPP) must be made available to existing clients on request and must be posted in a prominent location or on the therapist's (site's) website. Therapists (sites) must have a documented procedure to handle patients' requests:

- medical record access, inspection, and copy requests;
- disclosure restriction requests—when a patient asks you to limit sharing of their medical information with other covered entities;

- amendment requests—when a patient asks you to make a change to information in his/her medical record;
- accounting or disclosure requests; and
- confidential communication channel requests—when a patient asks to receive information in a specific way or at a specific location; for example, he/she may request not to be called at home for an appointment reminder (American Medical Association, 2013).

Counselors may wish to customize their Notice of Privacy Practices (NPP) to include a broader discussion of the limits of confidentiality, privilege, and privacy, including issues of imminent harm to self or others and other mandatory reporting duties. They may also wish to include a statement in the section related to psychotherapy notes which states that PHI and psychotherapy notes may be released in response to a complaint filed against the counselor. Another option is to use the model but cross-reference to the counselor's informed consent document (Wheeler, 2013).

For students preparing to become professional counsellors in Canada, health information privacy is protected under the Personal Information Protection and Electronics Documents Act (Office of the Privacy Commissioner of Canada, May, 2014). Since January 1, 2002, this act has applied to personal health information and the ways it is collected, used, or disclosed. Several provinces also have enacted laws in matters related to health care information, and these laws are substantially similar to the federal law.

Informed Consent

In counseling and psychology professions, ethical guidelines require that we disclose to clients some information about the benefits and risks of, and alternatives to, treatment procedures. Clients have a right to know what they are getting into when they are coming for counseling. In addition to being a proper and ethical way to begin counseling, there are legal concepts that require that informed consent be obtained from clients before counseling begins. A written informed consent form is a contract and a promise made by the mental health professional to perform the therapy competently. There are three basic legal elements of informed consent:

1. The client must be competent. Competence refers to the legal capacity to give consent. If, because of age or mental ability, a client does not have the capacity to give consent, the therapist should consult another person or a judicial body who can legally assume responsibility for the client.
2. Both the substance of the information regarding therapy and the manner in which it is given are important. The substance of the information should include the relevant facts about therapy. This information should be presented to the client in a manner that is easily understood.
3. The client must volunteer for therapy and must not be forced or coerced to participate. Some state licensing laws or regulations require that counselors provide written documents to clients (Remley & Herlihy, 2014).

The American Counseling Association *Code of Ethics* (2014) in Standard A.2.b details the elements that should be included in securing informed consent. These elements include the following:

- the purposes, goals, techniques, procedures, limitations, potential risks, and benefits of the counseling services;
- the counselor's qualifications, arrangements for continuation of services if necessary;

- the implications of diagnosis and the intended use of tests and reports;
- the role of technology and other pertinent information;
- fees and billing information;
- confidentiality and its limitations;
- clients' right to obtain information about their records and counseling plans; and
- clients' right to refuse any recommended services and be advised of the consequences of refusal.

In addition, Remley and Herlihy (2014) have identified elements that have been suggested by other writers. Some of these elements are summarized here:

- a description of the counselor's theoretical orientation or how the counselor sees the counseling process (Corey, Corey, & Callahan, 2011);
- information about the length and frequency of sessions, procedures for making and canceling appointments, policies regarding contact between sessions, and ways to reach the counselor or an alternative service in an emergency (Haas & Malouf, 1995);
- information about insurance, including that any diagnosis assigned will become a part of the client's permanent health record; what information will be provided to insurance carriers and how this limits confidentiality (Welfel, 2010); and a description of how the managed care system may affect the counseling process (Corey et al., 2011); and
- if applicable, a statement that sessions will be videotape or audiotaped, along with information that the client's case may be discussed with a supervisor (Corey et al., 2011).

Each field site should have in place written guidelines regarding informed consent, confidentiality, and privacy. The counseling student should review these with the client at the first session. Guidelines may vary somewhat because of different legal requirements in each state. They may also vary depending on whether the client is a minor or an adult. Consistent with our earlier statements about the importance of establishing and sustaining a therapeutic alliance, reviewing information in informed consent should be done in a manner which assists the client in the decision to proceed with the counseling. Counselors must achieve a balance between giving needed information and establishing rapport. Written disclosure statements can assist in the process of providing the detailed information needed. Many agencies have a written brochure that explains the counseling relationship and any limits to confidentiality and provide this to clients before their first appointment. This gives clients the opportunity to ask questions face-to-face with the counselor after they have received and thought about the information. Counselors should focus on developing rapport in a first session and, at the end, go over important details regarding the counseling relationship). A sample of an informed consent document (disclosure statement) is provided here.

SAMPLE INFORMED CONSENT AND DISCLOSURE STATEMENT

This form is intended to inform you about my background and to help you understand our professional relationship. I am a master's degree student in the Department of Counseling and Psychology at Blank University studying to be a professional counselor. I am not yet licensed by the state as a professional counselor. However, I am working under the direct supervision of a university faculty member and a site supervisor who are both licensed/certified by the state. The following information is provided about the site and my supervisors.

My internship placement is: Community Mental Health Center
1234 First St., Butler, PA
Phone number: 724-654-3210

Site Supervisor: Dr. John Smith   Phone number: 724-654-3211
University Supervisor: Dr. Elizabeth Jones   Phone number: 412-687-8675

Please read and understand this Informed Consent and Disclosure Statement and ask me about any parts that may be unclear to you. My university department requires that I have you sign this to acknowledge that I have provided you with this information. Please understand that you may end this agreement at any time.

My Background and Experience:

I graduated from the University of Pittsburgh in 2009 with a bachelor of arts degree in sociology. I worked as the student coordinator of freshman orientation during my junior and senior years. I worked as a college admissions and financial aid counselor for 2 years after earning my BA and began my graduate studies in counseling in 2011. I have enjoyed working with adolescents, adults, and families.

Counseling Philosophy:

A counseling relationship between a professional counselor and client is a professional relationship where the professional counselor assists the client in exploring and resolving difficult life issues. I believe in a collaborative approach while working with clients and will help each client develop his/her own individual counseling goals and plan to reach those goals. I follow a wellness model of mental health where the goal is to achieve positive mental health to the degree it is possible. I will adjust counseling techniques to best meet the needs of each client. I do align myself with cognitive behavioral theory and person-centered counseling theory.

Counseling may have both benefits and risks. Since counseling may involve unpleasant parts of your life, you may experience uncomfortable feelings. However, counseling has been shown to have many benefits. It can lead to better relationships, help solve certain problems, and decrease feelings of distress. Please understand there are no guarantees of what you will experience. I can assure you that my services will be conducted in a professional manner consistent with accepted ethical standards. Sessions are 50 minutes in duration. Some clients resolve their concerns after relatively few sessions, while others require many months or more to improve their life situations.

Clients are in complete control, and you may end our counseling relationship at any time and I will be supportive of that decision. If you have questions about procedures, please discuss them with me. You have the right to ask about any aspect of counseling or to decline any part of your counseling. You also have the right to request another counselor. If you are dissatisfied with my services, please let me know. If I am unable to resolve your concern, you may report your complaint to my supervisor here at the agency.

In an Emergency:

You may need help at a time when I am not available or cannot return your call. If you find yourself in a mental health emergency, please contact the agency or go to the emergency room and ask for the mental health professional on call. In the event that I become incapacitated and am unable to work, the agency will provide you with another counselor.

Confidentiality:

I will keep confidential anything you say to me with the following exceptions: you direct me to tell someone else; I determine you are a danger to yourself or others; I have reason to believe that a child or vulnerable adult is being neglected or abused; or I am ordered by a court to disclose information. Psychotherapy notes may also be released in the event of a complaint being filed against the counselor. Because of my training my supervisor may need information or audiotapes of my counseling for confidential supervision and training purposes. You have the right to refuse the taping of sessions.

Diagnosis:

If a third party such as an insurance agency is paying for part of your bill, I am normally required to give a diagnosis to that third party. Diagnoses are technical terms that describe the nature of your problems and indicate whether they are short-term or long-term problems. If I do use a diagnosis it will be from a book titled the *Diagnostic and Statistical Manual of Mental Disorders* (5th ed.; *DSM-5*). I have this book in my office and will be glad to make it available to you to learn more about what it says about your diagnosis.

The agency has provided you with information regarding privacy practices which comply with the Health Information Portability and Accountability Act (HIPAA); it outlines your rights to review, correct, and request transfer of files to other health care providers as well as keep your records secure.

Fees:

Information about policies and procedures regarding fees and any responsibilities you have regarding payment has been discussed with the mental health services coordinator at the agency prior to this appointment. Some managed care insurance policies limit the number of sessions they will pay for each year. If you exceed that limit, you may still receive services from me, but your plan will not reimburse you for the services and you will be responsible for any fees. Please refer to the materials that were provided to you for more information.

Signed Acknowledgment:

I have read and understand the statement and have had the opportunity to discuss it before revealing any personal information.

Client signature _____ Date _____

Parent/guardian signature _____ Date _____

Informed consent and confidentiality guidelines are handled differently in school settings. Most school-based field placements consider that school counseling services are an integral part of the educational program. Information about the counseling program is disseminated in a variety of ways so that parents and students understand the services provided and the confidentiality guidelines for school counselors. Some school districts have policies that require the counselors to obtain parents' permission before beginning the counseling of students; others require counselors to obtain parents' permission if they see students for more than a specified number of sessions (Glosoff & Pate, 2002).

Before the school year begins, the school's guidelines are typically posted in the student handbook, on the counseling department's web page, and in brochures in the counseling office. They also are discussed at the first meeting between the counselor and the student. Hanson (2009–2012) has developed a sample of a counseling confidentiality guidelines brochure and a sign-off sheet that the student counselor can review if the field site doesn't have one available.

Counseling students should review the guidelines in place in their field placement and be prepared to review these with the client in the initial session. Some field sites will include an authorization for student counselors or psychologists to see clients while being supervised and will include permission to audio- or videotape sessions for supervision. Other settings require a separate authorization for practice under supervision. Examples of authorization forms are included in the Forms section at the end of the book. The Parental Release Form (Forms 3.1a and 3.1b) can be used when initiating counseling with a child in a school, and the Client Permission to Record Counseling Session for Supervision Purposes (Form 3.2) should be used when initiating counseling with adults or children. These forms should be adapted for use by the counseling student according to the specific field site and university requirements.

Establishing a Therapeutic Alliance

The formation of a relationship with the client is the critical initial step in the therapeutic process. Essentially, it involves the processes of developing trust, caring, and respect between the counselor and client to foster the client's motivation to actively engage in the work of counseling. The building of rapport and collaboration begins the moment the counselor and client make contact. In your initial session, make sure that you greet the client and introduce yourself and walk to your office or counseling space with the student/client. Carl Rogers (1951), in proposing his theoretical approach to client-centered therapy, defined the core conditions for personality change to occur. They include accurate empathy, unconditional positive regard, and congruence. A more recent study of relationship variables in therapy suggests that the therapeutic relationship variables contribute to successful outcomes in counseling regardless of the theoretical approach and intervention strategies used by the practitioner (Norcross, 2002). These core conditions are important because they help clients feel safe, and clients who feel safe are trusting and free to be open. Clients who feel unsafe are often self-protective, guarded, and subdued (Cormier & Hackney, 2012). A summary of procedures and interventions that can promote rapport and the development of a positive therapeutic alliance follows:

- Facilitate the client's effort to begin treatment by clarifying how treatment will proceed and the roles of clinician and client.
- Support the client's decision to seek treatment, offer support and encouragement.

- Establish and consistently follow session guidelines (i.e., starting times, client participation, homework assignments, etc.).
- Discuss the client expectations for treatment, encouraging realistic hope.
- Develop with the client goals that reflect those hopes and expectations.
- Understand and value the client's perspective on the world.
- Communicate warmth, genuineness, and empathy for the client's concerns.
- Demonstrate congruence and genuineness in verbal and nonverbal messages.
- Engage the client in the therapeutic process.
- Acknowledge and build on successes and support networks that the person has already established (Seligman, 2004, pp. 30–31).

The Initial Session With the Client

In the initial contact with the client, the counselor sets the tone for the counseling work. The importance of the relationship conditions has been noted. The student counselor must also collect needed information from the client and help the client know what to expect in the ongoing counseling process. Counselors can proceed in two ways. Some counselors choose to start with a focus on relationship dynamics and focus solely on gaining an accurate sense of the client's world and communicating that understanding to the client. Other counselors use the first session as an intake session and collect needed information about the client. With either choice of beginning emphasis, information or relationship dynamics must soon be attended to. Cormier & Hackney (2012) have identified an underlying set of objectives for the initial session which are summarized here:

1. to reduce the client's initial anxiety to facilitate his/her talking;
2. to listen more than you talk;
3. to listen carefully and imagine the world he/she is describing; and
4. to be aware that your client's choice of topics gives insight into his/her priorities for the moment.

Structured and Unstructured Interviews

The initial interview with the client requires the counselor to make a determination as to the type of interview to conduct. Will it be a structured interview, an unstructured interview, or a semi-structured interview? According to Whiston (2009) there are advantages to all three types of interviews. The structured interview is one where the counselor has an established set of questions that he/she asks in the same manner with each client. This format is oftentimes used in agencies that require the same structure with each client. Furthermore, if the purpose of the interview is to screen clients to see if they are appropriate for the agency or clinic, then the structured interview is preferred.

The advantage of the unstructured interview is that it can be adapted to respond to the unique needs of the client. Similarly, if the purpose of the interview is to better understand the specifics of the individual client, then the unstructured interview may be preferred. Finally, the semi-structured interview is a combination of the structured and unstructured interviews, wherein certain questions are always asked but there is room for exploration and additional questioning. Whiston (2009) suggested several common guidelines for an initial interview:

- Assure the client of confidentiality and specify any limitations.
- Ask questions in a courteous and accepting manner.
- Use open-ended questions.
- Avoid leading questions.
- Listen attentively.
- Consider the client's cultural and ethnic background in structuring the interview.
- Adjust your approach to the individual client and be attuned to their comfort level.
- Avoid "chatting."
- Encourage clients to express feelings, thoughts, and behaviors openly.
- Avoid psychological jargon.
- Use voice tones that are warm and inviting yet professional.
- Don't rush clients to finish complex questions.
- If client responses drift from pertinent topics, gently direct them back to the appropriate topics.
- Vary your posture.

Basic and Advanced Helping Skills

Egan (2013) has presented and refined a three-stage structured, solution-focused approach to helping.

Stage 1—focuses on the current scenario: what is the client's story; what are the blind spots; what does the client want to change?

Stage 2—focuses on the preferred scenario: what are the possibilities; what are the priorities; to what does the client commit?

Stage 3—focuses on the strategy or getting-there phase: what strategies are possible; what strategies are the best fit; what is the plan to get there; what specific measureable change will happen in thoughts, feelings, and behaviors?

The basic skills of attending, active listening, making appropriate use of probes, and conveying empathy are used to explore the thoughts, feelings, and behaviors related to the client's current scenario. The skills of paraphrasing, reflecting feelings, clarifying, and summarizing also facilitate the counseling communication. The more advanced skills involve presenting a greater degree of challenge to the client. Advanced helping skills presented in the Egan model are interpretation, pointing out of patterns and connections, identification of blind spots and discrepancies, self-disclosure, confrontation, and immediacy. At each level the movement is from exploring to challenging to focusing and committing to change.

Another useful model regarding counseling performance skills is the microskills training model (Ivey, Gluckstern, & Ivey, 1993; Ivey, Ivey, & Zalaquett, 2010). This model identifies basic and advanced skills ranging from attending behaviors to skill integration and the development of one's own style and theory. Ivey has presented a useful representation of his model in the microskills hierarchy. It is visually presented as a pyramid (Ivey et al., 2010). The base of this pyramid of skills is ethics, multicultural competence, and wellness. Each skill level builds on this foundation and on each new level of microskills as presented. The skill levels progress from attending behaviors to the basic listening sequence of open and closed questions, client observation, encouraging, paraphrasing and summarizing, and reflection of feeling. The next level includes influencing skills which help clients explore personal and interpersonal conflicts. The skills of confrontation, focusing, reflection of meaning, interpretation, and reframing are at this level. The key skills of interpersonal influence—self-disclosure, feedback, logical consequences, information/psychoeducation, and directives—further build on the range of skills needed to successfully move the client from problem disclosure to goals to action. The microskills are intentionally used as the client is moved through a five-stage interview structure. The interview structure moves from relationship to story and strengths, and then to goals in the first three identified stages. Skillful use of attending behaviors and the basic listening sequence can guide the client through these stages. The fourth and fifth stages are "restorying" or describing your preferred story, and actions where you apply the identified influencing skills and the skills of interpersonal influencing. Clients restory their lives and move toward change and action (Ivey et al., 2010). This five-stage interview structure (relationship—story and strengths—goals—restory—action) can be applied to a wide range of theoretical approaches in counseling and psychotherapy. We have extrapolated specific basic and advanced skills from this model to help prepare counselors-in-training to become conscious of the range of skills implemented in their counseling sessions.

Procedural and Issue-Specific Skills

Procedural skills refer to the way the counselor manages the opening and closing of sessions. Does the session open easily and proceed to the ongoing work of the counseling? Or does it begin with chitchat about the weather or other content unrelated to the focus of the counseling work? Once the relationship with the client is established, ongoing interviews require that the counselor reinstates the relationship. This can be done with short statements helping the client to transition back into the counseling work. This can head off the possibility of spending too much time detailing how the week has gone. Ongoing sessions are characterized by more clinical information gathering and focusing in depth (Cormier & Hackney, 2012).

Procedural skills also refer to the way the counselor ends the session. A general guideline is to limit the session to a certain amount of time. With children sessions may be 20 to 30 minutes, with adults 45 to 50 minutes. Sessions rarely need to exceed an hour. Sommers-Flanagan and Sommers-Flanagan (2003) recommended (1) leaving enough time to close the session, (2) validating any concerns or self-disclosures the client has made during the session, (3) solidifying a follow-up appointment, and (4) giving the client a chance to ask questions or make a comment as the session ends. The counselor also sets the boundaries for ending the session, even though some clients may challenge these boundaries. For example, a client may abruptly end a session saying, "I'm done for today," or bring up a crisis just prior to the end of a session. Sommers-Flanagan and Sommers-Flanagan (2003) asserted that maintaining time boundaries is in the best interest of the client in the long run. In the first case the counselor acknowledges the client concern but is available for the full session, and in the second case he/she notes the timing of the crisis disclosure and reschedules the next session based on the agreed-on timing for the next appointment. The rare exception to this is if the client is desperately anxious to leave and when a client brings up a recent traumatic event or a serious threat against self or others.

Structuring the Initial Session

You may wish to open the counseling interview by structuring what the client can expect in the session. An example is:

> Hi Jane. We will have about an hour together today for you to let me know what brings you to counseling and some of the concerns you have and want to discuss. Whatever you discuss with me will be kept between you and me. This is called confidentiality. This is a very important part of the counseling. However, I must tell you that there are some exceptions to this. For example, if you tell me you are abusing a child or a vulnerable person, I'm mandated to report this as these actions are against the law in this state. Or if I was ordered by a court of law to provide information or if you were in a legal proceeding and requested I share information, I would have to comply. Finally, if you gave me information that gave me reason to think that there was a serious risk of harm to you or someone else, there would be some limits to the complete confidentiality of what we have discussed. Since I am a counselor-in-training I will be reviewing my work with my supervisor, who is also obligated to honor the confidentiality of what you talk about. Before we go on with our session and you let me know about your concerns, I want to be sure you understand this. Your safety and your privacy are important to me and to you. . . The rest of the session is for you to let me know about your concerns. I'm happy to answer any questions you may have. This is your time to talk about whatever you wish.

The initial contact with the client is a crucial point in the process of counseling. It provides the counselor with the opportunity to begin structuring the therapeutic relationship. Methods of structuring vary according to the counselor's style and theoretical approach to counseling. Ivey (1999) suggested a five-step process for the purpose of structuring the counseling relationship:

1. *Rapport and structuring* is a process that has as its purpose the building of a working alliance with the client to enable the client to become comfortable with the interviewer. Structuring is needed to explain the purpose of the interview and to keep the sessions on task. Structuring informs the client about what the counselor can and cannot do in therapy.
2. *Gathering information, defining the problem, and identifying the client's assets* is a process designed to assist the counselor in learning why the client has come for counseling and how he/she views the problem. Skillful problem definition and knowledge of the client's assets give the session purpose and direction.
3. *Determining outcomes* enables the counselor to plan therapy based on what the client is seeking in therapy and to understand, from the client's viewpoint, what life would be like without the existing problem(s).
4. *Exploring alternatives and confronting incongruities* is purposeful behavior on the part of the counselor to work toward resolution of the client's problems. Generating alternatives and confronting incongruities with the client assists the counselor in understanding more about client dynamics.
5. *Generalization and transfer of learning* is the process whereby changes in the client's thoughts, feelings, and behaviors are carried out in everyday life by the client.

Hutchins and Cole (1992) suggested that structuring also includes explaining to the client the kinds of events that can be expected to occur during the process of helping, from the initial interview through the termination and follow-up process. Some aspects of structuring will occur in the initial phase of the helping process (initial greeting; discussion of time constraints, roles, confidentiality), whereas other aspects of structuring may take place throughout the remainder of the helping process (clarification of expectations and actions both inside and outside the interview setting).

In summary, structuring the relationship entails defining for the client the nature, purpose, and goals of the counseling process and provides the client with information regarding confidentiality guidelines for their informed consent. Critical to the structuring process is the counselor's ability to create an atmosphere that enables the client to know that the counselor is genuine, sincere, and empathic in his/her desire to assist the client.

Closing the Initial Session

Remember that your goal in this first session is to understand, as fully as possible, the client's concerns from the client's point of view. Using the basic skills you have practiced in your classes, facilitate the telling of the story that the client brings about his/her circumstances. Understand the feelings, thoughts, and behaviors that are part of the client's concerns and communicate this understanding. At the same time that you are attuned to the concerns that the client presents, you are also observing how the client sees himself/herself in his/her world—what are the challenges, the strengths, the supports, the areas of confusion and intensity, and the client's interpretation of his/her experiences with others. In reflecting on the process through which the client tells of his/her concerns, you may have some hunches about the client's dynamics. How does the client present a picture of himself/herself as someone who can get his/her needs met in the world? Is the client likely to present one face to the world and feel quite differently on the inside? Is the client's narrative focused on how others have failed or misled him/her? By the completion of the first session, you will have formed the beginnings of a therapeutic relationship, you will be attuned to the client's concerns as he/she presents them, and you will have some tentative hunches about the client's dynamics and how this may assist or complicate a healthy resolution to his/her concerns.

Allow time before the end of the session to review additional informed consent information. Also allow time for the client to ask questions about the consent and/or about the session. You can end the session with a question about whether the client felt that his/her concerns had been understood. Or, if there is an issue that needs further exploration, you can ask the client to think further about this and you can begin the next session with this topic. You can also thank clients for being open to the counseling process and encourage them for being willing to look at their concerns and for being open to the changes they may need to consider to improve their situation.

Pretherapy Intake Information

Many agencies gather pretherapy intake information prior to the first counseling session. Typically this will include medical, psychological, and psychiatric data that focus on the history and outcomes of treatment. The Initial Intake Form (Form 3.3) is designed to provide the counselor or therapist with initial identifying data about the client. The Psychosocial History Form (Form 3.4) provides information to assess developmental history and the acuteness or chronicity of the current concerns. Data about the client are obtained directly from the client by the counselor at the initial interview in settings where a structured interview is preferred. Other agencies ask that the client fill in forms prior to the beginning of treatment, and this information is made available to the therapist prior to the initial session. Still other agencies have a separate intake interview by someone other than the counselor who will be providing the ongoing therapy. The counselor can refer to the pretherapy assessment information prior to writing an intake summary. Further assessment processes may be recommended based on the pretherapy information and the needs that were determined based on the initial session. Chapter 4 will provide a more extensive review of the intake interview which focuses on data collection. Other information regarding overall assessment and diagnosis procedures will also be found in that chapter.

Intake Summary

At the conclusion of the initial interview and intake process, the counseling student should include a brief description of the client during the session. Observations can include the client's physical appearance, ease in the session, the way the problems were verbalized, and the client's response to you (warmth, distance, eye contact, facial expressions). What are the ways, if any, that the client's race, ethnicity, and general cultural background may influence your perception and understanding. Finally, a summary of the initial session and pretherapy assessment should be written. Remember, this summary should be brief and represents your clinical hunches at this point. Cormier and Hackney (2012) identify several elements that can be included. The following elements can be included in the summary:

1. How do you understand the problem, and what outcome might you expect?
2. How does the intake information relate to the problem?
3. What strengths does the client bring to the counseling work?
4. What internal and external factors might complicate achieving the desired outcome?
5. What techniques and approaches to counseling might be helpful to this client?

Client Record Keeping

The keeping of client records is essential to the maintenance of professional and ethical practice. What is contained in a client's record is oftentimes unclear to the beginning counselor. We are providing you with two formats that are frequently used in agency settings.

Progress Notes

The specifics of the progress notes required may differ depending on whether the setting is clinical or nonclinical. The progress notes may also differ to reflect the counseling specialty pursued (addictions; career; college; marriage, couple, and family; mental health; school).

In clinical settings, the notes kept as part of the ongoing work of the agency are referred to as progress notes. These notes become part of the client's medical records and are protected by HIPAA federal guidelines. This information belongs to the client, and the client has the privilege that his/her information be kept confidential. This information is a legal document that can be subpoenaed. Records kept in agency or clinical settings typically include the counseling start and stop times, medications, modalities and frequency of treatment, results of tests, and progress notes which are a summary of diagnoses, functional states, symptoms, prognoses, and progress made. The two most frequently used formats for progress notes are DAP notes and SOAP notes (Gehart, 2013).

The DAP Format

DAP is an acronym for data, assessment, and plan. The notes are divided into three sections:

1. *The data or description section:* This section includes what happened in the session: interventions, clinical observations, symptom diagnosis, stressors. This can include both subjective and objective information. Subjective information includes themes of what the clients say about themselves, others, and their environment and situation. Objective information is what the counselor observes about the client's behavior and appearance. The counselor also records the interaction with the client, describing what took place and how it relates to the client's goals (Gehart, 2013).
2. *Assessment:* This is the interpretation section and includes the counselor's analysis and conclusion about the data. What do the data mean or suggest? Wiger (2013) identifies the following areas and types of information for this section: effects or results of this session, therapeutic progress, client's level of cooperation, client progress and setbacks, areas requiring more work, effectiveness of treatment strategies, completion of treatment plan objectives, changes needed to keep therapy on target, and need for diagnostic revision.
3. *Plan:* What happens next, or what is the follow-up (i.e., scheduled next session, homework, referral, change in treatment plan, or interventions for next session)?

The SOAP Notes Format

SOAP is an acronym for subjective, objective, assessment, and plan. The data collection is divided into subjective (S) and objective (O) parts.

The subjective part (S) contains information about the problem from the client's perspective or that of significant others. The entries here should be brief and concise. The client's perception of the problem should be clear to the outside reader when reading this section.

The objective part (O) consists of observations made by the counselor. The counselor's observations should be precise, descriptive, and factual. Report what can be seen, heard, smelled, counted, or measured. The phrase "is evidenced by" is helpful here.

The assessment (A) section demonstrates how the data are being interpreted and reflected on. This is a summary of the counselor's clinical thinking about the client's problem. This usually includes a *DSM* diagnosis. The counselor needs to have sufficient data to support the diagnosis.

The plan (P) section summarizes the treatment direction. This includes both the action plan and a prognosis (Cameron & Turtle-Song, 2002, pp. 288–290). Table 3.1 summarizes the SOAP notes format and provides examples.

Record Keeping and the School Counselor

Record keeping for the school counselor presents some complications that are different from those encountered by mental health counselors and psychologists. Merlone (2005), in a thorough review of laws regarding confidentiality and privilege, noted that most states do not grant privilege to school counselors. This has major implications for record keeping. The contradiction is that confidentiality is needed to properly assist students, but there is no legal protection of confidentiality. The Family Education Rights and Privacy Act, passed in 1979, defined the rights of parents and

Table 3.1   A Summarization of SOAP Definitions and Examples

Legend for Chart

A = Section
      B = Definitions
         C = Examples

Subjective (S)

What the client tells you
What pertinent others tell you about the client
Basically, how the client experiences the world
   Client's feelings, concerns, plans, goals, and thoughts
   Intensity of problems and impact on relationships
   Pertinent comments by family, case managers, behavioral therapists, etc.
   Client's orientation to time, place, and person
   Client's verbalized changes toward helping

Objective (O)

Factual: what the counselor personally observes/witnesses
Quantifiable: what was seen, counted, smelled, heard, or measured
Outside written materials received
   The client's general appearance, affect, behavior
   Nature of the helping relationship
   Client's demonstrated strengths and weaknesses
   Test results, materials from other agencies, etc., are to be noted and attached

Assessment (A)

Summarizes the counselor's clinical thinking
A synthesis and analysis of the subjective and objective portion of the notes
   For counselor: include clinical diagnosis and clinical impressions (if any).
   For care providers: how would you label the client's behavior and the reasons (if any) for this behavior?

Plan (P)

Describes the parameters of treatment
Consists of an action plan and prognosis
   Action plan: include interventions used, treatment progress, and direction.
   Counselors should include the date of next appointment.
   Prognosis: include the anticipated gains from the interventions.

Cameron, S. & Turtle-Song, I. (2002). Learning to write case notes using SOAP format. Table 1. A summarization of SOAP definitions and examples. *Journal of Counseling and Development, 8*(3), 286–292. Copyright 2002 by the American Counseling Association. Reprinted with permission.

students age 18 and older regarding access to student records. Student records were defined as a record maintained by the educational institution containing information directly related to the student. This definition does not include counselors' personal files if they are entirely private and not made available to others (Fischer & Sorenson, 1996). Common practice has become maintaining anecdotal notes in a personal notebook or folder securely kept on one's own person and not kept in the school. Swanson (1983) cautions that even though counselors' notes are not part of the school's record, they are subject to subpoena. Notes should be written in behavioral terms and avoid "any statements which could be defamatory" (p. 35). We have provided a Case Notes Form (Form 3.5) for practicum/internship students in school counseling to use to maintain their private notes about their clients. Other students who prefer a notes format other than DAP or SOAP notes may use the Case Notes format to monitor the progress of their clients and to prepare for supervision. Categories included in this format are presenting/current concern, key issues addressed, interventions, progress/setbacks, assessment, and objectives and plan.

American School Counselors Association's *Ethical Standards for School Counselors* (2010) provide both a rationale for student record keeping that protects student confidentiality and a rationale for organizing data about the scope of counseling practice. Documentation serves two major functions. First, accurate documentation is an integral part of providing professional counseling services which allow the counselor to keep track of pertinent information about specific students. These serve as a memory aid about the progress of the counseling, assist in any necessary referral processes, and meet the best practice guidelines of the professional school counselor. Second, documentation of all school counseling-related activities with students, teachers, parents; prevention programming; consulting; and non-counseling-related duties provides evidence to support the need for a school counseling program. This is a method of accountability and allows the school counselor to track the school counseling program's progress from year to year (Wehrman, Williams, Field & Schroeder, 2010).

The practicum/internship student in school counseling will be documenting all counseling-related activities on the Weekly Schedule/Practicum Log and Monthly Practicum Log (Forms 3.6 and 3.7). The Case Notes Form (Form 3.5) provides a structure for personal notes to aid in keeping track of work with specific students. Remember, case notes are considered your personal property and must not be shown to anyone or they become public property and can no longer be considered confidential. You can take your notes to court and read from them, but do not visually show them or turn them over to anyone (Hanson, 2009–2012). If you are working with a student at risk, you should take more detailed notes, separate from your case notes summary. These situations are usually when the student's safety is in question and you must inform others, such as parents, the administration, the school nurse, or someone in the legal system. Consult with your supervisor regarding the procedures in place at your practicum/internship site. Your more detailed notes should contain the following:

- the time and date you spoke to the student;
- exactly what the student said, "in quotes";
- interventions you did at the time—be specific;
- recommendations or suggestions you made to the student;
- follow-up calls you had with anyone—be specific (i.e., who, when, content of call, quote when significant);
- recommendations, referrals, and resources offered to parents; and
- other details you want in writing for future reference (Hanson, 2009–2012).

Hanson (2009–2012) also provides other useful forms such as the Record of All Students Seen, Individual Student Contact Sheet, Parent Contact Log, and a Support Group Log.

The taking of progress notes and case notes is an invaluable aid to the counselor-in-training. Session notes assist the counselor in focusing his/her attention on the most salient aspects of the counseling session. In addition, session notes can help the counselor to review significant developments from session to session.

WEEKLY SCHEDULE

Day of week	Location	Time	Practicum activity	Comment
Mon	UUC	9–10	Intake interview	1st session
			John W.	Problem exploration
		10–11	Individual counseling	5th session, taped
			Jane D.	Personal/social
		11–12	Ind. supervision	Reviewed reports
				Tape critique
		1–3	Group counseling	Eating disorder
			Co-lead	Group 3rd session
		3–4	Report writing	
		4–5	Testing	Interpreted
			Mary B.	Strong/Campbell
Wed	University	6–8	Group	Case presentation
			Supervision	Jane D.

Student counselor name _____

Week beginning _____ Ending _____

Figure 3.1

Documenting Practicum Hours

Because of national accreditation guidelines and state and university requirements, it is a necessary procedure to document both the total number of hours spent in practicum and the total number of hours spent in particular practicum activities. Two forms are provided here for your use in tracking the time spent on various activities. The Weekly Schedule/Practicum Log (Form 3.6) can be used in two ways. First, the weekly schedule can be used by the practicum student and the practicum supervisor to plan the activities in which the student will participate from week to week. Second, the weekly schedule can be used to document the weekly activities the student has already completed. An example of a completed Weekly Schedule is provided in Figure 3.1. The Monthly Practicum Log (Form 3.7) provides a summary of the number of hours of work per month in which the student has engaged in the activity categories established in the practicum contract. The student will calculate the number of hours spent in direct client contact and in indirect service and the total practicum hours. A file should be kept for each student for the duration of the practicum experience and turned in to the faculty supervisor after being signed by the site supervisor.

Summary

This chapter has presented a review of basic information and practices required to begin working with clients at your field site. Information regarding HIPAA and informed consent guidelines, as well as a sample informed consent and disclosure statement, was included. Forms for getting proper authorizations for recording sessions for supervision purposes are included in the Forms section at the end of the book. Basic and advanced counseling skills and procedural and structuring practices were reviewed. Guidelines for writing progress notes in clinical practice as well as guidelines for record keeping in a school setting were provided. The counselor-in-training must make certain that professional practices consistent with field site policies and procedures and the ethics of the counseling profession are followed when initiating counseling relationships.

Note

1 These sections were contributed by Megan Crucianni, MA, NBCC, LPC, part-time faculty in the graduate program in counseling at Marywood University, Scranton, Pennsylvania.

References

American Counseling Association (2014). *Code of ethics.* Alexandria, VA: Author.

American Medical Association. (2013). *HIPAA privacy and security toolkit: Helping your practice meet new compliance guidelines.* Retrieved from www.ama-assn.org/resources/doc/washington/hipaa.toolkit.pdf.

American School Counselors Association. (2010). *Ethical standards for school counselors.* Retrieved from www.schoolcounselor.org/asca/Media/asca/Resource%20Center/Legal%20and%Ethical%20Issues/Sample%Documents/EthicalStandards2010.pdf.

Cameron, S., & Turtle-Song, I. (2002). Learning to write case notes using the SOAP format. *Journal of Counseling and Development, 80*(3), 286–292.

Corey, G., Corey, M. S., & Callahan, P. (2011). *Issues and ethics in the helping professions* (8th ed.). Belmont, CA: Brooks/Cole/Cengage.

Cormier, S., & Hackney, H. (2012). *Counseling strategies and interventions* (8th ed.). Upper Saddle River, NJ: Pearson Education.

Egan, G. (2013). *The skilled helper: A problem management and opportunity development approach to helping* (10th ed.). Belmont, CA: Brooks/Cole.

Fischer, L., & Sorenson, G. P. (1996). *School law for counselors, psychologists and social workers* (3rd ed.). White Plains, NY: Longman.

Gehart, D. R. (2013). *Mastering competencies in family therapy: A practical approach to theory and case documentation.* Belmont, CA: Brooks/Cole.

Glosoff, H. L. & Pate, R. H., Jr. (2002). Privacy and confidentiality in school counseling. *Journal of School Counseling, 6*(1), 20–27.

Haas, L. J., & Malouf, J. L. (1995). *Keeping up the good work: A practitioner's guide to mental health ethics* (2nd ed.). Sarasota, FL: Professional Resource Exchange.

Hanson, S. (2009–2012). *Confidentiality and the school counselor.* Retrieved from www.school-counseling-zone.com/confidentiality.html.

Hutchins, D. E., & Cole, C. G. (1992). *Helping relationships and strategies.* Monterey, CA: Brooks/Cole.

Ivey, A. E. (1999). *Intentional interviewing and counseling.* Pacific Grove, CA: Brooks/Cole.

Ivey, A. E., Gluckstern, N., & Ivey, M. B. (1993). *Basic attending skills.* North Amherst, MA: Microtraining Associates.

Ivey, A. E., Ivey, M. B., & Zalaquett, C. P. (2010). *Intentional interviewing and counseling* (7th ed.). Belmont, CA: Brooks/Cole.

Merlone, L. (2005). Record keeping and the school counselor. *Professional School Counseling, 8*(4), 372–376.

Norcross, J. C. (Ed.). (2002). *Psychotherapy relationships that work.* New York: Oxford University Press.

Office of the Privacy Commissioner of Canada (2014, May). A basic overview of privacy legislation in Canada. Retrieved from www.priv.gc.ca/resources/fs-fi02_05_d_15_e.asp.

Remley, T. P., Jr., & Herlihy, B. (2014). *Ethical, legal, and professional issues in counseling* (4th ed.). Upper Saddle River, NJ: Pearson.

Rogers, C. (1951). *Client-centered therapy: Its current practice, implications and theory.* Boston: Houghton Mifflin.

Seligman, L. (2004). *Systems, strategies, and skills of counseling and psychotherapy.* Upper Saddle River, NJ: Merrill/Prentice Hall.

Sommers-Flanagan, J., & Sommers-Flanagan, R. (2003). *Clinical interviewing* (3rd ed.). New York: Wiley.

Swanson, C. D. (1983). The law and the counselor. In J. A. Brown & R. H. Pate Jr. (Eds.), *Being a counselor: Directions and challenges* (pp. 26–41). Monterey, CA: Brooks/Cole.

Wehrman, J. D., Williams, R., Field, J., & Schroeder, S. D. (2010). Accountability through documentation: What are best practices for school counselors? *Journal of School Counseling, 8* (38), 2–21. Retrieved from www.jsc.montana.edu/articles/v8n38.pdf.

Welfel, E. (2010). *Ethics in counseling and psychotherapy* (4th ed.). Belmont, CA: Brooks/Cole, Cengage.

Wheeler, A. M. (2013). Tick tock . . . beat the HIPAA/HITECH clock. American Counseling Association. Retrieved from www.counseling.org/docs/ethics/aca-hipaa-hitech-9-23-13-compliance-date.pdf?sfv.

Whiston, S. C. (2009). *Principles and applications of assessment in counseling* (3rd ed.). Belmont, CA: Brooks/Cole, Cengage.

Wiger, D. E. (2013). *Psychotherapy documentation primer* (3rd ed.). Hoboken, NJ: Wiley.

CHAPTER 4

ASSESSMENT AND CASE CONCEPTUALIZATION

The implementation of assessment practices appropriate to the counselor's specialization is a central skill in the practice of professional counseling. The standards of the Council for Accreditation of Counseling and Related Educational Programs (CACREP, 2009) require as part of the core curriculum that all specializations include instruction in "basic concepts of standardized and non-standardized testing and other norm referenced and criterion referenced assessment, environmental assessment, performance assessment, individual and group testing and inventory materials, personality testing and behavioral observation" (G.7.b). The specializations of addictions counseling and mental health counseling also require instruction in the use of the diagnostic classifications of the *Diagnostic and Statistical Manual of Mental Disorders* (*DSM*). The proposed 2016 *CACREP Standards*, Draft 2 (CACREP, 2013), include the use of assessments for diagnostic and intervention purposes (G.7.e); the use of assessment relevant to academic, career, personal, and social development (G.7.i); and the use of assessment results to diagnose developmental, behavioral, and mental disorders (G.7.l). The specializations of addictions counseling; clinical rehabilitation counseling; marriage, couple, and family counseling; and clinical mental health counseling will also require instruction in the *DSM* and International Classification of Disorders (ICD) diagnostic classification system. The practicum and internship experience provides the counselor-in-training with the opportunity to implement assessment and testing practices under supervision.

The task of counselors during the assessment process requires that they know what information to obtain and how to obtain it, and that they have both the ability to put it together in some meaningful way and the capacity to use it to generate clinical hunches. Such hunches, or hypotheses about client's problems, can then allow counselors and therapists to develop tentative ideas for planning and treatment (Cormier & Cormier, 1998). In the process of preparing the client for data-gathering and assessment activities, the therapist employs attending skills and facilitative therapeutic techniques. Remley and Herlihy (2014) describe the assessment process as a collaborative process between the counselor and the client where they work together to gain a better understanding of the client's problems. In the assessment process, clients have the right to understand what the process will involve, what its purposes are, and what the assessment will be used for.

It is through this initial contact and data-gathering process that the counselor is challenged to use his/her professional abilities through the application of appropriate interpersonal skills. The interviewer must demonstrate skills that promote the understanding of self and others in an attempt to gather relevant data about the client and his/her concerns. Like all other counseling skills, effective questioning requires the counselor to be sensitive to the client's emotional state, to demonstrate proper timing of questions, and to contain the questioning in an attempt to control the flow of information from the client. Questioning enables the counselor to gather information and to deepen the level of discussion with the client or to broaden its focus.

The following is a description and format of typical assessment activities occurring prior to and during the initial stages of counseling.

Initial Assessment

Many agencies gather assessment information about the client prior to the beginning of the first counseling session. Sometimes clients are asked to complete intake questionnaires and psychosocial history questionnaires on their own to bring with them to the initial counseling session. The Initial Intake Form (Form 3.3) and the Psychosocial History (Form 3.4) are examples. The psychosocial history provides more data than the initial intake and is invaluable in examining the acuteness or chronicity of the client's problem. Specific attention is directed toward the milestones or benchmarks in the client's developmental history that have implications for the treatment strategies to be employed in therapy. Other agencies conduct an initial intake assessment prior to assigning a client to a counselor. The intake interview is an information-gathering process rather than a therapeutic process. However, the use of basic counseling skills to create a facilitative interaction remains a priority. Frequently, someone other than the counselor conducts the interview and passes critical information on to the counselor. Regardless of who does the interview, it is essential that certain data be collected to provide the counselor with the information necessary to understand the client's presenting problem(s) and current life issues. Cormier and Hackney (2012) have proposed a helpful guide concerning the content of an intake interview. These areas of inquiry are the following:

- *Identifying data:* Name, address, phone number where client can be reached; age, gender, ethnic origin, race, partnered status, occupational and educational status, languages spoken, citizenship status.
- *Presenting issues—both primary and secondary:* Does it interfere with everyday functioning; how long has the concern existed; why has the client decided to seek counseling at this time?
- *Client's current life setting:* The client's typical day or week, living environment, important current relationships, financial stressors, current work or educational situation.
- *Family history:* Establish whether the client has a family of choice or biological family; age, order, and names of siblings and relationships between them; family distress or stability.
- *Personal history.*
- *Description of the client during the interview:* Appearance; the way the client related to you; areas of comfort or discomfort, warmth or distance; language use; mental status.
- *Summary and recommendations.*

When the client presents for counseling, he/she can bring concerns about emotional distress, overwhelming life circumstances, struggles to make complex life transitions, or any number of emotion-laden situations in which he/she is seeking help. Whatever the nature of the presenting concern, the situation occurs in the context of the client's whole life and worldview. Consequently, gathering information about family and personal history and contextual information about the client's current life can help both the counselor and the client become aware of some of the antecedents of the problem and of the possible complications in making the necessary changes for a healthy resolution. The counselor should be able to reassure the client about the benefits of reviewing this information. Some of the questions about family and personal history may elicit painful or emotionally uncomfortable memories. It is important to let clients know that they have choices about how much they want to disclose. This is a great deal of information to obtain. The counselor must move through the questions in a timely fashion but also be sensitive to areas of questioning that may be uncomfortable for the client. It is helpful to let the client know that the counseling process will occur over time, and any areas of concern that may be revealed in this intake process can be discussed with the counselor if the client so chooses.

Gathering Family History Data

Remember when you are gathering family history data that we live in a pluralistic society and there are many forms of family in our culture. There are many blended families, families of choice rather than biological families, single-parent families, and multigenerational families. When gathering family data, the counselor should pursue the following information:

- Begin by having the client let you know about the kind of family he/she grew up in. Then proceed to ask about the names, ages, and order of any brothers or sisters and, if siblings were present, whether they were biological, blended, or adopted.
- Inquire about parents and their relationship with one another and with the client and siblings. Ask about a history of distress or substance abuse.
- Ask about the stability of the family. Check about frequent moves, significant losses, and level of conflict, if any?
- Inquire about the client's current relationship with family members?

Gathering Personal History Data

In addition to gaining an accurate picture of family history, Cormier and Hackney (2012) suggested addressing the following categories of information to gather relevant data regarding personal history:

- Medical history: any significant illnesses or accidents or treatment for substance abuse.
- Educational history: progress through grade school, high school, and post–high school. Include extracurricular and peer relationships.
- Military service.
- Work history: where, when, what type, and for how long. Any job termination or job losses?
- Spiritual and religious history: any current beliefs and practices?
- Legal history: speeding tickets, fights, violence, bankruptcy.
- Substance use history: previous or current use of alcohol, drugs, or prescription drugs. How much and how often?
- Relationship history: when did client receive sexual information? Dating history? Any engagements and/or marriages and/or partnerships? Other serious emotional involvements prior to the present? Reasons previous relationships ended? Are there any children?
- Traumatic experiences: has the client been neglected or abused sexually, physically, or emotionally by anyone? Natural disasters? Oppression? Discrimination?

Obtaining Information From Others

Occasionally client information must be obtained from others (parents, therapists, teachers). The Initial Intake and Psychosocial History forms can be used for that purpose. The Elementary School Counseling Referral Form (Form 4.1) and the Secondary School Counseling Referral Form (Form 4.2) tend to include more data regarding the academic history of the student and his/her behavior and demeanor in school. The Elementary and Secondary School Counseling Referral Forms are designed to obtain appropriate precounseling data from sources other than the client. Typically, the professional making a referral of a school-age child for counseling or therapy is asked to describe and comment on his/her perceptions and knowledge of the pupil's current academic and social functioning.

At the completion of the intake assessment and the initial counseling session, the counselor should be prepared to write a summary of the presenting concerns and any connections that are noted that may connect the presenting problems with the background information that has been gathered. You may have recommendations for gathering additional assessment information; you may note whether anything in the client's history seems like a red flag, how you understand the problem, and how will you proceed. Be as concise as possible. Avoid elaborate inferences. Include only information that is directly relevant to the client and the counseling services to be recommended. Make sure *confidential* is stamped on the report.

Goals of Assessment

A helpful resource in understanding the goals of assessment and assessment interviewing is provided by Howatt (2000), who suggested that a number of goals need to be kept in mind when conducting an assessment interview. As the counselor is forming impressions of the client and his/her family background and personal history, the counselor is also developing a working relationship with the client and is making connections between the information and the problems and possible interventions. Additional probes and requests for more detail or examples should be consistent with the suggested goals of any assessment process. A summary of these goals includes the following:

1. to gather consistent and comprehensive information,
2. to identify a person's major strengths,
3. to identify the problem(s) that bring the client to counseling,
4. to prioritize problems,
5. to teach the inadequacy of a quick fix to problems,
6. to clarify diagnostic uncertainty,
7. to measure cognitive functioning,
8. to differentiate treatment assignments,
9. to develop rapport and create a healthy working environment, and
10. to focus on the therapeutic interventions.

Processes and Categories for Assessing Client Problems

When intake interviewing and initial assessment is concluded, the counselor shifts the focus of continuing assessment to obtaining a fuller understanding of the scope and degree of the problem/s the client is presenting. Cormier and Nurius (2003) suggested a variety of processes and categories which can be addressed when fully assessing the client's problems. This focus allows both the counselor and the client to appreciate and acknowledge the full range of concerns that the client brings and to prioritize the work of the therapy. An overview of these processes and categories for assessing a client's problems follows:

1. explanation of the purpose of assessment: rationale provided to the client;
2. identification of a range of problems: identify relevant issues to get "the big picture";
3. prioritization and selection of issues and problems: selecting the area of focus;
4. identification of present problem behaviors: affective, somatic, behavioral, cognitive, contextual, and relational;
5. identification of antecedents: sources of antecedents and effect on the problem;
6. identification of consequences: identify sources of consequences and their effect on problem behavior;
7. identification of secondary gains: variables that serve as "payoffs" to maintain problem behavior;
8. identification of previous solutions: identify previous solutions and their effect on the problem;
9. identification of client coping skills: identify past and present coping behaviors;
10. identification of the client's perception of the problem: describe the client's understanding of the problem; and
11. identification of problem intensity: client self-monitoring to identify the impact of the problem on the client's life.

Remley and Herlihy (2014) have suggested an approach to assessment from the perspective of the wellness model of mental health. As the scope of the problem is explored and clarified, the counselor can view the problem/s in terms of how this may effect the client's level of functioning in important areas of the client's life. In this model, the goal is for each person to achieve positive mental health to the degree possible. Mental health is seen as occurring on a continuum (Smith, 2001). The wellness orientation views mental health as including a number of scales of mental and emotional wellness in important areas of living. Counselors assess a client's functioning on a continuum ranging from dysfunction (very mentally ill) to highly functioning (self-actualizing) in the areas of

- family relationships, friendships, and other relationships (work/church, etc.);
- career/job;
- spirituality;
- leisure activities;
- physical health;
- living environment;
- financial status; and
- sexuality.

Counselors assess clients' current life situations and help determine which factors are interfering with the goal of reaching their maximum potential. Many persons are limited by physical disabilities or environmental conditions that cannot be changed. Consequently, counselors assist their clients in becoming as autonomous and successful in their lives as possible. Although counselors understand and use the *DSM* in diagnosis, the goal of counseling is to help the client accomplish wellness rather than to cure an illness.

Other approaches to assessment may include more emphasis on elements such as psychopathology, problem complexity, and resistance. Nelson (2002) suggested an eclectic selection model based on the premise that a single, one-dimensional approach is simply not appropriate for all clients who present for counseling and that individual clients can benefit from strategies that honor their particular needs and difficulties. As a result, Nelson suggested the following:

1. Identify initial counseling goals: How does the client want to benefit from counseling? What are the counselor's and client's time constraints for counseling?
2. Identify or rule out psychopathology: Does the client have a biological illness? Does the client demonstrate signs of clinical depression or other disorders that require a consultation with a physician or psychiatrist?
3. Determine problem complexity: Beutler and Harwood (1995) suggested that simple problems are found in clients who have had adequate support throughout life and need to address unwanted cognitive or behavioral symptoms related to situational life events. Complex problems stem from family-of-origin difficulties and often involve long-standing, complicated interpersonal difficulties that require greater analysis and time to address.
4. Assess resistance level: To what degree does the client resist the counselor's suggestions? Is it simply resistance to influence by an authority figure? Is it depression and a sense of hopelessness that trigger resistance?
5. Assess capacity and desire for insight: The counselor must assess the degree of insight a client is either capable or desirous of pursuing.

Thorough assessment of the potential interference or limitation in resolving the problems that the client brings to therapy helps both the counselor and the client to understand the boundaries, patterns, and intensity of those problems in the client's life.

Assessing the Client's Mental Status

Mental health counselors, counseling psychologists, and professional counselors routinely use the mental status examination. These professionals often find that to gain insight into the client's presenting condition, the client's mental status may need to be assessed. The mental status examination is, therefore, designed to provide the therapist with signs that indicate the "functional" nature of the person's psychiatric condition. In addition, the mental status examination can be used to provide the therapist with a current view of the client's mental capabilities and deficits prior to and during the course of treatment and is beneficial to the beginning therapist who lacks the clinical experience to quickly assess the client's mental status.

Many formats can be used to obtain a client's mental status. However, all formats have common areas that are routinely assessed. The following is an example of items fairly typically covered, with an explanation of material generally included. The Mental Status Checklist (Form 4.3) can be used by students in evaluating these common areas of assessment.

Mental Status Categories of Assessment

Appearance and behavior: This category consists of data gathered throughout the interview so that the person reading the narrative has a "photograph" of the client during the interview. Data are gathered by direct observation of the client. To assess a client's appearance and behavior, the counselor or therapist might employ the following questions: Is the client's appearance age appropriate? Does the client appear to be his/her stated age? Is the client's behavior appropriate to the surroundings? Is the behavior overactive or underactive? Is the behavior agitated or retarded? Is speech pressured? Retarded? Logical? Clear? What is the content of speech?

Attention and alertness: Is the client aware of his/her surroundings? Can the client focus attention on the therapist? Is the client highly distractible? Is the client scanning the environment? Is he/she hypervigilant?

Affect and mood: What is the quality of the client's affect? Is the client's affect expressive? Expansive? Blunted? Flat? Agitated? Fearful? Is the client's affect appropriate to the current situation?

Perception and thought: Does the client have false ideas or delusions? Does the client experience his/her own thoughts as being controlled? Does the client experience people putting thoughts in his/her head? Does the client experience his/her own thoughts as being withdrawn or taken away? Does the client feel that people are watching him/her? Out to get him/her? Does the client experience grandiose or bizarre delusions?

Sensory perception: Does the client hallucinate? Does the client experience visual, auditory, tactile, or gustatory false perceptions?

Orientation: Is the client oriented to persons, place, and time? Does the client know with whom he/she is dealing? Where he/she is? What day and time it is?

Judgment: Can the client act appropriately in typical social, personal, and occupational situations? Can the client show good judgment in conducting his/her own life?

Attention and concentration: Does the client have any memory disturbance?

Recent memory: Can the client remember information given a few minutes ago? (For example, give the client three or four things to remember and ask him/her to repeat back after several minutes.)

Long-term memory: Can the client remember or recall information from yesterday? From childhood? Can the client concentrate on facts given to him/her?

Abstract ability: Can the client recognize and handle similarities? Absurdities? Proverbs?

Insight: Is the client aware that he/she has a problem? Is he/she aware of possible causes? Possible solutions?

Diagnosis in Counseling

The use of diagnosis by counselors has been a controversial issue in the training of counselors (Ginter, 2001; Hohenshil, 1996; Ivey & Ivey, 1998). The controversy stems from the belief that in the counseling profession, counselors should follow the developmental model of treating clients with developmental concerns and should leave more severe cases to other trained professionals. In addition, it is felt that the use of diagnosis contradicts some of the more accepted models of counseling (i.e., client-centered, humanistic, etc.). However, it remains a fact that practicing counselors in schools, agencies, and mental health facilities are routinely asked to diagnose and treat clients who have severe mental health issues. This is especially true for counselors in private practice, who are routinely confronted with a managed care environment that requires the use of diagnosis for treatment consideration as well as for insurance coverage. In reality, this is nothing new. Every time a counselor treats a client, he/she is making a diagnosis when choosing and implementing therapeutic interventions. Whether it is through the use of the *DSM*, the highly formalized diagnostic system, or some other system, diagnosis is a reality for trained counselors.

Counselors are frequently asked to participate in collaborative mental health service teams that work together in planning, coordinating, evaluating, and providing direct service to clients.

Geroski and Rodgers (1997) suggested that because school counselors interact with a large number of children and adolescents on a daily basis, they are uniquely able to identify students who manifest particularly worrisome behaviors possibly consistent with significant mental health issues. The counselor is able to provide direct interventions and support services for some of these students. In a survey of the assessment and evaluation activities of school counselors (Ekstrom, Elmore, Schafer, Trotter, & Webster, 2004), results indicated that the most frequently performed assessment-related activity of school counselors was referring students to other professionals as appropriate. Hohenshil (1996) observed that it has become a necessity for all counselors to be skilled in the language of the *DSM*, regardless of their employment setting. Thus, to become a viable member of a collaborative mental health system, the counselor must at the very least become familiar with the language of the *DSM*. Remley and Herlihy (2014) agree that in today's world counselors must be knowledgeable of the current *DSM* and be able to talk with other mental health professionals about its contents.

DSM-5

Information on the *DSM-5* is included here to provide an overview of this classification and coding system. We believe that school, agency, college, career, and mental health counselors must become familiar with the *DSM-5*. Obviously, knowledge about the classification and coding is not a substitute for formal training in the *DSM-5*. The first step in determining a diagnosis is to carefully consider the criteria which must be met in order to form a diagnosis. Specific training and supervision are required. The information included in this text is offered as a resource and reference about changes to the coding and classification system. The *DSM-5* was published in May 2013, culminating a 12-year process of review. It has a goal of providing the best available description of how mental disorders are expressed and can be recognized by trained clinicians. It also has a goal of harmonizing two classification systems: the *DSM* and the ICD. The existing classifications in the *DSM-IV-TR* were reordered and regrouped into a new structure in the *DSM-5*. This reordering and reorganizing process assists with harmonizing it with the ICD. Classifications are now ordered according to developmental and life span considerations. (The order of diagnoses within classifications also follows developmental and life span considerations.) Classifications begin with diagnoses that manifest early in life (e.g., neurodevelopmental, schizophrenic spectrum, and other psychotic disorders), move on to diagnoses likely to manifest in adolescence and young adulthood (e.g., bipolar, depressive, and anxiety disorders), and then to those appearing in adulthood and later (e.g., neurocognitive disorders). The sections (diagnostic classifications) are also reordered to begin with neurological disorders, then groups of internalizing disorders, groups of externalizing disorders, and other disorders (American Psychiatric Association, 2013).

Another element which assists in the harmonization with the ICD is the coding system. In the United States, the Health Insurance Portability and Accountability Act (HIPAA) requires the use of ICD codes in diagnoses, and insurance companies also require this coding. ICD-9-CM codes correspond closely to the *DSM-IV* codes. However, ICD-10-CM codes are quite different and will be required to be in use beginning in October 2014. Therefore, the *DSM-5* codes include both the ICD-9-CM and the corresponding ICD-10-CM codes. ICD-10-CM codes are indicated in parentheses, for example, [309.0 (F43.21)].

The *DSM-5* defines a mental disorder as follows:

A mental disorder is a syndrome characterized by clinically significant disturbance in an individual's cognition, emotion regulation or behavior that reflects a dysfunction in the psychological, biological or developmental processes underlying mental functioning. Mental disorders are usually associated with significant distress in social, occupational, or other important activities. (p. 20)

Elimination of the Multiaxial Assessment System

The *DSM-IV* employed five axes to record biological, social, and psychological assessment of individuals. The first three axes were for recording mental and physical diagnoses; the fourth noted environmental problems, and the fifth provided an assessment of the client's level of functioning. The *DSM-5* has eliminated this multiaxial assessment system. The *DSM-5* has moved to a nonaxial documentation of diagnoses (formerly axes I, II, and III), with separate notations for psychosocial and contextual factors and disability. Psychosocial and environmental problems formerly identified on axis IV will use a selected set of Z codes contained in the ICD-10-CD. The Global Assessment of Functioning GAF has been dropped from the *DSM-5*. To provide a global measure of disability, the World Health Organization Disability Assessment Schedule (WHODAS) is included for further study. Clinicians will continue to list medical conditions that are important to the understanding of the individual's mental disorders.

Subtypes and Specifiers

In the formation of a diagnosis, first the diagnostic criteria are offered as guidelines. When the full criteria for a diagnosis are met, the application of disorder subtypes and/or specifiers are considered when appropriate. Subtypes and specifiers provide for increased specificity. *Subtypes* define mutually exclusive subgroupings within a diagnosis (American Psychiatric Association, 2013). An example of a diagnosis with a disorder subtype would be Adjustment Disorder with Depressed Mood [309.0 (F43.21)]. *Specifiers* are not intended to be mutually exclusive; therefore, more than one can be given. Specifiers can indicate severity (mild, moderate, severe, extreme), course (in partial remission, in full remission, recurrent), descriptive features (good/fair insight, poor insight, absent insight), and other specifiers as indicated in the manual. Subtypes and specifiers can be coded in the fourth, fifth, or sixth digit of the diagnostic code. However, the majority of subtypes and specifiers included in the *DSM-5* cannot be coded in the ICD-9-CM and ICD-10-CM systems. They are indicated by including the subtype after the name of the disorder (e.g., social anxiety disorder/social phobia, performance type is coded as [300.23 (F40.10)/performance type]. Not all disorders include the course, severity, or descriptive features as specifiers.

Other Specified and Unspecified Designation

The *DSM-5* replaces the previous NOS (not otherwise specified) with two options: *other specified disorder* and *unspecified disorder*. The "other specified/unspecified" disorder options have been included to allow for presentations that do not exactly fit the diagnostic criteria for disorders in each chapter. The "other specified" category indicates that the full criteria for a diagnosis within a diagnostic class are not met. The "other specified" designation is used when the clinician wants to indicate the specific reason that the presentation doesn't meet the criteria (American Psychiatric Association, 2013). An example of this diagnosis would be Other specified trauma- and stressor-related disorder [309.89 (F43.8)]. *If the clinician chooses not to specify the reason that* the criteria are not met for the disorder, then Unspecified trauma- and stressor-related disorder would be the diagnosis [309.9 (F43.9)].

DSM-5 *Codes and Classification*

The following codes are intended to be used in conjunction with the text descriptions for each disorder found in the *DSM-5*:

- Before each disorder name, ICD-9-CM codes are provided, followed by ICD-10-CM codes in parentheses.
- Blank lines indicate that either the ICD-9-CM or the ICD-10-CM code is not applicable.
- ICD-9-CM codes are to be used for coding purposes in the United States through September 30, 2014. ICD-10-CM codes are to be used starting on October 1, 2014 (American Psychiatric Association, 2013).

The final section (Section III) of the *DSM-5* is titled "Emerging Measures and Models," and includes the WHODAS 2.0, information and interview guidelines about cultural formulation, and a glossary of cultural concepts of distress.

The revision of criteria for the diagnosis and classification of mental disorders was completed in May 2013. The revised criteria for mental disorders can now be used for diagnosing mental disorders. At the time of this writing, text corrections, coding, and criteria updates for the *DSM-5* are ongoing. Clinicians will base their diagnostic decisions on the *DSM-5* criteria and then cross-walk their decisions to the appropriate ICD-9-CM code through September 2014. As of October 1, 2014, diagnostic decisions based on *DSM-5* criteria will be crosswalked to ICD-10-CM codes. There will be some instances where the *DSM-5* name of a disorder will be crosswalked to an ICD-10-CM code that has a different name. The new *DSM-5* disorders were assigned to the best available ICD codes. Because *DSM-5* and ICD disorder names may be different, the *DSM-5* diagnosis should always be recorded by name in the medical records in addition to listing the codes. The American Psychiatric Association will be working with the appropriate organizations to include new *DSM-5* terms in the ICD-10-CM and will inform clinicians and insurance companies when modifications are made.

We urge counselors-in-training to attend training opportunities to become informed and current in their understanding and application of the *DSM-5* criteria and classification revisions. Proper coding requirements for *DSM-5* and ICD-10-CM will be in place at the time of your internships and entry into full professional practice.

For a review of changes to classifications and diagnostic criteria, the student is referred to "Highlights of Changes From DSM-IV-TR to DSM-5," which may be accessed at http://www.dsm5.org/Documents/changes%20%from%20dsm-iv-tr%20to%20dsm-5.pdf.

Sharing Assessment Information With the Client

The process of assessment centers on gathering information from the client for the purpose of identifying the problem or problems that the client brings to the counseling session. The results of assessment activities enable the counselor to integrate the information he/she has gathered into the treatment planning process. It should be noted that assessment activities are primarily for the benefit of the client, enabling him/her to come to an understanding of his/her problems and to cope with real-life concerns. Patterson and Welfel (2000) discussed five components to the data-gathering and hypothesis-testing process of assessment which can be followed in assessment discussions with the client. The following is a summary of those components:

1. Understanding of the boundaries of the problem: Both the counselor and the client need to recognize the scope and limits of the difficulty the client is experiencing. It is important to know the problem boundaries in current functioning as well as the history and duration of the problem.
2. Mutual understanding of the patterns and intensity of the problem: Recognition on the part of the counselor and client that problems are not expressed at a uniform level all the time helps the client realize that understanding the pattern of the problem makes its causation clearer. Understanding the intensity of the problem helps the client to get a clearer sense of the dimensions of feelings and associated behavior.
3. Understanding of the degree to which the presenting problem influences functioning in other parts of the client's life: The aim is to learn how circumscribed or diffused the difficulty is and to clarify the degree to which it is compromising other unrelated parts of the client's experience.
4. Examination of the ways of solving the client's problem that he/she has already tried before entering counseling: This process aids understanding of the impact of the problem's history on the current status of the problem. It is also helpful in the selection of strategies for change.
5. Understanding of the strengths and coping skills of the client: This process helps in keeping a balanced perspective on the problem and aids in the client's realization that he/she has the resources to bring about the resolution of problems (pp. 121–123).

Gathering Additional Data

Many counselors supplement the intake information by administering additional structured assessments. These are usually related to the client's stated concerns such as substance abuse, depression, or anxiety. The use of these formalized questionnaires and instruments can be helpful in providing information about potential diagnoses (Cormier & Hackney, 2012). Examples of several widely used assessments are the Beck Depression Inventory II (BDI-II), the Zung Self-Rating Anxiety Scale, the Beck Anxiety Inventory (BAI), the Michigan Alcohol Screening Test (MAST), and the Alcohol Use Disorders Identification Test (AUDIT). When using tests in the assessment process, the student counselor should have completed formal coursework on testing and use the tests under the supervision of a qualified supervisor. Anastasi (1988) cautions counselors about their ethical responsibility to use multiple criteria for any decision making. Counselors should never use one test as the only criterion for making a clinical or educational decision. The counselor should also consider his/her clinical impressions and the client's reported behaviors and should consult the diagnostic criteria references before coming to any decision about treatment directions.

Assessing the Client's Progress

Assessment activities in counseling can take many forms. Regardless of the approach taken by the counselor, assessment needs to be viewed as an ongoing process that begins with the initial intake and culminates with the termination of counseling. All too often, the counselor learns that the presenting problem is only the tip of the iceberg, and new or more urgent needs arise during the therapy process. Viewing assessment as a continuous process enables the counselor to modify and adjust treatment plans, therapeutic goals, and intervention strategies as needed.

Some theorists encourage counselors to consider a variety of sources of data and information as continued assessment of progress is considered. According to Juhnke (1995), continuous assessment includes qualitative, behavioral, and client record-reviewing activities. Qualitative assessment activities can include role playing, simulations, and games. These methods are employed for the purpose of gathering additional data from the client. The use of qualitative methods in sessions provides for the processing of information and feedback to the client. Behavioral assessment examines the overt behavior of the client. According to Galassi and Perot (1992), behavioral assessment emphasizes the identification of antecedents to problem behaviors and of consequences that reduce their frequency or eliminate them. Indirect methods of behavior assessment might include talking to significant others about the client's issues and problems. Direct behavioral methods involve observing the client, administering behavioral checklists, and having the client self-monitor his/her behavior. A review of the client's records affords the counselor the opportunity to examine possible patterns of behavior. Likewise, it can provide the counselor with a history of the past therapy experiences of the client, as well as an understanding of the client's history in light of the client's presenting concerns. Assessment is not restricted to the use of objective, standardized, quantifiable procedures; rather, it includes interviewing, behavioral observation, and other qualitative methods.

Ongoing assessment also assists the counselor in evaluating the effectiveness of strategies used in the counseling process. Cormier, Nurius, and Osborne (2009) acknowledge the role and function of assessment in counseling as a crucial component in the selection of appropriate strategies for intervention. They assert that it is naive to think that a single theoretical framework or strategy is appropriate for all clients. Beutler and Harwood (1995) point out that research supports a departure from "one-size-fits-all" counseling approaches. They further assert that interventions that are based on specific client needs and problems, rather than on the preferred strategy of the counselor, tend to lead to better outcomes. Patterson (1997) argues that counseling would be beneficial when cases are conceptualized through a useful theory and when carefully selected techniques are used to address client-specific difficulties. The emergence of applying evidence-based treatment approaches is consistent with these points of view. Thus the areas of assessment are expanded to include an outcome-oriented review of client progress in relationship to selected interventions.

Monitoring of the client in therapy is a continuous process, beginning with the initial contact with the client and ending with therapy termination. Monitoring allows the therapist to understand how the goals and objectives of the therapy are being met as well as the direction of the therapy and the progress taking place during therapy. A cornerstone in assessment skills is the awareness, observation, and recognition of relevant data from which to formulate an accurate description and then an explanation of the client. Relevant data refer not only to specific content gleaned through a review of the records, the client's self-report, and anecdotes, incidents, and interaction shared by the client or others but also to process data such as how the client relates a story, what kind of affect is revealed, and what the client avoids talking about.

The counseling student must observe the emotions of the client and identify what would be relevant information in understanding the client's personal dynamic. This may include observations and inferences from the client's nonverbal behaviors. It may include the client's labeled or expressed emotions or the counselor's impression of the client's overall emotional state. The counseling student's ability to elicit, observe, and note relevant emotional data in the process of the counseling session contributes to the ability to formulate an accurate description of the client, which can then lead to potential explanations and hypotheses about the emotional development of the client and possible strength or problem areas.

As the counselor facilitates the client's telling of his/her story or concerns, she/he is also noticing patterns and themes in the way that the client describes himself/herself in relationship to the world, the recurring range of behaviors and thoughts chosen when confronted with problems, and the strengths in coping with a variety of situations. The counselor is also noting how the client interacts with the counselor; that is, is the client expansive or monosyllabic, selective or evasive in responses, emotionally responsive and open or cautious and suspicious?

This commentary emphasizes that a major element in establishing assessment skills is the recognition and selection of relevant data when beginning to form an impression, and then when monitoring the client's progress and sticking points as the counseling process unfolds. A helpful practice after each counseling session is to write brief notes about the client, in which you ask yourself the following:

1. What do I know about my client at this point in the counseling process? How does she/he think, act, and feel about who she/he is in the world as she/he sees it?
2. What would it be like to be in my client's shoes?
3. What are the influences that are currently contributing to my client's being who she/he is at this time in this circumstance?
4. What other information or observation would be helpful for me to understand this client?
5. What additional interventions, if any, may help my client progress toward healthier choices and actions?

The practice of writing such notes after each session helps the counseling student to develop assessment skills by regularly focusing on questions that will help in formulating a comprehensive explanation of the client and his/her issues. These questions can be incorporated into the assessment and plan sections of the case notes (Form 3.5). These notes can also be used in individual, group, or peer supervision, and the questions can be expanded or discussed as appropriate.

An adaptation of Kanfer and Schefft's (1988) discussion of monitoring and evaluating client progress suggests doing the following:

- monitoring and evaluating the client's behavior and environment from session to session;
- assessing improvement in coping skills by noting the client's use of the skills in relation to behavior and other activities;
- evaluating any change in the client's status or in his/her relationships to significant others that resulted from treatment;
- utilizing available data to review progress, to strengthen gains, and to maintain the client's motivation for completing the change process;
- negotiating new treatment objectives or changes in methods or the rate of progress if the evidence suggests the need for such changes; and
- attending to new conditions that have been created by the client's change and that may promote or defeat further change efforts.

Furthermore, Kanfer and Schefft (1988), in examining treatment effectiveness, suggest that therapists ask themselves the following questions:

■ Are the treatment interventions working? The therapist should note the client's progress with respect to therapeutic objectives, as compared to the baseline data gathered at the beginning of treatment (initial assessment).

■ Have other treatment targets been overlooked? By monitoring other changes and emergent problems, the therapist obtains cues for the necessity of renegotiating treatment objectives or treatment methods.

■ Is the therapeutic process on course? Individuals differ in their rate of progress, and plateaus may occur at various phases of therapy; these need to be scrutinized.

■ Are subsidiary methods needed to enhance progress or to handle newly emerged problems? Are there gaps in the client's basic skill level that need to be filled to make progress?

■ Are the client's problems and the treatment program being formulated effectively? Monitoring and evaluation by the therapist in process is crucial to successful treatment. Consultation with other professionals and colleagues is recommended (pp. 255–258).

Reporting Therapeutic Progress

The counselor-in-training may receive requests from other professionals to provide diagnostic information and reports of therapeutic progress, and to make recommendations regarding a client. The format for reporting the data will vary according to the specific requests that are made. Each progress report needs to be prepared in keeping with the request, the client, ethical standards regarding release of information, and the person to whom the report is sent. Therapeutic progress reports are often used by the agency or institution for the purpose of assisting in the development of treatment plans for placement of clients into appropriate programs and for providing information for the final disposition of a therapy case. A Therapeutic Progress Report (Form 4.4 at the end of the book) needs to include pertinent data about the method of treatment employed as well as the client's current status. Treatment recommendations are especially helpful to those who must make a final disposition of the case.

Implications

We have reviewed intake assessment guidelines, diagnosis, and continuing assessment recommendations. Basic to the discussion is the emphasis on the interplay between assessment and continuing review of the client's response to the counseling process. Thoughtful, thorough, ongoing assessment contributes to the counselor's ability to think through the case conceptualization and treatment planning process so that the client receives optimal benefit from the counseling services.

Case Conceptualization

The process of case conceptualization can be a daunting task for beginning counselors. Determining how to best conceptualize a case and following through with an appropriate treatment plan requires the counselor to thoughtfully consider the development of his/her own strategy. To assist in that process, we now provide a variety of methods and models of case conceptualization for your consideration.

Case Conceptualization Models

A case conceptualization or case formulation represents the clinical understanding of a client's concerns. It provides the counselor with a rationale and a framework for his/her work with a client (Sperry, 2010). Beton and Binder (2010) consider the conceptual frame to be the "linchpin of clinical practice" (p. 43). A conceptualization is a framework through which the counselor organizes his/her understanding of self, client, therapeutic interaction, and the process of helping that will be engaged. Counselors "observe, think and act based on the conceptual frame they are using" (Reiter, 2014, p. 4). Eels, Kendjelic, and Lucas (1998), in a study on case formulation skills, reviewed several systematic methods for constructing case formulations. A case formulation was defined as a hypothesis about the causes, precipitants, and maintaining influences of a person's psychological, interpersonal, and behavioral problems. The authors assumed that the primary function of a case formulation was to integrate rather than summarize descriptive information about the client. Four broad categories of information were found in most case formulation methods:

1. Symptoms or problems: This includes the patient's presenting concerns as well as problems apparent to the counselor but not to the client.
2. Precipitating stressors: This includes what triggered the current symptom or problems or increased the severity of a preexisting problem (i.e., divorce, job loss, illness, loss of social support).
3. Predisposing life events: This includes traumatic events or stressors occurring in the client's past which may have led to increased vulnerability.
4. Inferred mechanisms: This links together the information in the first three sections. This is the counselor's hypothesis about how psychological, biological, or sociocultural mechanisms contribute to the client's difficulties.

We are presenting the counseling student with three different conceptualization models which can facilitate the development of their clinical thinking skills. Each model brings a different focus in its application to understanding the counseling work. The first model, The "Linchpin" Model, requires that the counselor organize the case around one central underlying causal source. Another, the Inverted Pyramid Model requires that the analysis begins with identifying a broad array of client concerns and then progresses to the deepest level of motivation (from a theoretical perspective) that fuels and sustains the concerns. The final model, the Integrative Model, frames the symptom and diagnosis within the context of social and cultural elements that influence and sustain the dysfunction and how these elements can be effected by selected interventions. A review of each model is provided.

The "Linchpin" Model

Bergner (1998) suggested that using a linchpin concept would ideally culminate in the construction of an empirically grounded, comprehensive formulation for case conceptualization that would (a) organize all of the key factors of a case around one causal, explanatory source; (b) frame this source in terms of factors amenable to direct intervention; and (c) lend itself to being shared with the client to his/her considerable benefit. According to Bergner (1998), a clinical case formulation would embody the following characteristics:

1. *Organize facts around a linchpin:* Clients generally tend to provide a great deal of information about themselves, often above and beyond the data initially sought by the counselor. In addition to the presenting complaint, clients provide a wealth of information about their problem, including their emotional state, personal history, goals, expectations, and history of their concerns. However, in most cases, clients have not organized these data into a theory of their problem(s). Similarly, relevant information about such factors as personal beliefs and values, which can create problems, has been left out of their discussion. Organizing around a linchpin helps to organize all the information obtained but also identifies the core state of affairs from which all the client's difficulties spring. According to Bergner (1998), a linchpin, as the metaphor implies, is what holds everything together; it is what, if removed, might cause destructive consequences.
2. *Target factors amenable to intervention:* It is essential that the counselor look at factors that are currently maintaining the client's dysfunctional state and that are directly amenable to therapeutic intervention. The focus is to target the factors that currently maintain the problem and that permit translation into therapeutic factors.
3. *Share the data with the client:* The case formulation shared with the client results in (a) the client organizing his/her thinking about the problem, (b) the client identifying key or central maintaining factors in his/her dysfunction and making them the focal point of change efforts, and/or (c) maximizing the client's sense of control or power over what he/she is doing, sensing, and feeling. As a result, case formulation becomes a collaborative effort between the therapist and the client in an attempt to work through the client's problems.

The Inverted Pyramid Model

The inverted pyramid model was proposed by Schwitzer in 1996 and has been refined over a period of years. The purpose of this method is to identify and understand client concerns and to provide a diagram that visually guides the conceptualization process. Four steps are identified that proceed from theory-neutral clinical observations to systematically deeper theoretical understandings (Schwitzer & Rubin, 2012; Neukrig & Schwitzer, 2006; Schwitzer 1996, 1997).

Step I: *Problem identification.* The first step involves the exploration of the client's functioning, with emphasis on the inclusion of any potentially useful descriptive information about the client's particular difficulty. The clinician is advised to cast a wide net in listing client concerns.

Step II: *Thematic grouping.* The second step involves the process of organizing the client's problems into intuitively logical groupings or constellations. Thematic grouping entails grouping together those of the client's problems that seem to serve similar functions or that operate in similar ways.

Step III: *Theoretical inference about client concerns.* This moves from thematic groupings to theoretically inferred areas of difficulty (Schwitzer & Rubin, 2012). The third step requires that the counselor make inferences by applying selective general principles to his/her reasoning about a client's situation. Previously identified symptom constellations are refined further, as the inverted pyramid implies, allowing the counselor to progress down to deeper aspects of the client's problems. This honing-down process emphasizes a smaller number of themes that are unifying, central, explanatory, causal, or underlying in nature (Schwitzer, 1996). As a result, these themes can then be made a focus of treatment.

Step IV: *Narrowed inferences about client difficulties.* Finally, the unifying, causal, or interpretive themes inferred from the previous process are honed into existential, fundamental, or underlying questions of life and death (suicidal ideation or behavior), deep-rooted shame, or rage. This step will help the beginning counselor to apply a theoretical framework to the client's most threatening or disruptive difficulties. This moves to theoretical inferences about still-deeper areas of difficulty that provide still-deeper explanations.

Steps I and II use a pragmatic approach using theory-neutral clinical judgment. In steps III and IV the same theoretical orientation is applied to interpret or explain information collected in steps I and II. This model can use any theoretical orientation chosen as appropriate by the counselor.

The Integrative Model

The integrative model (Sperry & Sperry, 2012; Sperry, 2005a, 2005b, 2010) provides the theoretical understanding of the client and links the client's problem to an appropriate treatment plan. An important element in this case conceptualization model is the inclusion of the impact of culture on the client's symptoms and solutions. The integrative model has four components.

1. *What is the diagnostic formulation?* This focuses on the symptoms the client presents with in therapy. It includes whether it is an emergency or requires inpatient or outpatient treatment.
2. *What is the clinical formulation?* How did the symptoms develop, and how are they maintained? What is your understanding of the pattern of the client's symptoms?
3. *What is the cultural formulation?* How does the client's culture impact the symptom pattern? Culture can be based on ethnicity, gender, socioeconomic status, geographic region, religious beliefs, and any other factors which impact how people develop a sense of self.
4. *What is the plan of action?* What is the therapeutic model of the problem formation, and what is the theory of change to resolve the problem?

The therapist has a picture of what the symptom is and how it developed, as well as the larger systems impacting the client, and then develops a plan of action with the client. Approaching a case from a behavioral perspective would differ from approaching it from an existential or other theoretical perspective.

Each of these models can be applied to a variety of theoretical approaches which provide an understanding of how the process of development and change can be engaged. This way of thinking influences the selection of interventions which may result in healthier functioning for the client.

Summary

This chapter has presented the practicum/internship student with a review of assessment guidelines, diagnosis, and several case conceptualization models. The assessment of the client and his/ her problems and the way in which the counselor conceptualizes the problem are key aspects of any approach to counseling the individual. You have now begun working with clients. You are becoming more experienced in helping your clients disclose the problems which brought them to counseling and to understand, with them, the context in which they are trying to resolve their concerns. As a professional counselor you then frame the work based on your clinical understanding of how one can come to have these concerns and how one can accomplish the changes which allow healthier and more satisfying choices and behaviors. The counselor-in-training may find one case conceptualization model to be more useful during the practicum and may find another, perhaps more complex model to be appropriate once he/she has more experience. We assume that the counselor-in-training is working toward developing his/her own personal theory of counseling, which may be eclectic or may be a specific theory-based approach. The application of these case conceptualization models will assist the student in the process of refining his/her own approach to the practice of professional counseling. The variety of case conceptualization models just presented should enable counselors to choose a model that best fits their view of counseling. In addition, the models presented can be adapted to serve as a starting point for the development of the counselor's own way of viewing clients and their problems and then determining the best course of treatment. Following the completion of the case conceptualization process, the counselor must go on to decide how to set goals and plan effectively for the treatment of his/her client.

References

American Psychiatric Association. (2013). *Diagnostic and statistical model of mental disorders* (5th ed.) (*DSM-5*). Washington, DC: Author.

Anastasi, A. (1988). *Psychological testing* (6th ed.). New York: Macmillan.

Bergner, R. (1988). Characteristics of optimal clinical case formulations. *American Journal of Psychotherapy, 52*(3), 287–301.

Beton, E. J., & Binder, J. L. (2010). Clinical expertise in psychotherapy: How expert therapists use theory in generating case conceptualizations in interventions. *Journal of Contemporary Psychotherapy, 40*, 141–152.

Beutler, L. E., & Harwood, T. M. (1995). Prescriptive psychotherapies. *Applied and Preventive Psychology, 4*, 89–100.

Cormier, S., & Cormier, B. (1998). *Interview strategies for helpers*. Pacific Grove, CA: Brooks/Cole.

Cormier, S., & Hackney, H. (2012). *Counseling strategies and interventions* (8th ed.). Upper Saddle River, NJ: Pearson Education.

Cormier, S., Nurius, P. S. (2003). *Interviewing and change strategies for helpers*. Belmont, CA: Brooks/Cole.

Cormier, S., Nurius, P., & Osborne, C. (2009). *Interviewing and change strategies for helpers: Fundamental skills and cognitive behavioral interventions* (6th ed.). Belmont, CA: Brooks/Cole.

Council for Accreditation of Counseling and Related Educational Programs (CACREP). (2009). *CACREP standards*. Alexandria, VA: Author.

Council for Accreditation of Counseling and Related Educational Programs (CACREP). (2013). *Draft #2, 2016 CACREP standards*. Retrieved from www.cacrep.org/template/page/clm?id=141.

Eels, T. D., Kendjelic, E. M., & Lucas, C. P. (1998). What's in a case formulation? Development and use of a content coding manual. *Journal of Psychotherapy Practice and Research, 7*(2), 144–153.

Ekstrom, R. B., Elmore, P. B., Schafer, W. D., Trotter, T. V., & Webster, B. (2004). A survey of assessment and evaluation activities of school counselors. *Professional School Counseling, 8*(1), 24–34.

Galassi, J. P., & Perot, A. P. (1992). What should we know about behavioral assessment: An approach for counselors. *Journal of Counseling and Development, 75*(5), 634–641.

Geroski, A. M., & Rodgers, K. A. (1997). Using the DSM IV to enhance collaboration among school counselors, clinical counselors and primary care physicians. *Journal of Counseling and Development, 75*(3), 231–239.

Ginter, E. J. (2001). Private practice: The professional counselor. In D. C. Locke, J. E. Myers, & E. L. Herr (Eds.), *The handbook of counseling* (pp. 355–372). Thousand Oaks, CA: Sage.

Hohenshil, T. H. (1996). Editorial: Role of assessment and diagnosis in counseling. *Journal of Counseling and Development, 75*(1), 64–68.

Howatt, W. A. (2000). *The human services counseling toolbox*. Pacific Grove, CA: Brooks/Cole.

Ivey, A., & Ivey, M. B. (1998). Reframing DSM IV: Positive strategies from developmental counseling and therapy. *Journal of Counseling and Development, 76*, 334–350.

Juhnke, G. A. (1995). Mental health counseling assessment: Broadening one's understanding of the client and the client's concerns. *ERIC Digest*. Greensboro, NC: ERIC Clearinghouse on Counseling and Student Services.

Kanfer, F. H., & Schefft, B. K. (1988). *Guiding the process of therapeutic change*. Champaign, IL: Research Press.

Nelson, M. L. (2002). An assessment based model for counseling selection strategy. *Journal of Counseling and Development, 84*(4), 416–422.

Neukrig, E. S., & Schwitzer, A. (2006). *Skills and tools for today's professional counselors and psychotherapists: From natural helping to professional counseling*. Belmont, CA: Brooks/Cole.

Patterson, T. (1997). Theoretical unity and technical eclecticism: Pathways to coherence in family therapy. *American Journal of Family Therapy, 25*, 97–109.

Patterson, T., & Welfel, E. (2000). *The counseling process* (5th ed.). Pacific Grove, CA: Brooks/Cole.

Reiter, M. (2014). *Case conceptualization in family therapy*. Upper Saddle River, NJ: Pearson.

Remley, T. P., Jr., & Herlihy, B. (2014). *Ethical, legal, and professional issues in counseling* (4th ed.). Upper Saddle River, NJ: Pearson.

Schwitzer, A. M. (1996). Using the inverted pyramid heuristic. *Counselor Education and Supervision, 35*(4), 258–268.

Schwitzer, A. M. (1997). Using the inverted pyramid framework applying self psychology constructs to conceptualizing college student psychotherapy. *Journal of College Student Psychotherapy, 20*(2), 29–52.

Schwitzer, A. M., & Rubin, L. C. (2012). *Diagnosis and treatment skills for mental health counselors: A popular culture casebook approach*. Thousand Oaks, CA: Sage.

Smith, H. B. (2001). Counseling: Professional identity for counselors. In D. C. Locke, J. E. Myers, & E. L. Herr (Eds.), *The handbook of counseling* (pp. 569–579). Thousand Oaks, CA: Sage.

Sperry, L. (2005a). Case conceptualization: A strategy for incorporating individual, couple and family dynamics in the treatment process. *American Journal of Family Therapy, 33*, 189–194.

Sperry, L. (2005b). Case conceptualization: The missing link between theory and practice. *Family Journal: Counseling and Therapy for Couples and Families, 13*(1), 71–76.

Sperry, L. (2010). *Core competencies in counseling and psychotherapy: Becoming a highly competent and effective therapist*. New York: Taylor and Francis.

Sperry, L., & Sperry, J. (2012). *Case conceptualizing: Mastering the competency with ease and confidence*. New York: Taylor and Francis.

CHAPTER 5

GOAL SETTING, TREATMENT PLANNING, AND TREATMENT MODALITIES

This chapter focuses on cognitive skills, which represent the next step in forming an overall structure for the counseling process. Goal setting, treatment planning, and treatment modalities represent the action strategies the counselor intends to use to help the client move toward a healthier level of functioning. These two processes are interrelated.

Goal Setting in Counseling

Setting goals is a basic component of the treatment planning process. Failure to set goals inhibits the ability of the counselor and client to determine the direction of counseling, to assess the success of counseling, and to know when counseling should be concluded. The setting of goals is mutually determined by the counselor and client. The counselor's training and experience coupled with the client's experience with the issues and personal insight into problems enable the process of goal setting to provide direction to the counselor and client. Often the goals that are determined are affected by the client's openness to making the changes which might be necessary to achieve the desired outcome. In Chapter 3, both the Egan and the Ivey models of practice emphasized a progression beyond understanding clients' initial presentation of problems and concerns to identifying their preferred scenario or story. The clients are encouraged to work with the counselor to identify the kinds of changes or goals that might be necessary in order for them to move toward their preferred circumstances. However, some clients may stay overly long in the process of identifying problems and preferred scenarios and resist identifying the goals, which require personal changes.

Goals and the Stages of Change Model

The stages of change model proposed by Prochaska and Norcross (2010) provides a useful model to explain a client's resistance to change and goal setting. It also can provide useful information for planning treatment strategies to encourage the client to move forward in the process of making necessary personal changes. The stages of change model identifies six stages of change that a client progresses through as well as treatment strategies that can facilitate that progress. An overview of these stages and the implication each stage may have for treatment goals and the counseling process provides the counselor with a useful frame of reference when working with clients.

1. *Precontemplation:* The client is unaware of a need to change or doesn't want to change. Goals for those in this stage are process goals and would emphasize helping the client acknowledge the limitations of the current behaviors and identify elements which may be open to change.

2. *Contemplation:* The client is aware of a need to change and thinks about it but can't decide what to do about it. Clients can stay in this stage for years. Their ambivalence keeps them stuck. This can be about a job change, a relationship change, an education change—any number of important life issues. The counselor can encourage little action steps in the desired direction. Sometimes unexpected circumstances force a life change. Often clients stay stuck because they fear change and they must work on reducing the amount of anxiety they experience at even the thought of making a change.

3. *Preparation:* The client has decided to take some action in the near future and may have tried some action unsuccessfully. This is the time to set action goals with clients. Clients stuck in the previous stages benefit more from process goals.

4. *Action:* Clients are motivated to change and are taking action toward their goals. They also are likely to recognize the forces that may undermine the changes they are attempting. Some clients may terminate counseling when they reach this phase. Clients may be encouraged to return to therapy when anticipated undermining forces begin to surface or the counselor may suggest that clients reduce the frequency of sessions.

5. *Maintenance:* The client reaches his/her goals based on a solid action plan and maintains the change for at least six months. The focus is now on maintaining the gains and preventing relapse.

6. *Relapse and Recycling:* Those with serious clinical disorders and addictions issues can often have difficulties maintaining changes and may make several attempts to achieve maintenance (Prochaska & Norcross, 2010, pp. 492–495).

The change model is characterized as a cyclical model where clients spiral through change rather than moving through each stage in progression. When clients relapse, they may recycle back to a much earlier stage and require more process-type goals until they progress again toward maintenance. Prochaska and Norcross state that "each time relapsers recycle through the stages, they potentially learn from their mistakes and try something different the next time around" (p. 496). Identifying where your client falls in the process of change can help you work with the client to choose goals that are appropriate to your client and help you encourage the client to commit to fully engaging in the counseling process as part of the goals of therapy.

Types of Goals

The helping process involves two types of goals: process goals and outcome goals. Process goals relate to establishing the necessary conditions for change to occur. These include establishing rapport, providing a safe environment, and helping the client reveal his/her concerns. These goals are the responsibility of the counselor. Outcome goals are different for each client and are goals directly related to the client's changes. It is important to remember that goal setting is a flexible process open to modification and refinement. Outcome goals are shared goals that you and your client agree to work toward accomplishing. In this view, outcome goals form the basis for treatment plans in counseling. A summary of the elements proposed by Cormier & Hackney (2012, pp. 127–130), which are to be considered when identifying treatment goals, is offered for the counselor's consideration.

- The goals are culturally appropriate (Sue & Sue, 2008).
- The goals identify the behavior to be changed. What will the client do differently?

- The goals identify the conditions under which the change will occur. What are the situations in which the client will try the new behavior?
- The goals identify the level or amount of new behavior. What is a realistic amount of change?

The effectiveness of goal setting is determined to a large part by the ability of the counselor and client to choose goals that are relevant, realistic, and attainable and owned by the client.

Goal setting is the central focus in the solution-focused brief therapy approach to counseling (Corey, 2013). Solution-focused therapists believe people have the ability to define meaningful personal goals and that they have the resources required to solve their problems. In solution-focused therapy, the sessions begin with identifying what the client chooses to do in order to improve his/her situation (de Shazer, 1990). Prochaska and Norcross (2010) emphasize that goals are unique to each client and are constructed by the client as he/she defines a more satisfying future. From the first contact with clients, the counselor works to create a climate that will facilitate change and encourage clients to think about a range of possibilities for change. In solution-focused therapy, the emphasis is on small, realistic, achievable changes that can lead to additional positive outcomes. It is important for the beginning counselor to understand that structured goal setting aids the client in translating his/her concerns into specific steps needed to achieve his/her goals. Beginning counselors are cautioned to make sure that initial goals are modest and capable of being attained by the client with minimal effort.

Developing a Treatment Plan

Treatment planning is an essential part of the overall process of developing a coherent approach to counseling an individual. The presenting problem (or problems) has been explored and placed into the context of the client's life situation. Client strengths and limitations have been assessed. A conceptual frame for understanding the client's case has been hypothesized. Treatment goals have been identified. Now it is time to identify the range of interventions that will help the client move forward to achieve a healthier resolution of his/her problem(s). A treatment plan can include interventions specific to the individual counseling process. It can also include interventions such as a psychiatric assessment for needed medications, participation in a support or therapy group, getting a full medical check-up, and/or completion of homework outside of the counseling sessions. Treatment planning in counseling is a method of plotting out the counseling process so that both counselor and client have a road map that delineates how they will proceed from the point of origin (the client's presenting problem) to resolution, thus alleviating troubling and dysfunctional symptoms and patterns and establishing improved coping mechanisms and self-esteem. Seligman (1993) explains how treatment planning plays many important roles in the counseling process:

- A carefully developed treatment plan, fully grounded in research on treatment effectiveness, provides assurance that treatment with a high likelihood of success is being provided.
- Written treatment plans allow counselors to demonstrate accountability without difficulty.
- Treatment plans can substantiate the value of the work being done by a single counselor or by an agency and can assist in obtaining funding as well as providing a sound defense in the event of a malpractice suit.
- Use of treatment plans that specify goals and procedures can help counselors and clients to track their progress, can determine whether goals are being met as planned, and, if they are not, can allow them to reassess the treatment plan.

■ Treatment plans also provide a sense of structure and direction to the counseling process and can help counselors and clients to develop shared and realistic expectations for the process.

Gehart (2013) proposed a treatment planning process that establishes treatment across three phases of therapy: the initial phase (sessions 1–3), the working phase (sessions 4 and beyond), and the termination phase (the final sessions). The therapeutic tasks are process tasks that are the responsibility of the counselor. The goals and interventions are mutually determined by the counselor and the client. This model also includes a point at which therapy will conclude and allows the client to respond to the close of therapy with comments and concerns. This format may be used with the stages of change model, which also specifies the process goals associated with initiating therapy and identifies the action and maintenance stages as points where therapy may be concluded. Each of the three phases in the Gehart model include

■ therapeutic tasks which are treatment tasks across therapeutic models (i.e., establish therapeutic relationship, assess intra- and interpersonal dynamics, sustain working relationship);
■ client goals which are stated as behavioral goals specific to the client; and
■ interventions: each goal has two to three interventions associated with it.

In this treatment planning approach, goals are an integral part of the treatment plan and allow for continued assessment of treatment effectiveness.

Jongsma and Peterson (2006) identified six specific steps for developing a treatment plan. A summary of their steps includes the following:

1. Problem selection: During assessment procedures, a primary problem will usually emerge. Secondary problems may also become evident. When the problem selection becomes clear to the clinician, it is essential that the opinion of the client (his/her prioritization of issues) be carefully considered. Client motivation to participate in treatment can depend, to some extent, on the degree to which treatment addresses his/her needs.
2. Problem definition: Each problem selected for treatment focus requires a specific definition of how it is evidenced in the client. The *Diagnostic and Statistical Manual of Mental Disorders* (*DSM*) offers specific definitions and statements to choose from or to serve as an example for the counselor to develop his/her own personally developed statements.
3. Goal development: These goal statements need not be crafted in measurable terms but can be global, long-term goals that indicate a desired positive outcome to the treatment procedures.
4. Objective construction: Objectives must be stated in behaviorally measurable terms. Each objective should be developed as a step toward attaining the broad treatment goal. There should be two objectives for each problem, but the clinician can construct them as needed for goal attainment. Target attainment dates should be listed for each objective.
5. Intervention creation: Interventions are designed to help the client complete the objectives. There should be one intervention for every objective. Interventions are selected on the basis of client needs and the treatment provider's full repertoire.
6. Diagnosis determination: Determination of an appropriate diagnosis is based on an evaluation of the client's complete clinical presentation. The clinician must compare the behavioral, emotional, cognitive, and interpersonal symptoms that the client presents to the criteria for diagnosis of mental illness conditions as described in the *DSM*. The clinician's knowledge of *DSM* criteria and his/her complete understanding of the client's assessment data contribute to the most reliable and valid diagnosis (pp. 1–4).

Finally, Cormier, Nurius, and Osborne (2009) provided six guiding principles for use in the preparation of treatment plans that reflect client characteristics. These principles require attending to the cultural needs and preferences of the client which are an important element to be considered in treatment planning.

- Make sure your treatment plan is culturally as well as clinically literate and relevant; that is, the plan should reflect the values and worldview of the client's cultural identity, not your own.
- Make sure your treatment plan addresses the needs and impact of the client's social system as well as of the individual client, including (but not limited to) oppressive conditions within the client's system.
- Make sure your treatment plan considers the roles of important subsystems and resources in the client's life, such as family structure and external support systems.
- Make sure your treatment plan addresses the client's view of health and recovery and ways of solving problems. The client's spirituality may play a role in this regard.
- Consider the client's level of acculturation and language dominance and preference in planning treatment.
- Make sure the length of your treatment matches the time perspective held by the client.

We have provided a number of different formats for preparing a treatment plan. Some of the formats include a broad-brush approach and include interventions outside the one-to-one counseling process which can enhance and support the client's progress. This type of treatment plan would be appropriate when working with a client who has experienced chronic emotional distress or with a client who has multiple concerns, limited coping skills, and uncertain social support. For clients who are experiencing distress which is more a function of a current life situation, a treatment plan may focus more on the counselor–client process.

The counselor may wish to follow one of the previous mentioned guidelines for treatment planning or he/she may decide to combine elements of a variety of approaches. For example, he/she may first decide to determine if a broad-brush approach or counselor–client process approach is appropriate. The counselor may sequence the treatment across three distinct phases as suggested by Gehart (2013). Both process goals and outcome goals may be identified. Several interventions related to each goal can be identified; and consideration of how this approach may impact and be impacted by the client's cultural and social world view and identity can be discussed with the client.

A Review of Philosophy, Theories, and Theory-Based Techniques of Counseling

Beginning counselors are confronted with the struggle to integrate the knowledge base of their training program into a coherent method of counseling. From the very beginning of their training programs, students are encouraged to examine their own values and beliefs as they are exposed to the various philosophical and theoretical approaches to counseling. The necessity for students to develop their own "theoretical approach" to working with clients is stressed for the purpose of sensitizing students to the need for a consistent, well-thought-out approach to counseling. Spruill and Benshoff (2000) viewed the process of developing a personal theory of counseling as sequential. The initial phase emphasizes the examination of personal beliefs. Phase 2 emphasizes increasing the knowledge of counseling theories while integrating this knowledge with personal beliefs. Phase 3 emphasizes the development of a personal theory of counseling.

The following section will present an overview of critical questions, theory components, and techniques that will assist trainees in developing their own personal theory. This review is helpful to trainees in providing a framework for further refining their case conceptualizations, goal setting, and treatment planning skills.

Murdock (1991) proposed the following foundational questions to be considered when reviewing theories, and you can apply these questions to your own personal beliefs and philosophy.

- What is the core motivation of human existence?
- How is this core motivation expressed in healthy ways? What are the characteristics of a healthy personality?
- How does the process of development get derailed or stuck? What are the factors that contribute to psychological dysfunction?
- What stages of an individual's life are considered key to the development process?
- Does the theory restrict the focus to the individual, or does it include family, culture, and others?
- What is the relative importance of affect, cognition, and behavior in the theory?

Answering these questions aids students in examining the key issues addressed in theories of counseling. An important element in counseling practice is to have a way in which you explain how change toward healthier functioning can occur in relationship to the intervention strategies you choose to implement in the treatment plan.

Table 5.1 is provided to give the student a basic overview of the key points addressed in several theories of counseling and psychotherapy. Emphasis in this review section should focus on intervention strategies and goals and the ways your answers to the above questions are consistent with any of these theories.

Table 5.1 Overview of Theories of Counseling and Psychotherapy

Human Nature	Key Concepts	Intervention	Goals
Freud			
man as biological organism, motivated to fulfill bodily needs; ruled by unconscious; instincts driving forces behind personality	id, ego, superego; conscious, unconscious, preconscious; ego defense mechanisms; psychosexual stages; transference and free association	analysis of transference, countertransference and resistance; dream interpretation	make unconscious conscious; apply appropriate defenses
Jung			
man motivated to grow and develop toward individuation; growth as lifelong process; tendency toward wholeness; unification of opposing aspects in the psyche	principle of entropy and equivalence; personal and collective unconscious; extraversion and introversion; thinking, sensing, feeling, intuiting	dream interpretation; use of symbols; word association	understand data from personal unconscious; resolve inner conflict; balance and integrate

Table 5.1 (continued)

Human Nature	Key Concepts	Intervention	Goals
Adler			
inferiority feelings; free will to shape forces; unique style of life; strive for perfection, social interest	style of life; strive for superiority; birth order; early recollections	analysis of birth order; understanding style of life	development of socially useful goals; fostering social interest
Erikson			
potential to direct our growth throughout our lives; personality affected by learning, experience over heredity	psychosocial stages of development; epigenetic principle of maturation; personality development throughout the life span; identity crisis in adolescence	analyzing basic weaknesses caused by ineffectual resolution of developmental crisis; adaptation	correct unbalance; develop a creative balance; positive ego identity
Kelly			
optimistic; free to choose direction of our lives; development of constructs to view the world	anticipation of events; psychological processes directed by our constructs, ways of anticipating life events	assessment interview; self-characterization sketch; role construct repertory test	formulate new constructs and discard old ones
Skinner			
people shaped more by external variables than genetic factors; behavior controlled by reinforcement; responsible for developing our own environment	functional analysis; assessing frequency of behavior, situation in which it occurs, and reinforcement associated with the behavior	direct observation of behavior; reinforcement schedules, operant conditioning	behavior and environmental change
Bandura			
behavior controlled by the person through cognitive processes and environment through external social situations	process of observational learning; attention, retention, production, and motivation	direct observation of behavior; self-report inventories; physiological measures	change the learned behaviors seen as undesirable
Ellis			
tendency to think both rationally and irrationally; ability to develop self-enhancing thoughts, feelings, and behaviors	development of rational philosophy of life; testing one's assumptions and validity of beliefs	ABCD theory of change; cognitive, affective, and behavioral interventions	reduction of emotional stress and self-defeating behaviors

(continued)

Table 5.1   (continued)

Human Nature	Key Concepts	Intervention	Goals
Allport			
uniqueness of the individual personality; people guided by the present and future; conscious control of life	traits are consistent and determine behavior; personal dispositions; functional autonomy; stages of development; the proprium	personal document technique; study of values	identify personal traits; cope with the present, plan for the future
Horney			
man is unique; innate potential for self-realization; ability to solve our own problems	basic anxiety; neurotic needs; moving toward, away from, and against people	free association; dream interpretation; tyranny of the "shoulds"	realistic appraisal of abilities; flexibility in behaviors and attitudes
Fromm			
people can shape their own nature and destiny; innate ability to grow, develop, and reach their full potential	freedom versus security; interpersonal relatedness; basic psychological needs; character types	dream analysis, free association; interpretation of history, culture, and social events; clinical observation	realization of goals and potential; meaning in life; escape isolation and loneliness
Murray			
personality determined by needs and environment; grow and develop and change our society	personology; id, ego, superego; stages of development; complexes	Thematic Apperception Test; achievement and affiliation needs; techniques of assessment	to reduce tension; understand the role of needs in relation to behavior
Cattell			
deterministic; the regularity and predictability of behavior; influence of nature and nurture; innate traits	life records (L data), questionnaire (Q data), personality test (T data); factor analysis	common and unique traits; ergs and sentiment; stages of development	personality studied by multivariate approach; source traits of personality
Maslow			
humanistic and free will to choose how we satisfy needs and fulfill potential	hierarchy of needs; peak experiences; self-actualization	physiological needs, safety needs, esteem needs, belongingness, and love	realization and fulfillment of potential, talents, and abilities

Table 5.1   (continued)

Human Nature	Key Concepts	Intervention	Goals
Rogers			
optimistic; free will in determining, understanding, and improving oneself; innate tendency to grow and enhance	self-actualization tendency; organismic valuing process; conditions of worth; incongruency	unconditional positive regard; supportive dialogue; nonjudgmental therapeutic environment	to move toward self-actualization; responsibility for behavior
Existentialists			
optimistic, freedom, choice, self-determination; creation of meaningful life	self-awareness, uniqueness and identity; being in the world; anxiety as a fact of life	understand client's current experience; techniques to increase client's awareness; choosing for oneself	accept freedom and responsibility for actions; live an authentic life

Identifying Your Theory and Technique Preferences

In the previous section of this chapter, you have been asked to answer a number of questions regarding your values, beliefs, and views of humankind. Similarly, you have read over the above review of several major theories of counseling and psychotherapy. To extend your review process we are providing a Counseling Techniques List (Table 5.2), which can assist the you in identifying the techniques with which you are familiar and those which you would like to learn more about. Connecting the techniques to your theory base can also provide direction to your own developing personal or guiding theory.

The Counseling Techniques List (Table 5.2) provides a list of counseling and psychotherapy techniques which, while not all-inclusive, does represent techniques used by a broad spectrum of philosophical bases. The number of counseling techniques used by any one counselor varies. If a counselor reviews his/her tape recordings from several sessions with different clients, 10 to 15 different techniques may be identified that were used frequently with competence. An additional 10 to 15 may be identified that were used but with less frequency or, in some cases, with less professional competence. Suggestions for using the accompanying Counseling Techniques List are dependent on one's professional development. However, students have used the list primarily in two ways:

1. to check out and expand their knowledge about counseling techniques, and
2. to introspect into their own counseling, philosophical bases, and treatment approaches.

Please read the directions for completing Table 5.2. These directions should be read in their entirety before proceeding with the completion of the form.

Table 5.2 Counseling Techniques List

Directions

1. First, examine the techniques listed in the first column. Then, technique by technique, decide the extent to which you use or would be competent to use each. Indicate the extent of use or competency by circling the appropriate letter in the second column. If you do not know the technique, then mark an "X" through the "N" to indicate that the technique is unknown. Space is available at the end of the techniques list in the first column to add other techniques.

2. Second, after examining the list and indicating your extent of use or competency, go through the techniques list again and circle in the third column the theory or theories with which each technique is appropriate. The third column, of course, can be marked only for those techniques with which you are familiar.

3. The third task is to become more knowledgeable about the techniques that you do not know—the ones marked with an "X." As you gain knowledge relating to each technique, you can decide whether you will use it and, if so, with which kinds of clients and under what conditions.

4. The final task is to review the second and third columns and determine whether the techniques in which you have competencies are within one or two specific theories. If so, are these theories the ones that best reflect your self-concept? Do those techniques marked reflect those that are most appropriate, as revealed in the literature, for the clients with whom you want to work?

Extent of Use Key			
N = None	M = Minimal	A = Average	E = Extensive

Theory for Technique Key	
Ad = Adlerian (Adler, Dreikurs)	Ge = Gestalt (Perls)
Be = Behavioral (Skinner, Bandura, Lazarus)	PC = Person centered (Rogers)
CBT = Cognitive behavioral (Beck, Ellis, Meichenbaum)	Ps = Psychodynamic (Freud, Erikson)
Ex = Existential (May, Frankl)	Re = Reality (Glasser, Wubbolding)
FS = Family systems (Bowen, Satir, Minuchin)	SF = Solution focused (Berg, deShazur)

Technique	Extent of Use	Theory for Technique
ABC Model	N M A E	Ad Be CBT Ex FS Ge PC Ps Re SF
Acceptance	N M A E	Ad Be CBT Ex FS Ge PC Ps Re SF
Accurate empathic understanding	N M A E	Ad Be CBT Ex FS Ge PC Ps Re SF
Analysis of resistance	N M A E	Ad Be CBT Ex FS Ge PC Ps Re SF
Analysis of transference	N M A E	Ad Be CBT Ex FS Ge PC Ps Re SF
Analyze cognitive triad	N M A E	Ad Be CBT Ex FS Ge PC Ps Re SF
Analyze defense mechanisms	N M A E	Ad Be CBT Ex FS Ge PC Ps Re SF
Analyzing cognitive distortions	N M A E	Ad Be CBT Ex FS Ge PC Ps Re SF

Table 5.2 (continued)

Assertiveness training	N M A E	Ad Be CBT Ex FS Ge PC Ps Re SF
Assignment of tasks	N M A E	Ad Be CBT Ex FS Ge PC Ps Re SF
Avoid focus on symptoms	N M A E	Ad Be CBT Ex FS Ge PC Ps Re SF
Behavioral tasks	N M A E	Ad Be CBT Ex FS Ge PC Ps Re SF
Bibliotherapy	N M A E	Ad Be CBT Ex FS Ge PC Ps Re SF
Birth order	N M A E	Ad Be CBT Ex FS Ge PC Ps Re SF
Boundary setting	N M A E	Ad Be CBT Ex FS Ge PC Ps Re SF
Bridging compliments to tasks	N M A E	Ad Be CBT Ex FS Ge PC Ps Re SF
Change faulty motivation	N M A E	Ad Be CBT Ex FS Ge PC Ps Re SF
Change focused questions	N M A E	Ad Be CBT Ex FS Ge PC Ps Re SF
Change maladaptive beliefs	N M A E	Ad Be CBT Ex FS Ge PC Ps Re SF
Changing language	N M A E	Ad Be CBT Ex FS Ge PC Ps Re SF
Clarify personal views on life and living	N M A E	Ad Be CBT Ex FS Ge PC Ps Re SF
Classical conditioning	N M A E	Ad Be CBT Ex FS Ge PC Ps Re SF
Cognitive homework	N M A E	Ad Be CBT Ex FS Ge PC Ps Re SF
Cognitive restructuring	N M A E	Ad Be CBT Ex FS Ge PC Ps Re SF
Commitment to change	N M A E	Ad Be CBT Ex FS Ge PC Ps Re SF
Communication analysis	N M A E	Ad Be CBT Ex FS Ge PC Ps Re SF
Communication training	N M A E	Ad Be CBT Ex FS Ge PC Ps Re SF
Compliments	N M A E	Ad Be CBT Ex FS Ge PC Ps Re SF
Confrontation	N M A E	Ad Be CBT Ex FS Ge PC Ps Re SF
Co-therapy	N M A E	Ad Be CBT Ex FS Ge PC Ps Re SF
Detriangulation	N M A E	Ad Be CBT Ex FS Ge PC Ps Re SF
Disputing irrational beliefs	N M A E	Ad Be CBT Ex FS Ge PC Ps Re SF
Dramatization	N M A E	Ad Be CBT Ex FS Ge PC Ps Re SF
Dream analysis	N M A E	Ad Be CBT Ex FS Ge PC Ps Re SF
Dreamwork	N M A E	Ad Be CBT Ex FS Ge PC Ps Re SF
Early recollections	N M A E	Ad Be CBT Ex FS Ge PC Ps Re SF
Empty chair	N M A E	Ad Be CBT Ex FS Ge PC Ps Re SF
Enactments	N M A E	Ad Be CBT Ex FS Ge PC Ps Re SF
Encouragement	N M A E	Ad Be CBT Ex FS Ge PC Ps Re SF

(continued)

Table 5.2 (continued)

Exaggeration exercise	N M A E	Ad Be CBT Ex FS Ge PC Ps Re SF
Examine source of present value system	N M A E	Ad Be CBT Ex FS Ge PC Ps Re SF
Examining automatic thoughts	N M A E	Ad Be CBT Ex FS Ge PC Ps Re SF
Exception questions	N M A E	Ad Be CBT Ex FS Ge PC Ps Re SF
Experiential learning	N M A E	Ad Be CBT Ex FS Ge PC Ps Re SF
Experiments	N M A E	Ad Be CBT Ex FS Ge PC Ps Re SF
Explore quality world	N M A E	Ad Be CBT Ex FS Ge PC Ps Re SF
Explore subjective reality	N M A E	Ad Be CBT Ex FS Ge PC Ps Re SF
Exposing faulty thinking	N M A E	Ad Be CBT Ex FS Ge PC Ps Re SF
Family constellation	N M A E	Ad Be CBT Ex FS Ge PC Ps Re SF
Family-life chronology	N M A E	Ad Be CBT Ex FS Ge PC Ps Re SF
Finding alternative interpretations	N M A E	Ad Be CBT Ex FS Ge PC Ps Re SF
Flooding	N M A E	Ad Be CBT Ex FS Ge PC Ps Re SF
Focus on choice	N M A E	Ad Be CBT Ex FS Ge PC Ps Re SF
Focus on personal responsibility	N M A E	Ad Be CBT Ex FS Ge PC Ps Re SF
Focus on present problems	N M A E	Ad Be CBT Ex FS Ge PC Ps Re SF
Focus on what client can control	N M A E	Ad Be CBT Ex FS Ge PC Ps Re SF
Formulate first-session task	N M A E	Ad Be CBT Ex FS Ge PC Ps Re SF
Foster social interest	N M A E	Ad Be CBT Ex FS Ge PC Ps Re SF
Free association	N M A E	Ad Be CBT Ex FS Ge PC Ps Re SF
Genogram	N M A E	Ad Be CBT Ex FS Ge PC Ps Re SF
Genuineness	N M A E	Ad Be CBT Ex FS Ge PC Ps Re SF
Guided imagery	N M A E	Ad Be CBT Ex FS Ge PC Ps Re SF
Hypothesizing systemic roots of problems	N M A E	Ad Be CBT Ex FS Ge PC Ps Re SF
Identify and define wants and needs	N M A E	Ad Be CBT Ex FS Ge PC Ps Re SF
Identify basic mistakes	N M A E	Ad Be CBT Ex FS Ge PC Ps Re SF
Immediacy	N M A E	Ad Be CBT Ex FS Ge PC Ps Re SF
Internal dialogue	N M A E	Ad Be CBT Ex FS Ge PC Ps Re SF
Interpersonal empathy	N M A E	Ad Be CBT Ex FS Ge PC Ps Re SF
Interpretation	N M A E	Ad Be CBT Ex FS Ge PC Ps Re SF
In vivo exposure	N M A E	Ad Be CBT Ex FS Ge PC Ps Re SF

Table 5.2 (continued)

Keep therapy in the present	N M A E	Ad Be CBT Ex FS Ge PC Ps Re SF
Lifestyle assessment	N M A E	Ad Be CBT Ex FS Ge PC Ps Re SF
Logotherapy	N M A E	Ad Be CBT Ex FS Ge PC Ps Re SF
Maintain analytic framework	N M A E	Ad Be CBT Ex FS Ge PC Ps Re SF
Making the rounds	N M A E	Ad Be CBT Ex FS Ge PC Ps Re SF
Miracle question	N M A E	Ad Be CBT Ex FS Ge PC Ps Re SF
Natural consequences	N M A E	Ad Be CBT Ex FS Ge PC Ps Re SF
Negative reinforcement	N M A E	Ad Be CBT Ex FS Ge PC Ps Re SF
Objective empathy	N M A E	Ad Be CBT Ex FS Ge PC Ps Re SF
Objective interview	N M A E	Ad Be CBT Ex FS Ge PC Ps Re SF
Observational tasks	N M A E	Ad Be CBT Ex FS Ge PC Ps Re SF
Operant conditioning	N M A E	Ad Be CBT Ex FS Ge PC Ps Re SF
Plan for acting	N M A E	Ad Be CBT Ex FS Ge PC Ps Re SF
Positive reinforcement	N M A E	Ad Be CBT Ex FS Ge PC Ps Re SF
Progressive muscle relaxation	N M A E	Ad Be CBT Ex FS Ge PC Ps Re SF
Psychoeducation	N M A E	Ad Be CBT Ex FS Ge PC Ps Re SF
Recognizing and changing unrealistic negative thoughts	N M A E	Ad Be CBT Ex FS Ge PC Ps Re SF
Reflection of feeling	N M A E	Ad Be CBT Ex FS Ge PC Ps Re SF
Reframing	N M A E	Ad Be CBT Ex FS Ge PC Ps Re SF
Rehearsal exercise	N M A E	Ad Be CBT Ex FS Ge PC Ps Re SF
Reject transference	N M A E	Ad Be CBT Ex FS Ge PC Ps Re SF
Reorientation	N M A E	Ad Be CBT Ex FS Ge PC Ps Re SF
Reversal exercise	N M A E	Ad Be CBT Ex FS Ge PC Ps Re SF
Scaling questions	N M A E	Ad Be CBT Ex FS Ge PC Ps Re SF
Sculpting	N M A E	Ad Be CBT Ex FS Ge PC Ps Re SF
Self-evaluation	N M A E	Ad Be CBT Ex FS Ge PC Ps Re SF
Self-monitoring	N M A E	Ad Be CBT Ex FS Ge PC Ps Re SF
Shame-attacking exercises	N M A E	Ad Be CBT Ex FS Ge PC Ps Re SF
Social skills training	N M A E	Ad Be CBT Ex FS Ge PC Ps Re SF
Staying with the feeling	N M A E	Ad Be CBT Ex FS Ge PC Ps Re SF

(continued)

Table 5.2 (continued)

Stress inoculation training	N M A E	Ad Be CBT Ex FS Ge PC Ps Re SF
Subjective empathy	N M A E	Ad Be CBT Ex FS Ge PC Ps Re SF
Subjective interview	N M A E	Ad Be CBT Ex FS Ge PC Ps Re SF
Systematic desensitization	N M A E	Ad Be CBT Ex FS Ge PC Ps Re SF
Unbalancing	N M A E	Ad Be CBT Ex FS Ge PC Ps Re SF
Unconditional positive regard	N M A E	Ad Be CBT Ex FS Ge PC Ps Re SF

Adapted from Hollis, Joseph W. (1980). Techniques used in counseling and psychotherapy. In K. M. Dimick and F. H. Krause (Eds.), *Practicum manual in counseling and psychotherapy* (4th ed., pp. 77–80). Muncie, IN: Accelerated Development. Reprinted with permission. The Counseling Techniques List format was used. Theories and techniques listed have been updated and drawn from Corey, G. (2013). *Theory and practice of counseling and psychotherapy* (9th ed.). Belmont, CA: Brooks/Cole.

Be sure to reflect on the connections you have noticed between your answers to the questions posed about your values related to theory, the theories or aspects of theories you preferred on Table 5.1, and the techniques and theories you have identified on Table 5.2.

Extending the Counselor's Theory-Based Techniques

The practicum/internship student in mental health agencies is frequently confronted with the reality of having to use treatment methods capable of delivering low-cost, quality mental health services. The need to employ brief therapeutic strategies in counseling has exploded onto the scene as a result of our present-day managed care environment. Most health care companies today limit the number of outpatient visits for mental health concerns that members are allowed each year (Remley & Herlihy, 2014). School counselors as well may find some brief therapies that are appropriate to use with students, as students who require long-term counseling are usually referred to mental health agencies.

The following sections of the text are designed to provide counseling students with a sampling of the varied approaches to brief therapy. In some cases, students will be familiar with and have training in these models. In other cases, this section might provide students with their first exposure to models of brief therapy. In any case, students need to become familiar with and skilled in the implementation of brief therapeutic interventions and strategies.

Solution-Focused Brief Therapy

Solution-focused brief therapy is based on the research of de Shazer and associates (de Shazer, 1989, 1990; de Shazer & Berg, 1985), who developed a model of therapy that was intentionally brief by design and was based on "focused solution development." Some of the guiding principles of solution-focused therapy include the following:

1. the notion that the power of resistance need not be a part of effective therapy but can be replaced by cooperation;
2. the principle that solution-focused therapy is intended to help clients become more competent at living their lives day by day; accordingly, this conception involves normalizing behavior and the constructing of new meaning from behavior (Fleming, 1998); and

3. the belief that client–therapist interactions are directed by three rules: (a) if it ain't broke, don't fix it; (b) once you know what works, do more of it; and (c) if it doesn't work, don't do it again; do something else (de Shazer, 1990).

Solution-focused brief therapy differs from traditional approaches to therapy in a number of ways. The focus is not on the past but on the present and future. Behavior change is seen as the most effective approach to helping clients. De Shazer (1989, 1990) asserts that it is not necessary to know the cause of a problem to solve it and there is no necessary relationship between what caused the problem and how to solve it. Little attention is given to making a diagnosis, taking the client's history, or exploring the emergence of the problem (O'Hanlon & Weiner-Davis, 2003). An underlying assumption of solution-focused therapy is that people have the ability to resolve life's challenges but at times have lost their sense of direction or awareness of their competencies.

Treatment planning in solution-focused therapy is based on the understanding that clients must be customers for change and come to the realization of the existence of exceptions to their problems when they occur. Treatment plans become a source of documentation of treatment appropriateness, efficacy, and accountability (Fleming, 1998).

The client–therapist relationship is essential for the development of therapeutic interventions in solution-focused therapy. The therapeutic process works best when clients become involved, when they experience a positive relationship with the counselor, and when counseling addresses what clients see as being important (Murphy, 2008). According to de Shazer (1990), clients can be visitors, complainants, or customers, depending on both their views of themselves in relation to their problem and their willingness to take an active part in doing something to solve the problem. Customers are usually those individuals who are willing to do something about their problems. Customers are asked to do something and follow through by taking an active part in their own improvement. Similarly, what clients do to improve their situation between the time of the telephone call for an appointment and the first session can be important to the therapist in his/her search for exceptions to the problem. A client who is a complainant is one who describes a problem but is not able or willing to assume a role in constructing a solution. He/she generally expects the therapist to change some other person to whom he/she attributes the problem. The visitor client comes to therapy because someone else thinks the client has a problem. Both complainant and visitor clients have the potential to become customers based on skilled questioning and intervention (Corey, 2013). According to Fleming (1998), the underlying assumption of the solution-focused model is that clients come to therapy because they have a complaint, a problem, or both. Problems do not occur all the time. When clients choose to do something differently, in a way that does not involve the problem, problem behavior is less likely to occur, and exception behavior is more likely to be observed (de Shazer & Berg, 1985).

Both the client and the therapist construct exception behavior while exploring what happens when the problem does not occur (Gingerich, de Shazer, & Weiner-Davis, 1988). According to Fleming (1998), another guiding principle of solution-focused therapy is to help the client become more competent at living life day by day. Using the EARS (elicit, amplify, reinforce, and start again) approach, the therapist elicits dialogue about exception behavior and positive thoughts and behaviors that the client reports about himself/herself and others. This process helps the client progress toward goal attainment. Reinforcing what the client has done to improve the situation by attaching positive thoughts and behaviors to his/her goals helps the client realize that his/her action makes a difference.

De Shazer (1990) employed what he called the miracle question: "Let's suppose tonight while you're asleep a miracle happens that solves all the problems that brought you here. How would you know that this miracle really happened? What would be different?" The therapist uses exception questions and coping questions to get the client to examine his/her attempts at coping. The therapist believes that asking solution-focused questions helps clients become more aware of their resources and strengths and use them to make better choices for themselves. Finally, the focus of brief therapy is centered on specific, concrete, behavioral goals. Talking about goals and the steps taken to achieve them is essential for positive outcomes. Both the client and the therapist need to know where they are going and how they are going to get there for brief therapy to be successful. The therapy process involves five steps:

1. The client describes the problems.
2. The therapist and client develop goals as soon as possible.
3. The therapist and client explore the times when problems were less severe. They explore these exceptions and how they happened.
4. After each solution-building conversation, the therapist provides feedback, encouragement, and suggestions about what to do before the next session to further solve the problem.
5. The therapist and client evaluate the progress made by using a rating scale, and the client identifies what the next step will be (De Jong & Berg, 2008).

Strategic Solution-Focused Therapy

"What's the trouble?" "If it works, do more of it." "If it doesn't work, don't do it anymore. Do something different." These are some of the guiding principles of strategic solution-focused therapy. This method, developed by Quick (1998), combines the theories and procedures of brief strategic therapy (Fisch, Weakland, & Segal, 1982) and solution-focused therapy (de Shazer, 1985).

"What's the trouble?" and "Do something different" are principles derived from brief strategic therapy, a model developed at the Mental Research Institute in Palo Alto, California, in the 1960s and 1970s, which stressed the idea that people generally attempt to solve problems by doing what makes sense to them. In contrast, the "If it works, do more of it" principle comes from a model developed at the Brief Family Therapy Center in Milwaukee, Wisconsin, in the 1970s and 1980s.

The strategic solution-focused model integrates these parent models in two main ways: (a) by combining brief strategies of focusing on clarification of the problem with the solution-focused emphasis on elaboration of the solution, and (b) by blending the solution-focused emphasis on maintaining what works with the strategic emphasis on interrupting what doesn't work. Strategic solution-focused therapy is always tailored to the needs of the client. The following is a summary of some of the major principles and techniques of strategic solution-focused therapy as presented by Quick (1998).

The initial step in strategic solution-focused therapy is clarifying the client's complaint and identifying the highest-priority problem. The highest-priority problem is the problem to resolve to make the biggest positive difference in the client's life. The therapist wants to know the who, what, when, and where of what happened. Does the client's complaint result in a behavioral excess or deficit? The therapist's focus is to try to clarify what happened at this particular time that makes this problem an immediate issue. The therapist wants to clarify the client's expectations of how therapy is supposed to be helpful. Clarification of the primary problem is an important consideration throughout therapy. It is the therapist's job to find out from the client what problems or issues should be the focus in sessions.

The next step is the elaboration of the solution. "What will be different in the client's life?" "What will let the client know that things are moving in the right direction?" "What will be the first signs of change?" A focused inquiry invites the client to amplify the solution scenario, elaborating on what will be different as a result of lasting changes. When the solution has been elaborated, the therapist invites the client to describe how he/she has begun to make the positive changes happen. If the primary problem has been identified, the focus shifts to what will be different when that specific issue is resolved.

The next step is assessing what has already been done and suggested in previous attempts to solve the problem. "What has been done?" "What have you tried?" The therapist focuses on specific attempts at problem solution. The therapist looks for main themes among attempted solutions, particularly unsuccessful ones, in an attempt to avoid trying them again (Quick, (1998, pp. 527–529).

Near the end of the session, the therapist asks if the client wants feedback or input. The therapist will also compliment the client on realizations that he/she has made in the session. This suggestion component of therapy depends on what has or has not worked for the client. If things are working out, the suggestion may be to continue and amplify existing behaviors. On the other hand, if attempted solutions are not working, the suggestion may be designed to interrupt the behavior. General or specific suggestions may be offered to the client by the therapist.

"Keep doing what works for you, or do something different." It is important to remember that the needs of the client and the intervals between sessions are highly variable. Termination might include encouragement to continue doing what works or to slowly make additional changes.

Cognitive Restructuring Brief Therapy

This approach emphasizes the acquisition of new beliefs and thought patterns. The central notion is that clients build internal "schemas" of self and the world to organize their perceptions (Goldfried, 1988; Moretti, Feldman, & Shaw, 1990). Early experiences can lead to the development of negative schemas, which can affect one's perception of the self, world, and future. According to Beck (Beck, Rush, Shaw, & Emery, 1979), the counselor collaboratively helps the client to marshal evidence that disconfirms negative schemas.

Rational Emotive Brief Therapy

According to Steenbarger (1992), Albert Ellis, the founder of rational emotive therapy, took a different restructuring approach to brief therapy. The focus in rational emotive therapy is on identifying faulty beliefs as a link between activating events and emotional and behavioral consequences. Challenging, confronting, and disputing irrational beliefs is an attempt to reshape irrational thought patterns. Ellis, unlike Beck, relied on confrontation rather than on collaborative helping to get at the client's irrational thoughts.

Coping Skills Brief Therapy

This method represents a teaching approach to counseling in which clients learn to solve difficult life problems and cope with anticipated stresses (Steenbarger, 1992). The focus of this approach to brief therapy is on the use of cognition and behavioral methods in the development of life skills that promote self-efficacy (Bandura, 1977). Coping skills brief therapy relies heavily on in-session and between-session exercises.

Third-Wave Therapies

These therapies were born from the behavioral school of therapy. The first generation was traditional behaviorism. The second generation was cognitive behavioral therapy. The current "third-wave" generation includes contextual approaches to behavior (Hayes, 2005). The third wave has an existential component that assumes that suffering is a basic characteristic of human life. The change from behaviorism and cognitive behavioral therapy includes acceptance and mindfulness-based techniques. This third wave includes mindfulness-based therapy (MBT), mindfulness-based stress reduction (MBSR), mindfulness-based cognitive therapy (MBCT), acceptance and commitment therapy (ACT), and dialectical behavioral therapy (DBT).

Mindfulness-Based Therapy (MBT)

Mindfulness refers to a process that leads to a mental state of nonjudgmental awareness of the present-moment experience including one's sensations, thoughts, bodily states, consciousness, and the environment, while encouraging openness, curiosity, and acceptance (Bishop et al., 2004; Kabat-Zinn, 2003). The basic premise underlying mindfulness practices is that experiencing the present moment nonjudgmentally can counter the effects of stressors because excessive orientation to the past or future can be related to feelings of depression and anxiety (Hofman, Sawyer, Witt, & Oh, 2010). Some approaches to MBT, such as MBSR and MBCT, require that the therapist practice mindfulness meditation both personally and as part of the treatment protocol. However, to introduce into therapy mindfulness techniques such as watching the breath or labeling emotions, the therapist needs suitable instruction and supervision to try the techniques. Germer, Siegel and Fulton (2005) identify the key elements in mindfulness techniques as (1) awareness, (2) of present moment, (3) with acceptance.

Awareness: Awareness techniques involve a stopping or slowing down of our activity. For example, one can stop arguing on the phone by stopping and taking a deep conscious breath. Or one can slow down any activity to observe the activity in more detail such as mindful eating or mindful walking while attending to each detail. One can stop talking and remain silent. One can sit still, close one's eyes, and allow the mind to settle.

Awareness techniques involve observing. Observing as a mindful practice is not observing in an objective, detached manner but rather "calmly abiding" as a participant observer. In order to turn one's attention from any rumination to be able to observe, it is effective to focus on a particular object. The most common object of focus in mindfulness is the breath. As one shifts the focus of attention to the breath, you can begin to note the sensations, feelings, and thoughts that naturally arise. You can notice that your heart is pounding or that you forgot to make a doctor's appointment. Each mental event is there to be noted without judging, analyzing, or suppressing it. One notes only what it is that takes attention away from the breath. In the beginning, noticing the moment-to-moment experience is facilitated by labeling the experience, such as "thinking," "feeling," "fear," "anger," or "worry."

Awareness techniques include a return to awareness of the breath. Returning is the final awareness technique. When you notice you are distracted or absorbed by a thought, you "wake up," note what took your attention, and gently return awareness to the breath. Then watch where the mind wanders next. Waking up is a moment of mindfulness. Whenever necessary, you can return to the breath and anchor your attention.

Present moment: All mindfulness activities bring attention to the present. However, there are times when we need to focus on our goals to avoid making errors. An example would be if you feel angry while operating dangerous machinery. It would be dangerous to attend to your emotions. You must pour all your attention into the task at hand. Wise direction of attention to an activity in the present moment is a core mindfulness exercise. Mindfulness practice is training the attention to focus on present experience. If you are peeling an orange, notice the juice, the smell, the feel of the skin. If you are sitting with a young child as he/she plays, be there fully in the moment, attending to all your senses. Sometimes you will continue to think of other things, such as a work dilemma. A question for yourself is "Do you know where your attention is now?" Any instruction to return to the present moment is a mindfulness exercise.

Acceptance: Acceptance means to accept our experience without judgment or preference, with curiosity and kindness. Our acceptance is always incomplete and must be cultivated because we never really stop judging. A patient can be encouraged to "relax into" or "soften into" an experience. One can "breathe into" an aversive experience such as pain. Goldstein (1993) suggests using a mantra such as "It's OK, just let me feel this," or "Let it be."

Therapists can design mindfulness exercises by prescribing momentary breaks from activities, directing the client to anchor attention in the breath and notice the sensations, thoughts, and feelings that arise. For information regarding training and certification, access http://meditation-andpsychotherapy.org.

Mindfulness-Based Stress Reduction (MBSR)

MBSR is an approach developed by Jon Kabat-Zinn. It consists of several forms of mindfulness practice including formal and informal meditation practice as well as hatha yoga (Kabat-Zinn, 1990). Formal meditation practice consists of breathing-focused attention, body scan–based attention, shifting of the attention across sensory modalities, open monitoring of moment-to-moment experience, walking meditation, or eating meditation. Informal practice includes brief pauses involving shifting the attention to present-moment awareness. This package of mindfulness practices aims to enhance the ability to observe the immediate content of experience (Goldin & Gross, 2000). MBSR is provided in eight weekly group classes and one full day of mindfulness.

Mindfulness-Based Cognitive Therapy (MBCT)

MBCT is based on an integration of aspects of cognitive behavioral therapy for depression and components of the MBSR program. The focus of MBCT is to teach clients to become more aware of thoughts and feelings and to relate to them in a decentered perspective as "mental events" rather than as aspects of the self or as accurate reflections of reality (Teasdale et al., 2002). Mindfulness components from MBSR are combined with aspects of cognitive behavioral therapy which are designed to facilitate decentered views such as "Thoughts are not facts" and "I am not my thoughts." MBCT helps one see the patterns of the mind and know how to recognize when your mood begins to go down. It helps to break the connection between negative mood and negative thinking. You develop the ability to disengage from distressing moods and negative thoughts. MBCT has been demonstrated as effective in relapse prevention for patients in remission following three major depressive episodes. MBCT is provided in eight weekly group classes and one full day of mindfulness practice between weeks 5 and 7. Much of the work is also done at home between classes.

Acceptance and Commitment Therapy (ACT)

A basic assumption in ACT is that a person can take action without first changing or eliminating feelings. Acceptance-based approaches state that instead of only opting for change, a more effective approach is to accept and change. ACT suggests that both behavior and emotion can exist simultaneously and independently. For example, a patient may say, "I can't work today because I am too anxious about what the boss may say about my work evaluation." However, it is possible to go to work while feeling anxious. The goal of ACT is to help clients choose to act effectively (concrete behaviors as defined by their values) in the presence of difficult or disruptive "private" (cognitive or psychological) events (Dewane, 2008). In ACT the client accepts the effects of life's hardships, chooses directional values, and takes action. The theory holds that much of what we call psychopathology is the result of the human tendency to avoid negatively valued private events (what we think and feel). This is called *psychological inflexibility*. The goal of ACT is to "increase psychological flexibility—the ability to contact the present moment more fully as a conscious human being and to change or persist in behavior when doing so serves valued ends" (Hayes, Luoma, Bond, Misuka, & Lillis, 2006, p. 8). In ACT the aim is to transform our relationship with our difficult thoughts and feelings so that we no longer perceive them as symptoms. Instead, we learn to perceive them as harmless, even if uncomfortable, transient psychological events (Harris, 2006). ACT can be used with individuals, couples, and groups, as brief or long-term therapy with a wide range of clinical populations.

Psychological flexibility is achieved through six core processes:

Acceptance: This is taught as an alternative to experiential avoidance; for example, anxiety patients are taught to feel anxiety, as a feeling, fully and without defense.

Cognitive diffusion: ACT attempts to change the way a person interacts with or relates to thoughts. For example, a person could thank his/her mind for such an interesting thought or label the process of thinking ("I am thinking that I am no good").

Being present: ACT promotes ongoing nonjudgmental contact with psychological and environmental events as they occur. Language is used more as a tool to note and describe events than to predict and judge them.

Self as context: Self is a context for verbal knowing, not the content of that knowing. One can be aware of one's own flow of experiences without an attachment to them or an investment in what experiences occur. Mindfulness exercises and metaphors are used to foster this process.

Values: Values are chosen qualities of purposive action. ACT uses exercises to help clients choose life directions in family, career, spirituality, and other domains. Verbal processes which lead to choices based on avoidance, social compliance, and fusion are discouraged.

Committed action: This requires setting goals, guided by your values, and taking effective action to achieve them (Hayes et al., 2006, pp. 7–9).

Dialectical Behavior Therapy (DBT)

DBT is a combination of group skills training and individual therapy designed for the treatment of complex, difficult-to-treat borderline personality disorder (BPD; Linehan, 1993a, 1993b) and is currently used to treat other severe mental disorders such as substance dependence in persons with BPD; depressed, suicidal adolescents; and depressed elderly (Dimeff & Linehan, 2001). DBT is based on a motivational model which states "that (1) people with BPD lack important interpersonal self-regulation (including emotional regulation) and distress tolerance skills; and (2) personal and environmental factors often block and/or inhibit the use of behavioral skills that clients do have and reinforce dysfunctional behaviors" (p. 10). DBT combines basic behavioral strategies with Eastern mindfulness practices. The fundamental dialectic is between the radical acceptance and validation of the client's current capabilities and behavioral functioning and simultaneous attempts to help them change. Treatment includes structured skills-training group sessions, individual psychotherapy to address motivation and skills training, and regular phone contact with the therapist to support the use of coping skills. Therapists working with this client population often experience burn-out; consequently, therapist consultation and support are included in the model.

Acceptance strategies in DBT include mindfulness (attention to the present moment, a non-judgmental stance, focus on effectiveness) and validation. Change strategies include behavioral analysis of maladaptive behaviors and problem-solving techniques such as skills training, use of reinforcers and punishment, cognitive modification, and exposure-based strategies. Weekly group sessions emphasize skills in mindfulness, interpersonal effectiveness, distress tolerance/reality acceptance, and emotional regulation. Therapists who are DBT practitioners require extensive training and support in the use of this therapeutic approach. For more information regarding training and certification, access http://depts.washington.edu/brtc/dbtca/who-we-are/.

Summary

This chapter has added to the development of cognitive counseling skills for the counselor-in-training by reviewing resources focused on goal setting, treatment planning, and theory-based approaches to treatment. Several models and formats for applied practice in these cognitive areas have been presented as well as self-assessment questionnaires concerning theory and theory-based techniques to guide your progress toward developing your own theoretical approach to your counseling practice.

References

Bandura, A. (1977). Self-efficacy: Toward a unifying theory of behavioral change. *Psychological Review, 84*(2), 191–215.

Beck, A. T., Rush, A. J., Shaw, B. E., & Emery, G. (1979). *Cognitive therapy for depression.* New York: Guilford.

Bishop, S., Lau, M., Shapiro, S., Carlson, L., Anderson, N., Carmody, J., et al. (2004). Mindfulness: A proposed operational definition. *Clinical Psychology: Science and Practice, 11*(3), 230–241.

Corey, G. (2013). *Theory and practice of counseling and psychotherapy* (9th ed.). Belmont, CA: Brooks/Cole.

Cormier, S., & Hackney, H. (2012). *Counseling strategies and interventions* (8th ed.). Upper Saddle River, NJ: Pearson.

Cormier, S. Nurius, P. S., & Osborne, C. J. (2009). *Interviewing and change strategies for helpers* (6th ed.). Belmont, CA: Brooks/Cole.

De Jong, P., & Berg, I. K. (2008). *Interviewing for solutions* (3rd ed.). Belmont, CA: Brooks/Cole.

de Shazer, S. (1985). *Keys to solution in brief therapy*. New York: Norton.

de Shazer, S. (1989). Resistance revisited. *Contemporary Family Therapy, 11*(4), 227–233.

de Shazer, S. (1990). What is it about brief therapy that works? In J. K. Zeig & S. G. Gillian (Eds.), *Brief therapy: Myths, methods, and metaphors* (pp. 120–150). New York: Brunner/Mazel.

de Shazer, S., & Berg, I. K. (1985). A part is not apart: Working with only one of the partners present. In A. S. Gurman (Ed.), *Casebook of marital therapy* (pp. 97–110). New York: Guilford.

Dewane, C. (2008). ABC's of ACT. *Social Work Today, 8*(5), 34.

Dimeff, L., & Linehan, M. M. (2001). Dialectical behavior therapy in a nutshell. *California Psychologist, 34*, 10–13.

Dimick, K., & F. Krause (Eds.). (1980). *Practicum manual for counseling and psychotherapy*. Muncie, IN: Accelerated Development.

Fisch, R., Weakland, J. H., & Segal, L. (1982). *The tactics of change*. San Francisco: Jossey/Bass.

Fleming, J. (1998). Solution focused brief therapy: One answer to managed mental health care. *Family Journal, 6*(3), 286–295.

Gehart, D. R. (2013). *Theory and treatment planning in counseling and psychotherapy*. Belmont, CA: Brooks/Cole, Cengage.

Germer, C. K., Siegel, R. D., & Fulton, P. R. (Eds.). (2005). *Mindfulness and psychotherapy*. New York: Guilford.

Gingerich, W. J., de Shazer, S., & Weiner-Davis, D. (1988). Constructing change: A research view of interviewing. In E. Lipchik (Ed.), *Interviewing* (pp. 21–32). Rockville, MD: Aspen.

Goldfried, M. R. (1988). Application of rational restructuring to anxiety disorders. *Counseling Psychologist, 16*, 50–68.

Goldin, P. R., & Gross, J. J. (2000). Effects of MBSR in emotion regulation in social anxiety disorder. *Emotion, 10*(1), 83–91.

Goldstein, J. (1993). *Insight meditation: The practice of freedom*. Boston: Shambhala.

Harris, R. (2006). Embracing your demons. *Psychotherapy in Australia, 12*(4), 1–8.

Hayes, S. C. (2005). *Get out of your mind and into your life: The new acceptance and commitment therapy*. Oakland, CA: New Harbinger Publishing.

Hayes, S. C., Luoma, J. B., Bond, F. W., Misuka, A., & Lillis, J. (2006). Acceptance and commitment therapy: Model, processes and outcomes. *Behavior Research and Therapy, 44*, 1–25.

Hofman, S. G., Sawyer, A. T., Witt, A. A., & Oh, D. (2010). The effect of mindfulness-based therapy on anxiety and depression: A meta-analytic review. *Journal of Consulting in Clinical Psychology, 78*(2), 169–183.

Jongsma, A. E., & Peterson, M. (2006). *The complete psychotherapy treatment planner* (4th ed.). New York: Wiley.

Kabat-Zinn, J. (1990). *Full catastrophe living: Using the wisdom of your body and mind to face stress, pain and illness*. New York: Dell.

Kabat-Zinn, J. (2003). Mindfulness-based interventions in context: Past, present and future. *Clinical Psychology: Science and Practice, 10*(2), 144–156.

Linehan, M. M. (1993a). *Cognitive behavioral therapy of borderline personality disorder*. New York: Guilford.

Linehan, M. M. (1993b). *Skills training manual for treating borderline personality disorder*. New York: Guilford.

Moretti, M. M., Feldman, L. A., & Shaw, B. (1990). Cognitive therapy: Current issues in theory and practice. In R. A. Wells & V. J. Giametti (Eds.), *Handbook of psychotherapy* (pp. 217–238). New York: Plenum.

Murdock, N. (1991). Case conceptualization: Applying theory to individuals. *Counselor Education and Supervision, 30*, 355–365.

Murphy, J. J. (2008). *Solution-focused counseling in schools* (2nd ed.). Alexandria, VA: American Counseling Association.

O'Hanlon, B., & Weiner-Davis, M. (2003). *In search of solutions: A new direction in psychotherapy.* New York: Norton.

Prochaska, J. O., & Norcross, J. C. (2010). *Systems of psychotherapy: A transtheoretical analysis* (7th ed.). Belmont, CA: Brooks/Cole.

Quick, E. (1998). Doing what works in brief and intermittent therapy. *Journal of Mental Health, 7*, 527–534.

Remley, T. P., Jr., & Herlihy, B. (2014). *Ethical, legal, and professional issues in counseling* (8th ed.) Upper Saddle River, NJ: Pearson.

Seligman, L. (1993). Teaching treatment planning. *Counselor Education and Supervision, 35*(4), 287–298.

Spruill, D. A., & Benshoff, J. M. (2000). Helping beginning counselors develop a personal theory of counseling. *Counselor Education and Supervision, 40*(1), 70–80.

Steenbarger, B. N. (1992). Toward science-practice integration in brief counseling and therapy. *Counseling Psychologist, 20*(3), 403–451.

Sue, D. W., & Sue, D. (2008). *Counseling the culturally diverse: Theory and practice* (5th ed.). New York: Wiley.

Teasdale, J., Moore, R., Hayhurst, H., Pope, M., Williams, S., & Segal, Z. (2002). Metacognitive awareness and prevention of relapse in depression: Empirical evidence. *Journal of Consulting and Clinical Psychology, 70*(2), 275–287.

SUPERVISION IN PRACTICUM AND INTERNSHIP

CHAPTER 6

GROUP SUPERVISION IN PRACTICUM AND INTERNSHIP

The accreditation requirements of the Council for Accreditation of Counseling and Related Educational Programs (CACREP) for practicum and internship require that counseling students receive both individual and group supervision throughout the course of their field site–based experiences. Although these supervision processes may be conducted by both university-based faculty and field site–based supervisors, the focus on understanding and applying identified counseling skills is a common goal. In this chapter we focus on the practices and activities that are likely to be included in the group supervision classes during the practicum and internship.

Identifying Counseling Skill Areas

In this section we address the need for, the categories of, and the skills necessary for professional counselor development. Remley and Herlihy (2014) emphasize that a primary focus on counseling skills forms the basis for master's degree programs in professional counseling. They state that "although other courses are taught, all of the training emphasizes competency in individual and group counseling" (p. 31). The skill development framework presented here has been adapted from the work of Borders and Leddick (1997) and Borders and Brown (2005). Four broad skill areas have been identified as those within which self-assessment, peer consultation, supervisor assessment, goal identification, and evaluation can be implemented.

Skill Area One: Counseling Performance Skills

Counseling performance skills refers to "what the counselor does during the session" (Borders & Brown, 2005, p. 8) or his/her counseling behaviors. This includes use of basic and advanced counseling skills, use of theory-based techniques, procedural skills, and professional and issue-specific skills.

Basic and Advanced Counseling Skills

The basic skills identified in the Egan model (Egan, 2013) established the core conditions of genuineness, respect and empathy, attending, active listening, appropriate use of probes, paraphrasing, reflecting feelings, clarifying, and summarizing. The more advanced skills involve presenting a greater degree of challenge to the client. Advanced helping skills presented in the Egan model are interpretation, pointing out patterns and connections, identifying blind spots and discrepancies, self-disclosure, confrontation, and immediacy (Egan, 2013).

In the Ivey microskills model, the basic skill levels progress from attending behaviors to the basic listening sequence of open and closed questions, client observation, encouraging, paraphrasing and summarizing, and reflection of feeling. At the next level the skills of confrontation, focusing, reflection of meaning, interpretation, and reframing are added. Finally, the key skills of interpersonal influence—self-disclosure, feedback, logical consequences, information/psychoeducation, and directives—further build on the range of skills (Ivey, Ivey, & Zalaquett, 2010).

Theory-Based Techniques

This refers to the use of intervention techniques and strategies consistent with a chosen theoretical approach to case conceptualization and treatment planning.

Procedural Skills

This refers to the way the counselor manages the opening and closing of sessions and provides a transition from session to session.

Professional and Issue-Specific Skills

This refers to the way the counselor understands, integrates, and responds to issues related to professional ethics and the law, as well as the way the counselor responds to crisis-related situations.

Skill Area Two: Cognitive Counseling Skills

Cognitive counseling skills refer to the counselor's ability to think about the counseling session and to form a comprehensive explanation of the client and the client's issues (Borders & Brown, 2005). Related skills include the writing of intake summaries and case notes; assessment, diagnosis, and case conceptualization; and goal setting, treatment planning, and theory orientation.

Skill Area Three: Self-Awareness/Multicultural Awareness Skills

Self-awareness involves a counselor's recognition of how personal issues, beliefs, and motivations may influence in-session behavior as well as case conceptualization (Borders & Brown, 2005). Similarly, multicultural awareness involves a counselor's recognition of how personal issues, beliefs, and motivations may influence the worldview of the counselor and the worldview of clients from diverse cultures. We have adapted Skill Area Three to include multicultural awareness because this understanding also impacts the counseling process. Corey (2013) asserts that counselors have an ethical obligation to develop sensitivity to cultural differences and to help clients make decisions that are congruent with their own worldviews (p. 24). Goals must be defined that are consistent with the life experiences and cultural values of the client, not the therapist.

Self-Awareness Skills

This skill area starts with the recognition of how personal values and biases affect the counseling process and progresses toward the ability to integrate this awareness into the counseling process.

These skills are sometimes referred to as reflective skills and are defined as "the ability to examine and consider one's own motives, attitudes and behaviors and one's effect on others" (Hatcher & Lassiter, 2007, p. 53). Self-awareness skills help counselors to become aware of how their personal unresolved issues may get projected onto the client. This is called countertransference. Countertransference influences the way a counselor perceives and reacts to the client. Counselors can become emotionally reactive, respond defensively, or be unable to be truly present because their own issues are involved.

Multicultural Awareness Skills

The interrelationship between self-awareness and multicultural awareness is obvious. However, both these processes require ongoing work and focus as you develop as a counselor. The whole area of multicultural awareness and competency is receiving more and more emphasis as the profession matures and responds to the demands of recognizing the importance of understanding how diversity impacts the counseling relationship. Culture impacts gender relationships, authority relationships, communication patterns, expressions of formality/informality, family dynamics and expectations, ideas of power and privilege, and ideas about economic differences, to name a few. Cormier and Hackney (2012) note that achieving cultural competency does not happen overnight but is a long-term process. They recommend the following actions to develop multicultural awareness and skills:

- Become aware of your own culture and the impact it has on the counseling relationship.
- Become involved in cultures of people different from you.
- Be realistic and honest about your own range of experience and issues of power, privilege, and poverty.
- Educate yourself about dimensions of culture.
- Be aware of your own biases and prejudices.
- Broach cultural issues with the client: be willing to explore issues of diversity (pp. 12–13).

Skill Area Four: Developmental Level

Developmental level refers to the process of moving from being a novice counselor to becoming a professional counselor. This level is inferred based on how supervisees function on a continuum from dependence on the supervisor and the supervision process toward functioning at a collegial level with the supervisor. Developmental level as a skill area addresses the following elements:

- the ability to establish a working alliance with your supervisor,
- the ability to participate in an evaluation of your counseling practice,
- the ability to examine your work in a nondefensive manner,
- an openness to new learning and a continuing practice of refining your clinical thinking,
- an openness to reflecting on and examining your own dynamics as they relate to clients,
- an ability to reflect on and examine multicultural issues appropriate to your counseling practice,
- the ability to identify the strengths and weaknesses in your counseling practice, and
- an understanding of what you might need from supervision.

Self-Assessment in the Skill Areas

We suggest that the group supervision class in practicum begin with reviewing the skill areas and conducting a number of self-assessment activities. This allows the counseling student to become familiar with the skill development model that will form the framework for supervision processes throughout the practicum and internship. It also facilitates the process of forming specific goals for the counseling student to bring to the supervisor as they negotiate a supervision contract that will be the basis for both formative and summative evaluation. We have provided a number of self-assessment instruments and exercises in the Appendices and Forms sections at the back of the text. Appendix I includes the Supervisee Performance Assessment Instrument (Fall & Sutton, 2004), which allows the supervisee to do self-assessment in all skill areas. Other self-assessment instruments and exercises which focus on individual skill areas are Form 5.1: Counseling Techniques List; Form 6.1: Self-Assessment of Counseling Performance Skills; Form 6.2: Self-Awareness/Multicultural Awareness Rating Scale; and Form 6.3: Directed Reflection Exercise on Supervision.

At the completion of this self-assessment process, the counseling student should be able to identify specific goals in each skill area that will become the initial focus for both group and individual supervision.

A sample of a goal statement which can give focus and direction to the supervision process is provided below. Form 6.4 at the end of the text is available to be completed each time you reassess and move toward increased skill levels during practicum and internship.

SAMPLE SUPERVISEE GOAL STATEMENT (Form 6.4)

Directions: You should complete this and provide a copy to your individual and/or group supervisor at the beginning of supervision. This will assist you in forming the supervisory contract with your supervisor.

Student's name _____

Supervisor's name _____   Date submitted _____

Counseling Performance Skills:

1. Demonstrate the application of facilitative and challenging skills in client interviews.
2. In initial sessions with clients, be able to integrate giving informed consent and privacy information.
3. Be able to help client form goals about changes needed to improve and move toward healthier choices, behaviors, or feelings.

Cognitive Counseling Skills:

1. Complete initial intake processes and be able to write an intake summary.
2. Perform appropriate assessment and understand how this can be helpful in identifying the client's strengths and weaknesses.
3. Become skilled in writing case notes.

Self-Awareness/Multicultural Awareness Skills:

1. Actively examine any biases that would affect my counseling—especially in setting goals that are consistent with my client's worldview.
2. Increase my understanding and awareness of countertransference as it affects my counseling practice.
3. Increase my contact with clients and others whose culture I am not familiar with.

Developmental Level:

1. Decrease my self-consciousness about reviewing tapes of my counseling sessions.
2. Increase my confidence about asking questions (don't worry about seeming unskilled).
3. Be open to my supervisor's suggestions.

As the counseling student progresses from prepracticum to practicum to internship (final practicum) the focus of skill development in supervision shifts as the counseling student becomes more skilled in the practice of counseling. Figure 6.1 provides a visual schematic of this progression.

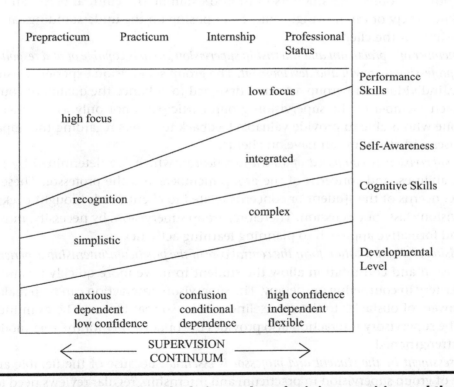

Figure 6.1   Schematic representation of relative goal emphasis in supervision and the shift in goal emphasis as the student progresses from prepracticum to completion of internship.

Concepts in Group Supervision

Concepts about the group supervision experience influence the kinds and range of activities, the process of supervisory and consulting interaction, and the nature of the teaching contract between the counseling student and the university professor. Such concepts provide the foundation of this experiential component of professional training.

This section presents a typical conceptual framework for group supervision that can be used as a reference for the student who is beginning the practicum and internship experience. Some concepts may be used as a point of departure for discussion, and others may be modified and/or challenged.

1. *Group supervision in counseling is a highly individualized learning experience* in which the counseling student is met at the level of personal development, knowledge, and skills that he/she brings to the experience. The student has the responsibility to bring in material about his/her counseling practice and to share any concerns related to practice.

2. *Group supervision facilitates an understanding of one's self, one's biases, and one's impact on others.* Whatever the theoretical orientation of counseling, practicum and internship students must personally examine those qualities about themselves that may enhance or impede their counseling. The group supervision experience provides the setting in which personal qualities related to counseling practice can be examined. Focus in supervision is directed not only toward determining the dynamics and personal meaning of the client but also toward examining how the student views others and how his/her behaviors and attitudes affect others. Counseling students must also examine the cultural biases and assumptions they, knowingly or unknowingly, may be imposing on the understandings and goals being established for the client.

3. *Each member of a practicum and internship supervision group is capable of and responsible for facilitating professional growth and development.* The group supervision experience usually involves dyadic, individual, and group activities designed to enhance the quality of counseling practice. Each member of the supervision group participates not only as a student but also as someone who is able to provide valuable feedback to others regarding the impact particular responses and attitudes can have on clients.

4. *Group supervision is composed of varied experiences,* which are determined by the particular needs, abilities, and concerns of the group members and the professor. These may be personal concerns of the student or concerns related to client needs brought back to the group supervision class for discussion. Therefore, group supervision, by necessity, must have a flexible and formative approach to planning learning activities.

5. *Supervision and consultation form the central core of the practicum/internship experience.* Intensive supervision and consultation allow the student to move more quickly toward competence and mastery in counseling or therapy. The supervisory interaction can help make the student more aware of obstacles to the counseling process so that they can be examined and modified. The supervisory interaction also provides the opportunity for the role-modeling process to be strengthened.

6. *Self-assessment by the student and professor is essential.* Because of the flexible and formative nature of group supervision in practicum and internship, regular reviews need to be made of how the group supervision experiences are meeting the learning needs of the student. Self-assessment allows the student to be consciously aware of and responsible for his/her own development and also provides information for the professor in collaborating on appropriate group supervision activities.

7. *Evaluation is an integral and ongoing part of the practicum/internship.* Evaluation in group supervision provides both formative information and summative information about how the counseling development goals of the student and professor are being reached. A variety of

activities support this evaluation process. Among these are self-assessment, peer evaluations, regular feedback activities, site supervisor ratings, and audio- and videotape review. The attitude from which evaluations are offered is characterized by a "constructive" coaching perspective rather than a "critical" judgmental perspective.

Group Supervision in Practicum

Group supervision course requirements are designed to support and monitor the evolving skill and knowledge base of the student. Practicum students are expected to spend a minimum of 1 1/2 hours per week in a group session with the university supervisor. This time can include didactic and experiential activities and will include some form of review of counseling practices.

In addition to attending the weekly group meetings, students are required to engage in a specified number of counseling sessions each week. These may be both individual and group sessions. Early in the course, the typical amount of required sessions would be fewer in number than in the middle and final phases of the course. A specific minimum number of sessions is required for the course. One-time sessions with clients, as well as a continuing series of sessions with a client, are specified. Accreditation guidelines require that students receive both individual and group supervision during the practicum. Guidelines and reference materials regarding individual supervision in practicum and internship will be reviewed in Chapter 7. Practicum students are expected to tape (audio and video) their counseling sessions. Of course, permission must be obtained from each client prior to taping the session (see Forms 3.1a, 3.1b, and 3.2 at the end of the book). The practicum site will have policies and procedures that must be followed to ensure the informed consent of the client. The tapes are to be submitted weekly to the university supervisor who is providing individual supervision to allow for sharing and evaluation. In some programs the same university supervisor provides both group and individual supervision. In other programs the student will have different university supervisors for group and individual supervision. Taped sessions can be reviewed in either group or individual supervision sessions, or both. Each tape should be reviewed by the student prior to submission and be accompanied by a written or typed critique (Form 6.5).

Every effort must be made to ensure the confidentiality of the counseling session. Be sure to check about the procedures at your field site regarding taping of sessions and the required safeguards and consents with regard to recording sessions for supervision purposes. When the tape has been reviewed and discussed with the student counselor, appropriate notes regarding counseling performance can be made for the counseling student's records. The tape(s) should then be erased.

A blank copy of a Tape Critique Form (Form 6.5) has been included in the Forms section for students' use. This form can be used to guide the student in developing a written review and analysis of taped therapy sessions. A sample of a completed Tape Critique Form is provided in Figure 6.2.

We are providing excerpts from a practicum syllabus to the counselor-in-training as a representative sample of course objectives and assignments in group practicum. Students should note that additional and varied requirements may be included in the practicum experience.

Jean Smith

Student counselor's name

Tom D. Session #3

Client I.D. & no. of session

Brief summary of session content:

Tom is citing his reasons for being unhappy in his job situation and reviewing all he has

attempted to do to make his boss like and respect his work.

Intended goals:

1. To help Tom explore all of his feelings and experiences related to the job situation.

2. To help Tom be able to assess and value his work from his own frame of reference

rather than his boss's.

Comment on positive counseling behaviors:

I was able to accurately identify Tom's feelings and to clarify the connection of feelings

to specific content.

Comments on areas of counseling practice needing improvement:

I sometimes became hooked into Tom's thinking about how to please his boss and would

work with him about problem solving in this way.

Concerns or comments regarding client dynamics:

_____

_____

Plans for further counseling with this client:

Continue weekly appointments; move focus back onto the client and try to identify other

ways he worries about approval.

_____

Tape submitted to _____

Date _____

Figure 6.2 Sample completed Tape Critique Form (Form 6.5).

SAMPLE OF COURSE OBJECTIVES AND ASSIGNMENTS IN GROUP PRACTICUM*

Course Objectives:

- To develop expertise in counseling, consulting, and guidance experiences
- To demonstrate an understanding of various counseling theories, techniques, and procedures
- To establish a facilitative and ongoing relationship with clients and on-site staff
- To demonstrate competence and skill in record keeping and case reporting
- To provide a safe place to share information about and reactions to your practicum experiences
- To define your professional identity as a counselor
- To develop skills in identifying and monitoring your strengths and growth edges
- To identify and examine personal issues that affect your work with clients
- To improve understanding of how multicultural issues interact with counseling practice
- To demonstrate an understanding of the ethical standards of the American Counseling Association (ACA) with respect to counseling practice.

Course Assignments:

- This course is a supervised practicum experience which focuses on case conceptualization, client assessment and evaluation, oral and written case reporting, and evaluation of counseling performance in individual intervention. Each section of the practicum uses a concerns-based developmental group supervision model. In this model, students are expected to openly discuss current cases and professional issues in counseling, develop their own personal counseling styles, and participate in giving and receiving feedback. The methods of instruction will include minilectures, demonstrations, group discussions, and student presentations.
- Precourse self-assessment: Write a 4- to 5-page paper assessing yourself as a developing counselor. The paper should include the following: (a) your strengths as a counselor-in-training, (b) growth edges, (c) learning goals for the semester, (d) countertransference issues requiring additional examination and work, and (e) theoretical orientation(s) to which you subscribe. The paper must be written using APA style.
- Clinical case presentation: Each student will make one major case presentation. An oral description of the client should briefly address the information listed below. The focus of the presentation should be on discussing the unanswered questions. For the case presentation, students must bring the most recent video- or audiotaped session cued for viewing. The case presentation should be 20 to 30 minutes. Furthermore, a case conceptualization paper summarizing the information on Intake Summary, Background Information, Clinical Impressions, Client–Therapist Match, Treatment, Client's Progress to Date, and Unanswered Questions will be submitted to the instructor on the assigned due date. The paper should be 8 to 10 pages in length. Grading will focus on relevance of content, depth of reflection, and quality of writing. The paper must be written using APA style.
- Postcourse self-assessment: Write a 4- to 5-page paper reassessing yourself since you have completed your first semester as a counselor trainee. Please make note of areas that are similar to and different from your initial assessment. The paper should include the following: (a) strengths, (b) growth edges, (c) learning goals for future training, (d) countertransference issues, and (e) theoretical orientation(s).

*Adapted from a syllabus by Megan Curcianni, MS, NCC, LPC, and Janet Muse-Burke, PhD, Department of Psychology and Counseling, Marywood University, Scranton, PA. Reprinted with permission.

Activities in Group Supervision

A typical class session in group supervision would begin by addressing any specific concerns a student has regarding his/her practicum. After immediate concerns are addressed, the practicum student might engage in any of the following:

- doing self-assessment and skill development orientation;
- role-playing problem situations with clients encountered at the practicum site;
- listening to and discussing various recorded counseling sessions;
- reviewing previously taped counseling sessions made by class members;
- discussing theories and techniques related to common problems and client work of concern to group members;
- giving and receiving feedback with peers regarding personal and professional interactions, including legal, ethical, and multicultural issues;
- participating in peer consultation group activities; and
- preparing and doing case presentations including assessments, case conceptualizations, goal setting, and treatment planning.

Peer Consultation

Peer supervision and consultation have been identified as a valuable adjunct to the supervision process. This modality is, however, recommended with some precautions. Peer supervision should be used only as a supplement to regular supervision in practicum. The peer consultant can promote skill development through ratings and shared perceptions, but it is important to make sure that any peer supervision activities that are initiated occur after group supervision has provided sufficient training and practice (Boyd, 1978). Peer supervision/consulting within the group supervision class with assigned peer dyads or small group consultation activities outside of class prepare counseling students to incorporate peer consultation activities into their ongoing work as a professional counselor. Peer collaboration has been referred to by a number of different terms in the literature (i.e., peer supervision, reflecting teams, peer consulting). For our purposes we will use the term *peer consulting*. The benefits of incorporating peer consultation into the group supervision process are that it

- fosters collegial supervision relationships;
- prepares the counseling student for continued use of peer consultation after the completion of training;
- fosters reciprocal learning, increased skills, and responsibility for self-assessment;
- decreases dependence on expert supervisors;

■ emphasizes helping each other achieve self-determined goals rather than focusing on evaluation; and

■ challenges the counselor to consider alternate perspectives (Benhoff & Paisley, 1996).

When involved in peer consultation activities, peers must assume a greater responsibility for providing critical feedback, challenge, and support to colleagues. As practicum students function as peer consultants, they are strengthening their own abilities to review their own work. A goal of peer consultation is enhanced self-awareness and a deeper understanding of the complexities of counseling (Granilla, Granilla, Kinsvetter, Underfer-Babulis, & Hartwood Moorhead, 2008). Suggested guidelines for peer consulting activities are as follows:

1. Comment on the case rather than solving it or giving advice.
2. Speak tentatively and speculatively about possible meanings or interpretations.
3. Ask questions and express curiosity.
4. Avoid judgment (Winslade & Monk, 2007).

Peer consultation can use directed feedback for tape review, goal setting, case conceptualization, and theoretical orientation. It works best when applying structured supervision tools. After a particular counseling skill has been introduced, modeled, and practiced within the group context, peer rating of tapes can be implemented. We suggest that the peer critique of tapes be structured to focus on the rating of specific skills. For instance, the target skills might be identified as one or more of the facilitative skills such as basic empathy, use of open-ended questions, or concreteness. Other target skills could be the recognition and handling of positive or negative affect or the effective use of probes. The Peer Rating Form (Form 6.6) and the Interviewer Rating Form (Form 6.7), used to structure the use of peer rating activities, have been included in the Forms section.

Another approach to improving the use of functional basic skills is to teach students to identify their dysfunctional counseling behaviors and then to minimize those behaviors (Collins, 1990). Instead of rating functional skills, peer reviewers can measure the incidence of dysfunctional skills such as premature problem solving or excessive questioning in their review of counseling tapes. The goal would be for the counselor to decrease or eliminate dysfunctional counseling behaviors in actual sessions. Collins (1990), in a study of the occurrence of dysfunctional counseling behaviors in both role playing and real client interviews of social work students, identified the following as dysfunctional behaviors:

■ poor beginning statements: the session starts with casual talk or chitchat instead of engagement skills;

■ utterances: the counselor's responses consist of short utterances or one-word responses such as "uh-huh," "yeah," "okay," or "sure"; two different types of utterance responses rated were utterances (alone) and utterances (preceding a statement);

■ closed questions: the counselor asks questions that require one-word answers by clients, such as yes or no or their age or number of children;

■ *why* questions: the counselor asks statements starting with the word *why*;

■ excessive questioning: the counselor asks three or more questions in a row without any clear reflective component to the questions (reflective component refers to restating content the client has expressed in his/her statements to the counselor);

■ premature advice or premature problem solving: the counselor gives advice that is considered premature, that is, advice given in the first 10 minutes of the session or after the first interview, judgmental statements, or problem solving where the counselor is doing the work for the client; and

■ minimization: the counselor downplays the client's problem, gives glib responses, or offers inappropriate comments such as "Life can't be all that bad."

Another structured peer reviewing process could be implemented using Form 6.1 (at the end of book), the Self-Assessment of Counseling Performance Skills. Instead of applying this to a self-assessment, the peer consultant group could use these items to rate counseling tapes presented by members of the group supervision class. The student who has a tape under review could choose the items for which he/she wants to receive feedback.

Borders (1991) has presented a Structured Peer Group Supervision Model (SPGS) which is based on a case presentation approach. In this model the counselor provides a brief summary of a client and therapy issues. The counselor then provides a sample of a counseling session (audio or video recording). The counselor then identifies questions about the client or the taped session and requests feedback. The peers are assigned roles, perspectives, or tasks for reviewing the taped session.

The peers may perform *focused observations* on a skill, such as how well the counselor performs a confrontation, or on one aspect of a session, or on the relationship between the counselor and the client. Another assigned task may be *role taking*. Peers may be asked to take the perspective of the counselor, the client, or some significant person in the client's life.

Similarly, structured learning activities could focus instead on self-awareness or multicultural awareness questions posed by the counseling student who is requesting feedback. Several other strategies which may be included using the SPGS model will be suggested for use in the internship seminar.

Evaluation of Practicum in Group Supervision

Formative Evaluation

Assessment is provided by the supervisor at various times throughout the practicum. Continuing assessment of the student's work occurs regularly during weekly individual and/or group supervision sessions both at the field site and in the university setting. This regularly occurring feedback to the practicum student about his/her work is called formative assessment. The supervisor is constantly assessing the student on a variety of skills, abilities, and cognitions. These evaluations can range from comments about a counseling technique to dialogue about a case conceptualization. These formative evaluations are usually verbal, and the supervisor often keeps notes on the content and process of the supervision. In group supervision, a number of assignments, both written and verbal, are assigned and evaluated as completed. Group interaction which involves peer consultation and audiotape review is observed and assessed related to the appropriate skill areas which were the focus. Evaluations from individual supervision are integrated into group supervision evaluations to determine the final grade in practicum.

Summative Evaluation

Summative evaluation is usually provided at the midpoint and completion of practicum. The supervisor can give a narrative report of the student's progress, or he/she can use a standardized assessment instrument. The Supervisee Performance Assessment Instrument can be found in Appendix I. It can be used for self-assessment, collaboration between the supervisor and the supervisee to identify new goals for supervision, and/or supervisor assessment of the supervisee. Form 7.5 (Supervisor's Final Evaluation of Practicum Student) rates the student on recommended skill levels for transitioning into internship.

Transitioning Into Internship

The final evaluation in practicum serves two purposes. First, it serves as a decision point about whether the student is recommended to proceed into the internship phase of training. We must note that if there is a concern about the student's abilities to practice counseling with clients, the student should have been receiving supportive and honest formative assessments along the way. The student's group and individual supervisors would have collaborated and met with the student to discuss any ways that the situation could be remedied. Most programs have a procedure in place to address this situation. Second, summative evaluation in practicum provides the opportunity for the student to advance into the internship with a clearer identification of the skill development goals which he/she will pursue at the next level of training. Group supervision and individual supervision evaluations are both reviewed as part of the practicum student's final grade and evaluation.

Recommended Skill Levels for Transitioning Into Internship

Each training program will have considered the criteria related to the skill levels which must be met in order to recommend that the counselor-in-training proceed on to the internship. We are proposing the following skill levels as a guide for making this recommendation. The practicum student

1. consistently demonstrates the use of basic and advanced helping skills;
2. has the ability to appropriately use additional theory-based techniques consistent with at least one theoretical framework;
3. demonstrates skill in opening and closing sessions and managing continuity between sessions;
4. demonstrates knowledge and integration of ethical standards into practice;
5. has cognitive skills of awareness, observation, and recognition of relevant data to explain some client dynamics;
6. writes accurate case notes, intake summaries, and case conceptualizations;
7. recognizes how several of his/her personal dynamics may impact a client and the counseling session and demonstrates sensitivity to cultural differences; and
8. demonstrates moderate to low levels of anxiety and moderate to low levels of dependency on supervisor direction during supervision sessions.

Group Supervision in Internship

CACREP accreditation guidelines stipulate that the internship student be provided an opportunity to become familiar with a variety of professional activities and resources in addition to direct service. They further require that the internship student receive an average of 1 1/2 hours per week of group supervision throughout the internship by program faculty or a student supervisor under the supervision of a faculty member. The student's counseling performance and ability to integrate and apply knowledge will receive formative and summative evaluation as part of the internship (CACREP, 2009). The guidelines of the Canadian Counselling and Psychotherapy Association's Council on Accreditation of Counsellor Education Programs require that students complete a 400-hour final practicum where students receive regularly scheduled individual supervision by qualified field site supervisors in collaboration with program faculty. A group supervision experience is not stipulated (Canadian Counselling and Psychotherapy Association, 2003). At the internship (final practicum) level, students will be further refining and progressing in their counseling practice of understanding and analyzing client concerns and implementing appropriate counseling interventions.

Hatcher and Lassiter (2007), in their article on practicum competencies in professional psychology, identified several levels of competence to apply to the progression of developing competencies in training. They proposed the following levels:

1. Novice (N): Novices have limited knowledge, understanding, and abilities in analyzing problems and implementing intervention skills. Distinguishing patterns and differentiating between important and unimportant details are limited. They do not yet have well-formed concepts about how clients change toward healthier functioning.
2. Intermediate (I): Students at this level have gained enough experience to recognize important patterns and can select interventions to respond to the presenting concerns. They understand and intervene beyond the surface level more typical of those at the Novice level, but generalizing diagnosis and intervention skills to new situations and clients is limited and supervisory support is needed.
3. Advanced (A): At this level, the student has more integrated knowledge and understanding of client processes and can recognize recurring patterns and select appropriate intervention strategies. Treatment plans and case conceptualization are based on more integrated knowledge, and this understanding influences treatment actions taken. The student is less flexible than the proficient practitioner (the next level of competence) but has mastery and can cope with and manage a broader range of clinical work.

Internship students can reflect on this description of progressing toward proficiency when reviewing their own skill levels as they complete their practicum experience. In general, most students will have developed some confidence and skills in establishing therapeutic relationships with their clients, and they will be seeking a broader range of theory-based techniques that are consistent with their concepts of how people change to become healthier in their emotional and functional life situations. The focus of group supervision in internship shifts toward cognitive counseling skills with a concurrent integration of self-awareness/multicultural awareness and professional understanding into the counseling process.

The group supervision seminar in internship generally includes assignments which allow counselors-in-training to demonstrate how their clinical thinking skills are applied to their counseling practice. A typical seminar includes assignments such as the following:

■ Case Conceptualization Presentation and Paper: Students are to present a case from their internship practice that outlines the presenting problem, psychiatric history, medical history, family history, educational/occupational history, mental status, assessment, diagnostic impressions, and treatment plan and goals and includes a sample of progress notes.

■ Integrative Paper: Students will write a double-spaced, typewritten paper presenting their integrated approach to counseling. The paper is to be written in two parts. In Part I, students are to cover their philosophical, theoretical, and practical view of (a) human health and dysfunction, (b) the role of the counselor, (c) the goals and methods of therapeutic change, and (d) the process of therapeutic change. In Part II, students are to present an illustrative case from their internship practice. A counseling case presentation is to be written, including a description of the case from intake through termination (including a prognostic statement).

■ The student will demonstrate the application of cultural diversity skills by showing the following competencies in counseling practice reviews:

Awareness of and respect for clients' cultural differences

Orientation to learning more about the client's culture as needed

Application of multicultural competencies to case conceptualization, diagnosis, interventions, and prevention work

Group Supervision Models in Internship

Bernard and Goodyear (2014) define group supervision as "the regular meeting of a group of supervisees (a) with a designated supervisor; (b) to monitor the quality of their work; and (c) to further their understandings of themselves as clinicians, of the clients with whom they work, and of service delivery in general" (p. 181). As the members of the supervision group move from novice to more advanced levels of skill, they typically interact at first with a focus on conceptualization and intervention and slowly move to more sharing regarding personalization.

The SPGS Model

This model, proposed by Borders (1991), was reviewed earlier in the section on peer consultation groups in practicum. This approach is similarly effective at the internship level. When using this model with novice counselors, the supervisor provides more direction and structure. When using this model with more advanced supervisees, the supervisees take on more responsibility. The supervisor serves as the moderator for the group and assures they stay on task. Then the supervisor takes on the role of process commentator and offers feedback about group dynamics. The supervisor then summarizes the initial feedback and discussion and asks the presenting counselor if his/her supervision needs were met.

Lassiter, Napolitano, Culbreth, and Ng (2008) proposed an expansion of Borders's format to include a multicultural-intensive observer role for a peer responder. This person focuses on cultural matters represented in the session, including issues of cultural differences and assumptions, privilege, and power differentials.

Another variation would be to ask an observer to watch the session by developing a *descriptive metaphor*. Borders found this useful when the issue was the interpersonal dynamics between the counselor and the client, or when the counselor felt "stuck." A suggestion would be for the observer to think of a road map and describe the direction the counselor is taking, or to think of the session as a movie and describe each actor's part in the drama.

For a focus on cognitive counseling skills, the counselor question and the peer assignment are on theoretical perspectives regarding

1. the assessment of the client,
2. the conceptualization of the issue or problem,
3. the goals of counseling,
4. the choice of intervention, and
5. the evaluation of progress (Borders & Brown, 2005, pp. 62–63).

After the counselor presents the taped segment of the counseling session, the group members give feedback from their theoretical perspectives. The presenting counselor then summarizes the feedback. This process facilitates the development of cognitive counseling skills and gives the supervisor the opportunity to observe the complexity and accuracy of the theoretical perspectives which are offered.

The Structured Group Supervision (SGS) Model

The SGS Model (Wilbur, Roberts-Wilbur, Hart, Morris, & Betz, 1994) begins with a supervisee making a "plea for help." This plea includes information about the case and often a sample from the session. The supervisee then specifically states what he/she needs help with. The supervision group members then ask questions about the information presented to clear up any faulty assumptions or missing information. These are informational and clarifying questions. The supervisor monitors this so that group members don't offer premature feedback. The group members are given a few moments to think about how they would handle whatever was sought in the plea for help. Then, in orderly fashion, each member offers what he/she would do "if this were my client," or "if I had your concern." The supervisee remains silent but may take notes. This continues until there is no more feedback. At the conclusion of this feedback process, there is a 10- to 15-minute break in which the supervisee can think about the feedback. Group members do not converse with the supervisee during this break. After the break, the supervisee responds to the group by addressing each member to say what feedback was helpful and what feedback was not helpful and why. This is presented in a way that does not infer that the feedback was right or wrong but focuses more on the cultural fit, style of therapy, or history with the case. Depending on the needs of the group, the supervisor may summarize or discuss the process or reframe an issue to invite the group to look at it in another possible way. Comments on the group process or comments about the case are offered as "something to think about." Supervisees are affirmed for being open and taking the risk in allowing themselves to be vulnerable.

Evaluation in Group Supervision of Internship

Your internship grade will be determined by your university supervisor in collaboration with your field site supervisor and given upon the completion of your internship contract. Documentation of your internship hours will be done by the site supervisor. Evaluations from your individual supervisor are an important part of your final evaluation because they reflect how you integrate and put into practice with clients the various elements in the skill areas. Several evaluation instruments have been provided in the Forms section for use by the site supervisor. The collaboration between your faculty supervisors and your site supervisor is essential for summative evaluation of your progress toward the completion of the internship. Your faculty group supervisor will be evaluating your cognitive performance skills based on weekly group counseling participation and completion of cognitive counseling skill assignments. Formative evaluations will be based on observations of performance in the four identified skill areas which were the focus of peer group interactions. Students in internship should be practicing at the intermediate, advanced, or professional levels of performance. Students performing at the novice level in any skill area would require notification and appropriate remediation action.

For summative evaluations the group supervision faculty supervisor will review and evaluate the intern's case conceptualization presentations; review and evaluate the Integrative Paper, which articulates the guiding theory used by the intern; and observe how the intern integrates cognitive skills and self-awareness/multicultural awareness skills into practice during the seminar. Form 7.6 can also be used by the group supervisor to evaluate counseling practice.

Evaluations from your individual site supervisor and/or your individual faculty supervisor are an important part of your midpoint and final evaluations because they reflect how you integrate and put into practice with clients the various elements in the skill areas. Several evaluation instruments have been provided in the Forms section for use by your individual supervisor(s). The collaboration between your group supervisor and your individual supervisor(s) is essential for summative evaluation of your progress toward the completion of the internship. A successful completion of the internship indicates that the intern has demonstrated adequate competency in counseling performance and professional skills, cognitive counseling, self-awareness/multicultural awareness, and collaboration in supervision to be recommended for certification as an entry-level professional counselor.

Summary

In this chapter we have presented a skill-based model to be used as a framework for both group and individual supervision during practicum and internship. The skill development areas of counseling performance and professional skills, cognitive counseling skills, self-awareness/multicultural awareness skills, and developmental level in supervision were reviewed. Self-assessment activities were presented to guide counselors-in-training in the articulation of their supervision goals. Sample course objectives and assignments which are typically included in both group practicum and group internship seminars were included. A variety of learning activities and peer consultation approaches which could be included in the group supervision process were suggested. Finally, formative and summative evaluation practices were reviewed.

References

Benhoff, J. M., & Paisley, P. O. (1996). The structured peer consultation model for school counselors. *Journal of Counseling and Development, 74*(3), 304–318.

Bernard, J. M., & Goodyear, R. K. (2014). *Fundamentals of clinical supervision* (5th ed.). Upper Saddle River, NJ: Pearson.

Borders, L. D. (1991). A systematic approach to peer group supervision. *Clinical Supervision, 10*(2), 248–252.

Borders, L. D., & Brown, L. L. (2005). *The new handbook of counseling supervision.* Mahwah, NJ: Lahaska.

Borders, L. D., & Leddick, G. R. (1997). *Handbook of counseling supervision*. Alexandria, VA: Association for Counselor Education and Supervision.

Boyd, J. (1978). *Counselor supervision: Approaches, preparation, practices*. Muncie, IN: Accelerated Development.

Canadian Counselling and Psychotherapy Association. (2003). *Accreditation manual*. Retrieved October 2013 from www.ccpa.accp.ca/en/accreditation/standards.

Collins, D. (1990). Identifying counseling dysfunctional skills and behaviors. *Clinical Supervisor, 8*(1), 67–69.

Corey, G. (2013). *Theory and practice of counseling and therapy* (9th ed.). Belmont, CA: Brooks/Cole, Cengage Learning.

Cormier, S., & Hackney, H. (2012). *Counseling strategies and interventions* (8th ed.). Upper Saddle River, NJ: Pearson.

Council for Accreditation of Counseling and Related Educational Programs (CACREP). (2009). *CACREP standards*. Alexandria, VA: Author.

Egan, G. (2013). *The skilled helper: A problem management and opportunity development approach to helping* (10th ed.). Belmont, CA: Brooks/Cole.

Fall, M., & Sutton, J. M., Jr. (2004). *Clinical supervision: A handbook for practitioners*. Boston: Allyn and Bacon/Pearson.

Granilla, D. H., Granilla, P., Kinsvetter, A., Underfer-Babulis, J., & Hartwood Moorhead, H. J. (2008). The structured peer consulting model for school counselors. *Counselor Education and Supervision, 48*(1), 32–47.

Hatcher, R. L., & Lassiter, K. D. (2007). Initial training in professional psychology: The practicum competencies outline. *Training & Education in Professional Psychology, 1*, 49–63.

Ivey, A. E., Ivey, M. B., & Zalaquett, C. P. (2010). *Intentional interviewing and counseling* (7th ed.). Belmont, CA: Brooks/Cole.

Lassiter, P. S., Napolitano, L., Culbreth, J. R., & Ng, K. M. (2008). Developing multicultural competence using the structured peer group supervision model. *Counselor Education and Supervision, 47*, 164–178.

Remley, T. P., Jr., & Herlihy, B. (2014). *Ethical, legal, and professional issues in counseling* (4th ed.). Upper Saddle River, NJ: Pearson.

Wilbur, M. P., Roberts-Wilbur, J., Hart, G., Morris, J. R., & Betz, R. L. (1994). Structured group supervision (SGS): A pilot study. *Counselor Education and Supervision, 33*, 262–279.

Winslade, J. M., & Monk, G. D. (2007). *Narrative counseling in schools*. Thousand Oaks, CA: Corwin.

CHAPTER 7

INDIVIDUAL SUPERVISION IN PRACTICUM AND INTERNSHIP

Role and Function of the Supervisor in Practicum and Internship

According to the *Code of Ethics* of the American Counseling Association (ACA), "the primary obligation of the counseling supervisor is to monitor the services provided by other counselors or counselors in training. Counseling supervisors monitor client welfare and supervisee clinical performance and professional development" (ACA, 2014, F1.a). In addition, supervisors are trained in supervision methods and techniques and regularly pursue continuing education in supervision and counseling. Regulating boards are beginning to require that counseling professionals who provide supervision receive supervision training and certification. Bernard and Goodyear (2014) identify the purpose of supervision as twofold:

1. to foster the supervisee's professional development—a supportive and educational function; and
2. to ensure client welfare—the gatekeeping function is part of the monitoring process.

Supervisors are considered to be master practitioners who, because of their special clinical skills, training, and experience, have been identified by the field site to monitor and oversee the professional activities of the counseling student. University supervisors share a similar role in promoting applied skills but have an indirect or liaison relationship to the field site (Ronnestad & Skovholt, 1993). The function of the supervisor has been variously described in the literature. Dye (1994) suggested that supervision should provide high levels of encouragement, support, feedback, and structure. Psychotherapy supervisors undertake multiple levels of responsibility as teachers, mentors, and evaluators (Whitman & Jacobs, 1998). Supervisors are variously described as role models for a specific theoretical approach, as agents of professional development as supervisees progress through the stages of acquiring advanced skills, and as teachers, counselors, or consultants in the supervisory process (Bernard & Goodyear, 2014). The role that the supervisor takes with the counselor depends, optimally, on the developmental level of the counselor (Pearson, 2000). Beginning-level counselors tend to be uncertain about their counseling effectiveness and skills and tend to need a great deal of support. Intermediate-level counselors tend to fluctuate in their levels of confidence. High-level counselors are more consistent in their confidence and skill level. Practicum students are likely to move through the developmental levels idiosyncratically, usually at the beginning or intermediate levels. Some move more rapidly than others. Some progress, reach a plateau, then progress again. Some stay at the beginning levels. Some progress, encounter a new situation and regress, then stabilize and progress again. The supervisor often structures the supervision in ways consistent with the developmental needs of the practicum student.

Administrative and Clinical Supervision

The most controversial area of supervision lies in the contrast between clinical functions and administrative supervision functions. Clinical supervision functions emphasize counseling, consultation, and training related to the direct service provided to the client by the counselor trainee. Administrative functions emphasize work assignments, evaluations, and institutional and professional accountability in services and programs. For example, when clinical supervision is the emphasis, the counselor trainee's development of clinical skills is the focus of the supervisor–supervisee interaction. Feedback is related to professional and ethical standards and the clinical literature. In contrast, when administrative supervision is the focus, issues such as keeping certain hours, meeting deadlines, following policies and procedures, and making judgments about whether work is to be accomplished at a minimally acceptable level are emphasized. Feedback is related to institutional standards. Ideally, it is recommended that the same person should not provide both clinical supervision and administrative supervision. Realistically, this is not always the case. Therefore, separate meetings should be scheduled for clinical and administrative supervision.

The counselor trainee can expect to receive both clinical and administrative feedback. However, the emphasis of this chapter is directed toward clinical supervision and the intervention, assessment, and evaluative techniques related to a clinical supervisory situation. The student may want to reflect on the proportion of clinical to administrative supervision that he/she is receiving in practicum and internship.

The Supervisor–Supervisee Relationship

In clinical supervision, the importance of developing a working relationship with the supervisor cannot be overstated. The consensus of supervision researchers and theorists is that "good supervision is about the relationship" (Ellis, 2010, p. 106). Good supervision happens when supervisors are genuine, real, and present with their supervisees. In many ways it is similar to the process that goes on in good therapy (Majcher & Daniluk, 2009). Thus, counseling students should assess their own attitudes, biases, and expectations as they enter into the supervisory process.

The supervisee typically brings a number of predictable sources of discomfort to the supervision process. Common sources of discomfort are

- anxieties about evaluation by the supervisor,
- feelings related to negative self-evaluation (i.e., I am flawed; I have done something wrong), and
- issues of transference (i.e., a negative transference in which he/she perceives the supervisor to be more critical or punitive than actually is the case; or a positive transference in which the supervisor is idealized) (Bernard & Goodyear, 2014).

Concerns over performance and evaluation by supervisors can lead to a defensive stance on the part of the student. It is not uncommon for trainees to react by criticizing their supervisors, and therefore becoming resistant to supervisory feedback and evaluation. Borders (2009) emphasized that a safe environment that demonstrates mutual respect is necessary for a supervisee to be open to feedback and be willing to learn and change. Kaiser (1997), in discussing the supervisor–supervisee relationship, suggested that supervision takes place in the context of the relationship between the supervisor and supervisee. Kaiser cited the following three components of the relationship: "the use of power and authority, creation of shared meaning, and creation of trust" (p. 16). It is essential that the counselor trainees recognize that supervisors do have power over them, primarily because they will be evaluating the trainees' work. Thus, trainees need to be open and honest with their supervisors to gain effective guidance and feedback. Similarly, the creation of shared meaning between supervisor and supervisee is related to understanding and agreement between the two parties. The degree to which understanding and agreement are obtained determines how the two parties can communicate. Finally, the creation of trust between supervisor and supervisee develops out of the creation of shared meaning and the building of confidence in the mutual understanding between the two parties. Bordin (1983) characterized the supervisor–supervisee relationship as a working alliance or a "collaboration to change" which consists of an agreement on goals, an agreement on tasks necessary to achieve these goals, and an affective bond which develops between them. Scott (1976) emphasized the importance of establishing a collegial relationship within the supervisor–supervisee interaction. The relationship is characterized by balance and a shared responsibility for understanding the counseling process. A disruption in this balance or an inability to establish collegiality should be open areas of discussion to identify learning problems. A general rule is that disruptions in the supervisor–supervisee relationship always take precedence.

Direct supervision of clinical work is perhaps the most important element in the training of a counselor or psychotherapist. Supervision is more than a didactic experience. It includes intensive interpersonal interaction with all of the potential complications that such relationships can include. Research has documented the importance of the supervisor–supervisee relationship. Several studies have related success in supervision to the quality of the relationship between the supervisor and the supervisee (Alpher, 1991; Freeman, 1993; Ladany, Ellis, & Friedlander, 1999). Relationship qualities of warmth, acceptance, trust, and understanding are defined as fundamental to positive supervision. Good supervision must integrate both task- and relationship-oriented behavior. In positive supervision experiences, a critical balance exists between relationship and task focus. In negative supervision experiences, the total emotional focus is on the negative relationship. The literature cited in the foregoing section may provide the counselor-in-training with sufficient rationale and motivation to consider the supervisor–supervisee relationship as an important area on which to focus during supervision. Relational concerns and conflicts clearly detract from the amount of learning in supervision.

What Is "Lousy" Supervision?

The literature on supervision is replete with articles that focus on the qualities and practices of good supervisors. However, there is a paucity of information dealing with ineffective supervision. Magnuson, Wilcoxon, and Norem (2000) published an article titled "A Profile of Lousy Supervision: Experienced Counselors' Perspectives." The article is a result of a study of 10 experienced clinical supervisors who were asked to respond to a number of prompts (e.g., "I am interested in knowing about things you might have experienced in supervision that hindered your learning and professional development"). In addition, participants were asked to describe or characterize lousy supervision. The following is an overview and summary of that study. According to the authors, the data yielded two broad categories of findings: (a) overarching principles of lousy supervision and (b) general spheres of lousy supervision. The following are statements and comments that reflect the participants' opinions regarding lousy supervision.

Overarching Principles

Unbalanced: This is an overemphasis on some elements of supervisory experiences, excluding others.

Developmentally inappropriate: This is the failure to recognize or respond to the dynamics and changing needs of supervisees.

Intolerant of differences: This is the failure to allow the supervisee the opportunity to be innovative; supervisors were impatient, rigid, and inflexible.

Poor model of professional or personal attributes: This includes boundary violations, intrusiveness, and exploitation.

Untrained: The supervisors had inadequate training and a lack of professional maturity and were uncomfortable assuming supervisory responsibilities.

Professionally apathetic: The supervisors were lazy and not committed to the growth of the supervisees.

General Spheres

Organization and administrative: This includes a lack of supervisory guidelines, the neglect of initial assessment procedures to identify supervisees' needs, a lack of continuity between sessions, and ineffective group supervision.

Technically and cognitively unskilled practitioners, unskilled supervisors, and unreliable resources: This includes a lack of therapeutic and developmental skills, a reliance on a single model of supervision, and a disregard for supervisees' approach to counseling.

Rational/affective: This includes failing to humanize the supervisory process, being overly critical and providing little positive feedback, and having the inability to address personal concerns that hampered supervision.

These characteristics of a lousy supervisor are important to consider when approaching supervision. Unfortunately, ineffective supervisory methods become known after the supervision process has begun. However, it is important to note that supervisees who experience such inappropriate and nonprofessional supervisors should consult with their on-campus supervisor (or liaison), who can provide guidance in coping with the situation or reassign the supervisee to another supervisor.

Approaches to Individual Supervision

The counselor-in-training often approaches clinical supervision with mixed feelings. On the positive side, supervision can be regarded as a helpful, supportive interaction that focuses on validating some practices. On the negative side, supervision can be regarded as an interaction that will expose inadequacies and leave the student with even more feelings of incompetence. Both sets of expectations coexist as the student approaches supervision. The tendency, particularly in the early stages of supervision, is for the student to work at proving himself/herself as a counselor so that the negative feelings of inadequacy will diminish. Generally, the initial phases of supervision are spent establishing a working alliance between the supervisor and supervisee. This holds true for the various approaches to supervision that might be implemented. To reduce the counseling student's anxieties about supervision and to facilitate the creation of a working alliance, we believe a preview of how supervision could be implemented is in order.

Bernard and Goodyear (2014) identify three major categories of clinical supervision models: models grounded in psychotherapy theory, developmental models, and process models. Each of these categories contains several different approaches to supervision. We will present one model from each category to provide the counseling student with an overview of the models of supervision she/he might encounter.

Models Grounded in Psychotherapy Theory: The Psychodynamic Model

Psychodynamic supervision falls within the category of psychotherapy theory-based models. In this supervision approach the supervisor models a key competence (relationship) that is considered foundational for psychodynamic therapy (Bernard & Goodyear, 2014). In the psychodynamic model, "counselor supervision is a therapeutic process focusing on the intrapersonal and interpersonal dynamics in the supervisee's relationship with client, supervisors, colleagues, and others" (Bradley & Ladany, 2001, p. 148). Goals in this approach are to attain awareness of and acquire skills in the use of dynamics in counseling. The supervisee might expect to focus on a parallel process, that is, the idea that similar dynamics occur in the counselor–client dyad and the supervisor–supervisee dyad. Another focus might be on the interpersonal dynamics between the supervisee and the client, where the supervisor teaches the supervisee by modeling effective interpersonal dynamics. A third focus might be on the interpersonal dynamics occurring in the counseling situation. Here the supervisor brings attention to how internalized feelings, thoughts, and meanings are affecting the thoughts and meanings of the supervisee and the client.

Other psychotherapy theory-based models are cognitive-behavioral, humanistic-relational, or systemic models. The advantage of these theory-based models is the modeling provided to supervisees who wish to master a particular theoretical approach to counseling (Bernard & Goodyear, 2014).

Developmental Models: The Integrated Developmental Model

This model falls within the developmental category of models. These models are organized around the needs of the supervisee based on his/her state of professional development. The integrated developmental model (Stoltenberg, 1981; Stoltenberg & McNeill, 2010) describes counselor development as occurring through four phases:

Level 1. Supervisees have limited training or experience and have high motivation and anxiety.
Level 2. Supervisees are making the transition from dependent and imitative and needing structure and support to more independent functioning. This usually occurs after practicum.
Level 3. Supervisees are focusing on a more personalized approach to practice.
Level 4. Supervisees' focus is on integrating practice across the domains of treatment, assessment, and conceptualization.

Stoltenberg and McNeill (2010) identified eight domains of professional functioning: intervention skills competence, assessment techniques, interpersonal assessment, client conceptualization, individual differences, theoretical orientation, treatment plans and goals, and professional ethics. Counseling students can identify themselves as being at a specific level of professional development and anticipate the supervision focus within and across the eight domains. As the supervisee moves forward to each new level, the structures of self–other awareness (cognitive and affective); motivation as reflected in interest, investment, and effort expended in clinical training and practice; and autonomy as reflected in the degree of independence the supervisee shows are characterized by changes. For example, at Level 1 the counselor focuses on himself/herself and what feelings, thoughts, and behaviors he/she is experiencing, with less focus on the client. Motivation is high, and autonomy is low. At Level 2 the focus shifts toward the dynamics of the client, and this shift moves back and forth, causing confusion and varying motivation levels; the counselor will show more autonomy but fall back into dependence on the supervisor. At Level 3 the fluctuations stabilize, and the counselor moves toward a more personalized approach with the self–other focus in balance, motivation consistent, and autonomy more prevalent. At Level 4, all domains of practice are integrated, and underlying structures are stable, with high levels of autonomy. The supervisor uses Facilitative Interventions, Authoritative Interventions, or Conceptual Interventions to facilitate progress to the next stage of development (Bernard & Goodyear, 2014, pp. 35–38).

Other developmental models are the Loganbill, Hardy, and Delworth model, which identifies the three recurring stages of stagnation, confusion, and integration as the supervisee deals with eight developmental issues; the Reflective Model; and the Life Span Model.

Process Models: The Discrimination Model

The discrimination model (Bernard, 1979, 1997) is a widely used model of supervision. The model falls in the category of supervision process models. Models in this category can be used in any psychotherapy orientation and are compatible with developmental models. In the discrimination model, the supervisor can take the roles of teacher, counselor, or consultant. The teacher role is taken when the supervisee needs structure and includes instruction, modeling, and feedback. The counselor role is taken when the supervisor wants to enhance the supervisee's reflectivity about his/her own dynamics. The consultant role is more collegial and supports the supervisees' trust in their own work and in their ability to work on their own (Bernard & Goodyear, 2014). The focus can be on any one of three foci:

- intervention, or what the supervisee is doing in the session, what skill levels are being demonstrated;
- conceptualization, or how the supervisee understands what is occurring in the session; and
- personalization, or how the supervisee practices a personal style of counseling while attempting to keep counseling free of his/her personal issues and countertransference responses.

In this model, the supervisor has great flexibility in how each focus area is approached. For example, the supervisor may take the role of teacher when addressing a situation where the discussion is about how an ethical standard such as the "duty to warn" may apply to a client. In another situation, the supervisor may take on the role of counselor when the focus is on self-awareness and the supervisor is helping the counselor identify his/her feelings of anxiety when a client talks about acting out. When the supervisor takes the role of consultant, the supervisor and counselor may discuss the benefits of a variety of intervention approaches as the counselor decides how best to proceed with treatment. The supervisor at any given moment may be responding in one of nine different ways. The supervisor may respond from any role within each area of focus depending on the needs of the supervisee. Supervisors are more likely to use the teacher role with novice supervisees. Supervisors of beginning supervisees might focus more on intervention and conceptual skills, while supervisors of more advanced students may focus more on personalization issues. Other process models of supervision include the events-based model and the systems approach to supervision model.

The approaches to supervision that have been reviewed are those that are most likely to be experienced by the counseling student. Because the trainee will probably have more than one supervisor during the field experiences, it is likely that he/she may be working with a university supervisor who utilizes the discrimination model approach to supervision while simultaneously working with a field site supervisor who utilizes a cognitive behavioral approach to supervision. The trainee is advised to be open to any one of the approaches to supervision by recognizing the goals and advantages of each type of supervision.

The Triadic Model of Supervision

The triadic model of supervision has been recommended as an acceptable method of providing individual supervision according to the accreditation standards of the Council for Accreditation of Counseling and Related Educational Programs (CACREP, 2009). The author of this text is familiar with the variation of the triadic model of supervision that was used by the University of Pittsburgh Counselor Education Program during her tenure there. The model was proposed and articulated by C. Gordon Spice, PhD (professor emeritus in the Department of Psychology in Education, University of Pittsburgh). Spice and Spice (1976) recommended that the triadic supervision model be used in peer supervision practice for counselors-in-training. Triadic supervision has been described as being a bridge between individual and group supervision. It is the term for supervision with one supervisor and two supervisees. The model has received significant research since it was adopted as an acceptable form of individual supervision by the Council for Accreditation of Counseling and Related Educational Programs (CACREP, 2001).

In the triadic model of supervision, three roles are designated: the role of supervisor, the role of supervisee, and the role of observer/commentator. For supervision of practicum/internship students, the field site or university supervisor takes the role of supervisor. In this role the supervisor reviews the counseling student's work sample (a video- or audiotape, case presentation, or clinical notes together with a tape). The supervisor then gives feedback to the supervisee regarding (a) what is particularly well done in the work sample, (b) what has need for improvement, and (c) what is unclear or confusing in the work sample. An example of this feedback is as follows: The supervisor states, "Your use of the basic empathy skills and confrontation skills was excellent. I particularly liked the way you confronted the client about the contradiction between his values and his behaviors. It didn't come across as blameful. You do need to review your use of questions. Too many questions in a row sound more like an interrogation. What I'd really like to focus on in this supervisory session is the theoretical approach you have in mind in working with this client. It is not clear to me how you see his concerns in relationship to making better decisions and healthier choices." Discussion then follows, with clarification and expansion of the possible ways of viewing the client as the topic.

The supervisee provides the work sample, and the peer observer/commentator focuses on the communication and interpersonal dynamics going on between the supervisor and the supervisee. Before the close of the supervisory session, the observer shares his/her comments about what he/she observed in the interaction. An example of the observer's comment is as follows: To the supervisee, "I noticed that you seemed a bit defensive when the supervisor asked you to clarify what you meant when describing better decisions." Or "The two of you seemed to be going all around the subject of the client's concerns, but you never gave specifics."

The two supervisees can alternate taking the roles of supervisee or observer/commentator. When they alternate by taking the role of supervisee in one session and the role of observer/commentator at the next supervisory session, this is referred to as the single-focus form. If the session is in a 90-minute time frame, the supervisees may switch roles midway through the session so that each student has the opportunity to present his/her work for feedback. This is referred to as the split-focus form (Nguyen, 2004).

When using a split-focus 90-minute time frame, Stinchfield, Hill, and Kleist (2010) describe a process where the role assigned to the peer is that of observer/reflector and the peer engages in silent reflection and inner dialogue while observing the supervisor–supervisee process. This is followed by the peer then engaging in outer dialogue with the supervisor about what was reflected on. At the same time, the presenting supervisee moves into the reflective role and must listen and reflect on the outer dialogue taking place. The session then continues with supervisees switching roles for the second half of the session.

Use of this framework can have many variations for supervision. For example, the peer can be asked to adopt the perspective of the client and track thoughts and feelings as the session is being presented and then share these observations with the supervisee. Or the peer can role-play the client when the supervisor is demonstrating to the supervisee the use of a specific intervention (Lawson, Hein, & Getz, 2009). Bernard and Goodyear (2014) have identified factors which may enhance the success of triadic supervision:

- Allot 90 minutes each week so that a split-focus form can be used.
- Thoughtfully consider the pairing of supervisees. The success of this model depends on the compatibility of the supervisees paired together.
- Have a distinct role for the nonpresenting supervisee.
- Orient the supervisees to the model.
- Supplement with individual supervision—particularly when addressing personal growth issues and evaluation.
- Train supervisors in the use of the model to allow the supervisor to be aware of the needs of more than one supervisee and to be flexible and creative with the choice of strategies (Oliver, Nelson, & Ybanez, 2010).

The use of the triadic model can facilitate a deepening of the supervisory process and provide an opportunity to summarize the interaction process. Benefits associated with the use of triadic supervision include reports that supervisees value the special relationship developed with their supervisee cohort, that it allows for more diversity of perspectives, and that supervisees report a benefit from vicarious learning when a peer is the focus of the session (Lawson, Hein, & Stuart, 2009). Practicing professional counselors can also use this model when meeting for collegial peer supervision in the workplace.

The Clinical Supervision Process

We have noted previously the parallels between clinical supervision and the counseling process. Clinical supervision, similar to counseling practices, begins with informed consent.

Informed Consent in Supervision

The ACA *Code of Ethics* (2014) offers standards regarding supervision practices in counseling. The Association for Counselor Education and Supervision (ACES), in response to counseling supervisors' requests for more specific guidelines regarding supervision practices, developed and approved *Best Practices in Clinical Supervision* (ACES, 2011). Many of the apprehensions and concerns about the clinical supervision process can be mitigated by providing a formal structure for the process. The supervisee should be informed about the structure, processes, and evaluation practices that will be offered by the supervisor. This formal structure is facilitated by providing a Supervisor Informed Consent and Disclosure Statement to the supervisee at the initial supervision session. The informed consent can facilitate the development of a professional relationship and rapport between the supervisor and supervisee. It provides the supervisee with the opportunity to understand the supervisor and, when possible, make a voluntary choice between supervisors. We are offering a sample statement which is consistent with the best practice guidelines and has been adapted from several sources (Fall & Sutton, 2004; Haarman, 2009; Remley & Herlihy, 2014; Bernard & Goodyear, 2014; Kitchener & Anderson, 2011).

SAMPLE OF A SUPERVISOR INFORMED CONSENT AND DISCLOSURE STATEMENT

Jane Doe
Student Services Supervisor
Anywhere School District

Purpose: The purpose of this form is to provide you with essential information about the supervision process you are about to begin. The information provided conforms with best practices guidelines and ensures that you understand our professional relationship and my background.

Professional Disclosure:

I earned my M.Ed. in School Counseling from a CACREP-approved university program and am a certified K–12 counselor in my state and a National Certified School Counselor. I earned a post-master's Educational Specialist degree (Ed.S.) in School Counseling and am a certified student services supervisor in my state. I am a member of ACA, ASCA, and ACES and practice according to the ethical codes of my profession. I have additional training in crisis response and solution-focused brief therapy. I have been a school counselor for 20 years—10 years as an elementary school counselor and the last 10 years as a high school counselor and counseling supervisor. My general areas of competence in school counseling include crisis response, intervention, referral, and follow-up; social skill development group leadership; short-term counseling for academic, personal, and career-related concerns; and psychoeducational guidance and consultation.

The Supervision Process:

As your supervisor I am responsible to meet your professional development needs as a counselor-in-training while protecting the welfare of clients. Although the focus of supervision will be on you and your professional skill development, a primary concern will be client care. The benefits of receiving individual supervision are the potential growth and development of your professional skills as a counselor. The risks are the feelings of discomfort you may experience as you disclose any deficits or personal concerns as they relate to your counseling practice. Ours is a professional supervisor–supervisee relationship, and I will honor and respect the boundaries of this relationship. Our relationship can be congenial and collegial, but private social interactions will be considered inappropriate.

As your supervisor I follow a supervision model that employs the roles of teacher, counselor, and consultant within a developmental context. In the teacher role, I will help you learn and practice counseling techniques and skills. In the counselor role, I will attend to the development of your reflective skills concerning the interaction between your personal dynamics and those of your clients. Your dynamics will be a focus as they relate to client concerns and cultural considerations. Ethically, I cannot provide you with therapy as part of supervision but will encourage and refer you to continue personal work in therapy when appropriate. The consultant role is used to discuss areas of uncertainty or approaches to case conceptualization. The skill areas we will focus on in supervision are (1) counseling performance skills, which includes professional and ethical components; (2) cognitive counseling skills, which include how you think about, gather information about, and analyze your cases; (3) self-awareness and multicultural awareness skills, which help you examine personal dynamics such as transference and countertransference and personal values and biases which may impact your counseling practice; and (4) developmental level, which relates to your response to supervision and the level of needs you bring to supervision.

You will be taping your counseling sessions for review in supervision. We will also be using case note review, live observation, role-playing, case conceptualizations, and other modalities in our sessions. Supervision will require that you reflect on your counseling sessions, yourself as a counselor, and the profession of counseling.

Practical Issues:

We will meet for 1 hour per week with regularly scheduled appointments. You should have a new tape available for review each week after the first two sessions of practicum/internship. If our appointment is cancelled for any reason, you should call and reschedule for another time that same week.

I will keep a record of our weekly sessions and suggest that you do the same. The records belong to me, but they are available for you to review at any time. I will destroy them 1 month after the completion of your practicum/internship.

I will provide you with both formative and summative feedback and evaluation throughout your practicum/internship. I will regularly give you feedback concerning your strengths and weaknesses as a counselor. I will provide a written summative evaluation at the midpoint and end of your practicum/internship. Evaluation will be based on the responsibilities, goals, and objectives established in the supervisory contract and consistent with identified skill areas and the format of your university program. I will complete university-required forms which document your practice hours in practicum/supervision. I will make recommendations to your university supervisor which will be considered in the grade you receive from your university supervisor.

Legal and Ethical Issues:

My services as your supervisor will be given in a professional manner consistent with accepted ethical standards. It is important that you agree to act in an ethical manner as outlined in ACA and ASCA ethical codes and follow laws and regulations related to confidentiality, reporting of abuse, and the duty to warn. You will inform me immediately if these situations become a concern. You will always act in a manner that will not jeopardize, harm, or be potentially damaging to clients.

All information that you share with me concerning yourself or your clients will be kept confidential with several important exceptions:

- You or your client are a danger to yourself or others.
- I have reason to suspect child, vulnerable adult, or elder abuse on the part of you or a child.
- You direct me to share information.
- I am ordered by a court or laws to disclose information.
- I must defend myself against a legal action or formal complaint that you or your client has filed against me.
- Your progress requires me to bring your name up to your university field site liaison.

If you are dissatisfied with the supervision, please let me know. If we can't resolve your complaints, you may follow procedures established by your university field site liaison.

If you must reach me by phone, you can call me at _____ Home (emergency only) _____ Office

If it is an emergency and I can't be reached, please call Dr. _____ , Director of Student Services, at _____.

If you have questions concerning the information in this statement or other questions about supervision, you may ask about them at any time.

Please sign and date this form

_____   _____

Supervisee name and date   Supervisor name and date

Forming a Supervision Contract

A second formal structuring process is accomplished by negotiating a goals statement. ACES's best practices policy (2011) recommends developing a mutually negotiated goals statement when possible. In addition to an informed consent statement, Cobia and Boes (2000) recommend a second document which is a formal plan for supervision. They conceptualize this as an individualized learner plan. It would include mutually agreed-upon goals for supervision, competencies to be learned and evaluated, and the responsibilities of both the supervisor and supervisee. We are providing a Sample Supervision Contract consistent with best practices guidelines and recommendations from several sources (ACES, 2011; Kitchener & Anderson, 2011; Remley & Herlihy, 2014; Cobia & Boes, 2000; Haarman, 2009; Bernard & Goodyear, 2014).

SAMPLE SUPERVISION CONTRACT

Purpose: The purpose of the supervision is to monitor client services provided by the supervisee and to facilitate the professional development of the supervisee. This ensures the safety and well-being of our clients and satisfies the clinical supervision requirements of _____ University and _____ school/agency.

Supervisor's Responsibilities:

- The supervisor agrees to provide face-to-face supervision to the supervisee for 1 hour per week at a regularly scheduled time for the fall/spring practicum/internship semester as required by _____ University.
- The supervisor will complete forms required by the university concerning hours, completion, verification, and evaluation of the supervisee's practicum/internship and make appropriate contact with the university liaison concerning the supervisee's progress.
- The supervisor will make a recommendation as to the student's grade, but responsibility for the final grade rests with the university.
- The supervisor will review audiotapes, case notes, and other written documents; do live observations; and co-lead groups as part of the supervision format.
- The supervision sessions will focus on professional development, teaching, mentoring, and the personal development of the supervisee.
- Skill areas will include counseling performance skills and professional practices, cognitive counseling skills, self-awareness/multicultural awareness, and developmental level in supervision.
- The supervisor will provide weekly formative evaluations, document supervision sessions, and provide summative evaluations based on mutually agreed-on supervision goals. Evaluation will be offered within the skill categories listed above and will be consistent with university guidelines.
- The supervisor will practice consistent with accepted ethical standards.

Supervisee's Responsibilities:

- Uphold the ACA *Code of Ethics*.
- Prepare for weekly supervisions by reviewing audiotapes and framing concerns to be the focus of the supervision session.
- Be prepared to discuss and justify the case conceptualization made and the approach and techniques used.
- Reflect on your own personal dynamics and any multicultural issues which may surface in your sessions.
- Review any ethical dimensions which may be important in your sessions.
- Contact your supervisor immediately in any crisis situations involving harm to self or others or abuse of a child, vulnerable adult, or elder.

■ Keep notes regarding the supervision sessions.
■ Provide the supervisor with videotapes to be reviewed prior to the supervision session.

Supervision Goals and Objectives:

Goal 1: Solidify my use of basic and advanced counseling skills in intake sessions and continuing sessions.

Objective: Demonstrate skill in doing initial sessions, including addressing HIPAA and informed consent components.

Objective: Close sessions well by summarizing and allowing time for questions and transitions into the next session.

Objective: Demonstrate skill in preparing initial intake summaries and writing case notes.

Goal 2: Use assessment information and components of the client's story to form case conceptualizations which can help me think clinically about my client's needs.

Objective: Integrate more assessment information into the intake summary to form accurate diagnoses.

Objective: Apply two different case conceptualization models to cases.

Objective: Apply a preferred theoretical approach to explaining how change may occur when thinking of intervention strategies and techniques with specific clients.

Goal 3: Increase my awareness of personal and multicultural dimensions in my practice.

Objective: Examine counseling sessions to recognize instances where my issues may be complicating how I understand the client's concerns.

Objective: Pay particular attention to how any goals identified for the client may be influenced by multicultural elements.

Goal 4: Decrease my level of anxiety and self-consciousness when being supervised.

Objective: Allow time at the end of supervision sessions to review the session and identify points of anxiety and self-consciousness.

Objective: Attend to developing a supervisor–supervisee working alliance by focusing on mutually identified tasks and techniques.

The supervision contract will be revised at specified times or as competencies are established and new goals and objectives become appropriate. Form 7.1 at the end of the text provides a form to be used for initial and subsequent supervision contracts. Supervisee self-assessment practices within the four skill areas have been presented in Chapter 6 as well as a sample goal statement (Form 6.4). The completed Supervisee Goal Statement should be brought to the initial individual supervision session to assist in identifying mutually agreed-on goals in the supervision contract.

The Supervision Session Format

There are probably as many supervision session formats as there are supervisors. However, most sessions include

■ review of taped sessions,
■ a critical review of specific aspects of the counselor's practice,

- a focus on areas which could benefit from encouragement or redirection,
- a discussion of how the clinical thinking relates to techniques and interventions used,
- a focus on areas in which reflection on personal dynamics or multicultural elements may be needed, and
- attention to the ethical underpinnings of practice.

Fall and Sutton (2004) recommend that the supervisee be given guidelines about how to do advanced preparation for the supervision session. These guidelines include how to develop an agenda for what the supervisee would like to focus on during supervision. They suggest identifying:

What content will be the focus? New cases, previous cases, self-awareness/cultural awareness, ethical or crisis issues, personal theory, and technique development.

What process will be the focus? How is what you are doing with the client helpful? What am I not getting about this client? Are there resources I could research that may help me with this client? Why do I feel exasperated/relieved when the session with this client ends? Are the goals we have established really the client's goals? I am not comfortable with proceeding as you have advised me with this client.

What is your priority for topics to be covered in the session?

What do you need from the supervisor, and what modality will you use (case notes, audio-recording, role-playing, self-report, etc.)?

The session proceeds with the supervisee taking responsibility for identifying his/her needs and the supervisor clarifying concerns and responding to the agenda as appropriate. The supervisor may want to add to or amend the agenda. The supervisor keeps notes of content, process, priority of supervisee needs, and modality and intervention (teacher, counselor, consultant) used. (See Form 7.2 at the end of the book.) The supervisee may take notes during or after the session. Form 7.3 at the end of the book provides a format for these notes. The supervisee can make note of any changes or new understandings that will be incorporated into work with a particular client or applied generally in his/her counseling practice. Form 7.4 can be used by the site supervisor to evaluate taped sessions provided by the supervisee.

Supervising the Developing Counselor-in-Training

The individual supervisor mentors and facilitates the process of the counseling student evolving from a beginning professional helper to become a professional counselor who is prepared to accept the rights and responsibilities of the profession. The sequence has been characterized as moving from dependence and a need for teaching and instruction to becoming a collaborator in the process of understanding the counseling work. It has been described as progressing through increasingly complex levels of practice where one is initially focused on one's own implementation of skills and processes to the level where one can fully integrate all the elements of counseling practice as understood through the frame of one's own personal theory of counseling. The process has been evaluated as progressing from novice status, where the trainee has limited knowledge and understanding of intervention skills and limited knowledge of how a client moves to better functioning, to intermediate levels, to advanced levels where the supervisee has deeper knowledge of the complexity of intervention and concepts and has the ability to manage many aspects of clinical work. At the proficient psychologist level the trainee has advanced to be flexible across all areas of functioning, and work is based on more integrated knowledge which guides therapeutic action. Supervision goals and processes also evolve to support the progress of the counselor-in-training toward full professional status. The levels of progress and needs in supervision are a determinant for appropriate supervision interventions and are one aspect of evaluation of the counselor-in-training. For example, to progress from practicum to internship may require that the supervisee is functioning at level 2 or intermediate or as having less dependence on the supervisor in the teaching role. These descriptors are based on the supervisor's observations and clinical judgment about how the supervisee functions in the supervision process. Supervision in practicum tends to focus on learning and applying assessment, basic conceptualization, and basic and advanced counseling skills.

As the counselor-in-training progresses to internship, individual supervision serves the unique training function of facilitating the integration of the various components of counseling training in one course. The supervisor introduces a variety of activities and processes that intertwine the following components:

1. forming a therapeutic relationship;
2. facilitating the client's healthy emotional development;
3. viewing the client and the counseling process through the lens of several theoretical perspectives;
4. identifying personalization or self-awareness related to values, beliefs, understanding, and the internal trigger points related to the counseling process;
5. identifying cultural components which are part of the counseling process;
6. integrating ethical principles into the professional identity of the counselor;
7. fostering maturation of the supervision process;
8. encouraging the development of a personal theory of counseling; and
9. supporting the developmental and/or remedial goals of counseling by consulting with others who also influence the healthy development of the client.

What makes the focus on these various components more powerful, in the context of supervision, is that the awareness, understandings, and insights are examined in direct relationship to the counselor's actual behavior with clients. Managing the supervision process so that these goals (awareness, understanding, and insight) are realized is quite complex. When the supervisor and counselor-in-training mutually understand the full range of components that are part of the supervisory process, less resistance is likely to occur when the supervision moves beyond just focusing on learning diagnostic and interaction skills. The counseling student's self-assessment within each of the skill components provides a preparation for understanding the complexities and subtleties of professional counseling practice. When the counselor trainee is in the beginning phase of preparation—at the clinical practice level of prepracticum and practicum—the trainee needs "an environment with large amounts of support, direct instruction, and structure, and minimal amount of challenge and personal exploration" (Pearson, 2001, p. 174). As the trainee progresses to internship, he/she is likely to be at the intermediate or advanced level of development. The needs of the intern fluctuate between feeling dependent and wanting autonomy, and focusing on his/her own practices while wanting to improve awareness of client relationship dynamics. The supervisor generally reduces the amount of direct instruction and the degree of structure, provides a challenge relative to support, and begins to examine the counselor's personal reactions to clients. The supervisee is encouraged to influence getting what he/she needs and wants from supervision by self-assessment, forming specific goals within the skill areas, and preparing for supervision sessions by forming an agenda related to his/her practice concerns. The supervisor prepares for the supervision session by reviewing any audiotapes, live observation, co-leading, or written case material which may be relevant to the session. The supervisor uses strategies which are appropriate to the developmental level of the supervisee.

Evaluation of Individual Supervision in Practicum and Internship

Assessment is provided by the supervisor at various times throughout the practicum and internship. Continuing assessment of the student's work occurs regularly during weekly individual supervision sessions both at the field site and in the university settings.

Formative evaluation includes verbal commentary about the work accomplished within the supervision session and includes identifying strengths and areas which need improvement. Sessions are organized around specific goals and objectives in the supervision contract, and evaluations are based on observation, discussion, and evidence of improved performance within the goals and objectives. Feedback will be based on regular observation of counseling sessions (via audio recording and live) and review of clinical documentation. Supervision notes can be shared with the supervisee when considered appropriate by the supervisor and at the request of the supervisee. The Supervisor's Formative Evaluation of Supervisee's Counseling Practice (Form 7.4) can also be used to provide feedback after several sessions if a structured format is preferred by the supervisor.

Summative evaluation will be given at the midpoint and the end point of the practicum/internship semesters. These assessments are important because they influence major educational, regulatory, and credentialing consequences. The assessment requires thoughtful attention to identifying the forms and competencies that will be included. We are including examples and forms which could be considered for use by sites and programs. Our formats are organized around the skill areas identified in the text.

Summative Evaluation in Practicum

The midpoint evaluation should reflect the supervisor's assessment of overall progress thus far in the term. It is an important evaluation point because it allows the supervisor to identify whether there are any concerns about recommending that the supervisee to go on to internship. It also provides an opportunity to identify remediating possibilities for those who are not progressing. For practicum students who are meeting or exceeding expectations, this becomes an opportunity to affirm elements of their practice and to renegotiate aspects of the supervision contract as appropriate. We are providing a sample of a narrative evaluation which is a format which can be used for the midpoint evaluation.

SAMPLE OF A MIDPOINT NARRATIVE EVALUATION OF A PRACTICUM STUDENT

Supervisor name _____

Supervisee name _____   Date _____

The purpose of this evaluation is to provide feedback about your progress toward becoming a professional counselor as demonstrated in the skill areas that have been the focus of our supervision. The evaluation is based on my observations of your practice, the conversations about your work, and my notes about the content and process of our supervision sessions.

Counseling Performance Skills:

Use of basic and advanced counseling, procedural, and professional skills: You are able to form solid therapeutic relationships with a variety of clients by your genuine warmth and accurate empathy toward understanding their concerns. You begin the session smoothly and integrate privacy and informed consent information into initial sessions. A variety of helping skills are appropriately used to assist the clients' framing of their story and identification of areas which need change. You sometimes hurry the process toward an action plan without fully exploring feelings associated with thoughts and actions which may be triggered. More attention to the stage of change in which the client presents may be helpful in directing your efforts to move the counseling progress forward. In all, being able to stay with and explore the client's feelings as they relate to thoughts and actions is an area for you to identify goals for your next supervision sequence. You may also want to identify theory-based techniques that would broaden your range of intervention possibilities.

Cognitive Counseling Skills:

We have focused on the areas of writing an intake summary, clinical notes, assessment, and goal setting thus far in supervision. Initially it was difficult for you to identify and connect relevant information to become confident that you could do this in a professional manner. The goals and objectives set for these areas have been met, although you still depend on me for feedback and approval about these functions. I would recommend that you set goals for increasing your case conceptualization skills and attend to the interrelationship of how you view a case clinically and how you conduct your sessions and the documentation that supports your work.

Self-Awareness/Multicultural Awareness:

You have become more attuned to how your personal background and values and unexamined biases may impact your counseling practice—particularly when setting goals and staying with feeling content. Continued attention to this aspect of your work is recommended. This site has many clients who come from life situations and cultural backgrounds that are very different from yours. Staying open to and aware of the worldview of these clients is an important part of being an effective and helpful counselor.

Developmental Level:

Your comfort level in supervision has noticeably increased. You regularly review your work, come to supervision with appropriate concerns, and take personal risks in revealing counseling practices which need to be improved. You also examine how your personal issues impact the counseling process. You have become less self-focused about your counseling and are able to focus more on client dynamics.

For the final evaluation of the practicum student, we are providing two assessment formats. First, you may use the Supervisee Performance Assessment Instrument (SPAI) developed by Fall and Sutton (2004). A copy of the SPAI can be found in Appendix I at the end of the book. We are also providing an evaluation tool for use at the end of the practicum experience which is based on the criteria suggested in Chapter 6 as required for proceeding into internship (see Form 7.5, Supervisor's Final Evaluation of Practicum Student). Documentation of practicum hours on the Weekly Schedule/Practicum Log (Form 3.6) and the Monthly Practicum Log (Form 3.7) must be signed by the site supervisor and turned in to the university supervisor along with the final practicum supervision evaluation.

Summative Evaluation in Internship

We have provided a sample of a narrative midterm evaluation in practicum. A similarly organized narrative could be used for the midterm intern evaluation. The narrative is organized within each skill area, and progress as demonstrated in relationship to goals and objectives is noted. Comment should also include assessment about how this progress meets or exceeds expectations in progressing toward a successful completion of internship requirements for professional practice.

An alternative evaluation process could be implemented which is similar to a work performance review utilized in the corporate world. In this process, both the supervisor and supervisee prepare an evaluation of the supervisee's performance in each of the skill categories based on how the supervisee has made progress toward meeting the goals and objectives established in the supervision contract. Each goal or objective is evaluated based on the categories of 1 = no progress; 2 = does not meet expectations; 3 = meets expectations; 4 = exceeds expectations; 5 = outstanding. After progress in the skill categories has been evaluated, comments are made about overall progress and new objectives are suggested. When the supervisor and supervisee meet for evaluation (approximately 30 minutes), they compare each review for areas of agreement and differences. Future goals and objectives are discussed in relationship to the evaluation. These goals are accepted or revised and committed to. In the case of a supervisee who is falling behind in a skill area, remedial recommendations are established. The site supervisor will have been in contact with the university site liaison person. These recommendations may include additional on-campus supervision, formal writing about the personal theory of counseling in response to specific theory development questions, and/or personal counseling or therapy. The remedial necessities will be part of an overall policy of the university program and determined and implemented by the university supervisor.

The final summative evaluation of the counseling intern assesses whether the supervisor believes that the supervisee has achieved entry-level status as a practicing professional counselor. The professional literature describes the necessary skills in a variety of ways. For example, Fouad et al. (2009) developed a list of competencies for psychologists which identified readiness for entry to practice in several skill areas. In the skill area of intervention, the essential component was "independent intervention planning, including conceptualization and intervention planning specific to case and context" (p. S19) with the behavior anchors of ability to establish rapport with a wide variety of clients, use of good judgment in crises, and effective delivery of interventions. Engels et al. (2010) have developed an extensive list of competencies that parallel the CACREP standards. Chapters cover generic counseling competencies as well as those specific to the specialization areas (e.g., clinical mental health counseling, school counseling). Many summative evaluation forms used by universities and others have chosen a representative sample of similar competency items within specific categories which have been identified as consistent with generic counseling competencies. Form 7.6 at the end of the text (Supervisor's Final Evaluation of Intern) provides an evaluation instrument with a list of criteria within each skill area that can be rated using a 5-point Likert scale. A rating of 3 would signify that the intern possesses adequate competence on each item rated. Supervisors working with counselor trainees in a specialization (i.e., career counseling; marriage, couple, and family counseling) can add on items from the specialization by referring to items in the competency areas in the work of Engels et al. Form 12.3 (Evaluation of Intern's Practice in Site Activities) provides a shorter final evaluation form based on activities performed at the practicum site.

Documenting Internship Hours

CACREP standards require that the intern successfully complete a 600-hour supervised internship which provides the counselor-in-training the opportunity to perform under supervision a variety of activities that a regularly employed staff member in that setting would be expected to perform—with 240 hours of direct service to clients, including group work. The remaining 360 hours are in other professional activities including documentation and record keeping, assessment, information and referral, staff and professional development, planning, and others depending on the site and specialization. The Canadian Counselling and Psychotherapy Association (2003) requires a 400-hour advanced practicum with 200 hours of direct service (140 with individual clients and 40 with groups). Forms 12.1 and 12.2 at the end of the book provide a format for the weekly and summary logs of internship hours which will be signed by the site supervisor and given to the faculty supervisor upon completion of the internship. Other forms to be completed at the end of the internship will be provided in Chapter 12.

Summary

In this chapter we have described several approaches to supervision which the counselor-in-training may experience. Information was provided about the triadic model of supervision with several examples of practice applications. Examples and formats for a supervisor's informed consent and disclosure statement and a supervision contract which are consistent with ACES best practice guidelines were included. Finally, a variety of formative and summative evaluation processes, samples, and forms were included. A review of this chapter should provide the counselor-in-training with an understanding of what to expect in the individual supervision component of the practicum/internship.

References

Alpher, V. (1991). Interdependence and parallel processes: A case study of structured analysis of social behavior in supervision and short term dynamic psychotherapy. *Psychotherapy, 29*(2), 218–231.

American Counseling Association. (2014). *Code of ethics*. Alexandria, VA: Author.

Association of Counselor Education and Supervision (ACES). (2011). *Best practices in clinical supervision*. Retrieved from www.acesonline.net/wp/content/uploads/2010/10/ACES-Best-Practices-in-clinical-supervision-document-FINAL.pdf.

Bernard, J. M. (1979). Supervision training: A discrimination model. *Counselor Education and Supervision, 19*, 60–68.

Bernard, J. M. (1997). The discrimination model. In C. E. Watkins (Ed.), *Handbook of psychotherapy supervision* (pp. 310–327). New York: Wiley.

Bernard, J. M., & Goodyear, R. K. (2014). *Fundamentals of clinical supervision* (5th ed.). Upper Saddle River, NJ: Pearson.

Borders, L. D. (2009). Subtle messages in clinical supervision. *Clinical Supervisor, 28*, 200–209.

Bordin, E. S. (1983). The working alliance model of supervision. *Counseling Psychologist, 11*, 35–42.

Bradley, L. J., & Ladany, N. (2001). *Counselor supervision: Process and practice*. Philadelphia, PA: Brunner/Routledge.

Canadian Counselling and Psychotherapy Association. (2003). *Accreditation manual*. Retrieved from www.ccpa.accp.ca/en/accreditation standards.

Cobia, D. C., & Boes, S. R. (2000). Professional disclosure statements and formal plans for supervision: Two strategies for minimizing risk of ethical conflicts in post-master's supervision. *Journal of Counseling and Development, 78*, 293–296.

Council for Accreditation of Counseling and Related Educational Programs (CACREP). (2001). *Accreditation manual* (2nd ed.). Alexandria, VA: Author.

Council for Accreditation of Counseling and Related Educational Programs (CACREP). (2009). *Accreditation standards*. Alexandria, VA: Author.

Dye, A. (1994). Training doctoral student supervisors at Purdue University. In J. E. Myers (Ed.), *Developing and directing counselor education laboratories* (pp. 130–131). Alexandria, VA: American Counseling Association.

Ellis, M. V. (2010). Bridging the science and practice of clinical supervision: Some discoveries, some misconceptions. *Clinical Supervisor, 29*, 95–116.

Engels, D. W., Minton, C. A. B., Ray, D. C., Bratton, S. C., Chandler, C. K., Edwards, N. A., et al. (2010). *The professional counselor: Portfolio, competencies, performance guidelines, and assessment* (4th ed.). Alexandria, VA: American Counseling Association Press.

Fall, M., & Sutton, J. M., Jr. (2004). *Clinical supervision: A handbook for practitioners*. Upper Saddle River, NJ: Pearson.

Fouad, N., Grus, C. L., Hatcher, R. L., Kaslow, N. J., Hutchings, P. S., Madson, M. B., et al. (2009). Competency benchmarks: A model for understanding and measuring competence in professional psychology across training levels. *Training and Education in Professional Psychology, 3*(4, Suppl.), S5–S26.

Freeman, S. C. (1993). Reiteration on client centered supervision. *Counselor Education and Supervision, 32*, 213–215.

Haarman, G. (2009). *Clinical supervision: Legal, ethical and risk management issues. Course workbook*. Brentwood, TN: Cross Country Education.

Kaiser, T. L. (1997). *Supervisory relationships*. Pacific Grove, CA: Brooks/Cole.

Kitchener, K. S., & Anderson, S. K. (2011). *Foundations of ethical practice, research, and teaching in psychology and counseling* (2nd ed.). New York: Taylor & Francis/Routledge.

Ladany, N., Ellis, M. V., & Friedlander, M. L. (1999). The supervisory working alliance, trainee self-efficacy, and satisfaction. *Journal of Counseling and Development, 77*, 447–455.

Lawson, G., Hein, S. F., & Getz, H. (2009). A model for using triadic supervision in counselor preparation programs. *Counselor Education and Supervision, 48*, 257–270.

Lawson, G., Hein, S. F., & Stuart, C. L. (2009). A qualitative investigation of supervisees' experiences of triadic supervision. *Journal of Counseling and Development, 87*, 449–457.

Magnuson, S., Wilcoxon, S. A., & Norem, K. (2000). A profile of lousy supervision: Experienced counselors' perspectives. *Counselor Education and Supervision, 39*, 189–202.

Majcher, J. A., & Daniluk, J. C. (2009). The process of becoming a supervisor for students in a doctoral supervision training course. *Training and Education in Professional Psychology, 3*, 63–71.

Nguyen, T. V. (2004). A comparison of individual supervision and triadic supervision. *Dissertation Abstracts International, 64*(9), 3204A.

Oliver, M., Nelson, K., & Ybanez, K. (2010). Systemic processes in triadic supervision. *Clinical Supervisor, 29*, 51–67.

Pearson, Q. (2000). Opportunities and challenges in the supervisory relationship. *Journal of Mental Health Counseling, 22*, 283–294.

Pearson, Q. (2001). A case in clinical supervision: A framework for putting theory into practice. *Journal of Mental Health Counseling, 23*(2), 174–183.

Remley, T. P., Jr., & Herlihy, B. (2014). *Ethical, legal, and professional* issues *in counseling* (4th ed.). Upper Saddle River, NJ: Pearson.

Ronnestad, M. H., & Skovholt, T. M. (1993). Supervision of beginning and advanced graduate students of counseling and psychotherapy. *Journal of Counseling and Development, 71,* 396–405.

Scott, J. (1976). Process supervision. In J. Scott (Ed.), *A monograph on training supervisors in the helping professions* (pp. 1–10). Retrieved from www.eric.govcontentdelivery/servlet/ERICServlet? accno-ED126398.

Spice, C. G., & Spice, W. H. (1976). A triadic method of supervision in the training of counselors and counseling supervisors. *Counselor Education and Supervision, 15,* 251–258.

Stinchfield, T. A., Hill, N. R., & Kleist, D. M. (2010). Counselor trainees experiences in triadic supervision: A qualitative exploration of transcendent themes. *International Journal for the Advancement of Counselling, 32,* 225–239.

Stoltenberg, C. D. (1981). Approaching supervision from a developmental perspective: The counselor complexity model. *Journal of Counseling Psychology, 28,* 59–65.

Stoltenberg, C. D., & McNeill, B. W. (2010). *Supervision: An integrative developmental model for supervising counselors and therapists* (3rd ed.). New York: Routledge.

Whitman, S. M., & Jacobs, E. G. (1998). Responsibility of the psychotherapy supervisor. *American Journal of Psychotherapy, 52*(2), 166–176.

SECTION IV

PROFESSIONAL PRACTICE TOPICS

CHAPTER 8

SELECTED TOPICS ON ETHICAL ISSUES IN COUNSELING

The importance of ethics education in counselor training has been cited by all credentialing bodies in counselor training. It is required that counseling ethics be addressed in core and specialized areas of the curricula. Codes of ethics address a broad range of behavior in counseling and psychology. Most important, they serve to educate counseling and psychology practitioners about the responsibilities inherent in their professional practice and serve to protect clients from unethical practices. Seligman (2004) suggested that having knowledge of and familiarity with those ethical standards, and abiding by them, is essential to sound clinical practice. The many reasons include the following:

- Ethical standards give strength and credibility to the mental health profession. Ethical guidelines help clinicians make sound decisions.
- Providing clients with information on when clinicians can and cannot maintain confidentiality, as well as other important ethical guidelines, affords clients safety and predictability and enables them to make informed choices about their treatment.
- Practicing in accord with established ethical standards can protect clinicians in the event of malpractice suits or other challenges to their competence.
- Demonstrated knowledge of relevant ethical and legal standards is required for licensing and certification as a counselor, psychologist, or social worker.

Fowers (2005) similarly states that ethics codes serve four functions:

- They establish integrity for the profession by providing an assessment of what is or is not morally acceptable.
- They serve an educational and role socialization function.
- They incur public trust because professionals can be held accountable for actions that do not meet standards.
- They serve an enforcement value in developing licensing requirements and legal sanctions.

Definitions: Ethics, Morality, and Law

Ethics are "moral principles adopted by an individual or a group to provide rules for right conduct" (Corey, Corey, & Callahan, 2011, p. 14). Huber and Baruth (1987) noted that "ethics is concerned with the conduct of human beings as they make moral decisions" (p. 37). Ethics are normative in nature and focus on principles and standards that govern relationships between individuals, such as between counselors and clients.

Morality refers to principles concerning the distinction between right and wrong or good and bad behavior. Morality used normatively refers to a code of conduct that applies to all who can understand it and govern their behavior by it. No one should ever violate a moral prohibition or requirement for non-moral considerations (Gert, 2012).

Law is defined as a rule of conduct prescribed or recognized as binding by a controlling authority (*Webster's Ninth New Collegiate Dictionary*, 1988).

Ethical Codes for Counselors

Ethical codes are the written set of ethical standards for the professional mental health provider. Ethical codes represent "aspirational goals, or the maximum or ideal standards set by the profession, and they are enforced by professional associations, national certifying boards and government boards that regulate professions" (Corey, Corey, & Callahan, 2011, p. 14). Each profession (psychology, social work, counseling, etc.) has a code specific to its particular client relationships. The codes are both national and regional. Mental health professionals have an obligation to behave in ways that do not violate these codes. Violations of the standards by a mental health worker can result in sanctions or loss of licensure.

The primary obligation of mental health professionals is to promote the well-being of their clients, and ethical codes were developed to protect the integrity of this process. They allow mental health professionals to police their own members, thus reducing the need for government regulation of the profession. These codes are normative in nature in that they prescribe what mental health professionals ought to do. Before you begin your practicum and internships, we urge you to review again the codes of ethics relevant to your area of specialization in your counseling program. We are providing you with a list of websites to access these codes.

Websites for Ethical Codes and Related Standards for Professional Organizations

American Association of Marriage and Family Therapy: www.aamft.org

American Association of Pastoral Counselors: www.aapc.org

American Counseling Association: www.counseling.org

American Mental Health Counselors Association: www.amhca.org

American Psychological Association: www.apa.org

American School Counselors Association: www.schoolcounselor.org

Association for Multicultural Counseling and Development: www.amcdada.org/amcd/default.cfm

Canadian Counselling and Psychotherapy Association: www.ccpa.ca

Canadian Psychological Association: www.cpa.ca

Code of Professional Ethics for Rehabilitation Counselors: www.crccertification.com

NAADAC—The Association for Addiction Professionals: www.naadac.org/membership/code-of-ethics

National Board for Certified Counselors: www.nbcc.org

National Career Development Association: www.ncda.org/aws/NCDA/asset_manager/get_file3395

Codes of Ethics: Similarities

Codes of ethics for counseling professionals are found in the American Counseling Association (ACA) and its divisions, national certification boards (the Council for Rehabilitation Counseling Certification, the National Board of Certified Counselors), state licensure laws, and ACA specialties (rehabilitation, school, career, college, mental health, community, marriage and family, and career counseling), the American Psychological Association (APA), as well as the Canadian Counselling and Psychotherapy Association and the Canadian Psychological Association. A variety of state psychological associations and several international associations also have published codes of ethics. The proliferation of ethical standards and codes has the potential of creating confusion for professional counselors (Herlihy & Remley, 1995). However, similarities across the codes can be identified.

- All major professional associations stipulate that clients have the right to safeguarded confidentiality with limitations in some situations. Limits to confidentiality are based on state laws, provincial laws, and the professional codes of ethics. Clients must be notified at the start of counseling of any exceptions to confidentiality.
- The issue of competence is addressed across ethical codes. You must practice within the areas for which you have received training and/or certification. Seek supervision and training before trying an intervention on your own. As a student counselor, you should discuss and consult with your supervisor about when and how to incorporate a new technique into your practice.
- The practice of establishing multiple relationships is addressed across all professional associations' ethical codes. First, *ALL ETHICAL CODES PROHIBIT SEXUAL INTIMACY OF ANY KIND WITH CLIENTS*. When counselors have a "connection with a client in addition to the therapist-client relationship, a secondary relationship exists" (Welfel, 2010, p. 217). These have been referred to as dual relationships, multiple relationships, or nonprofessional relationships. None of the codes refers to nonsexual relationships as unethical, but most warn against them. If such a relationship is entered into, it must be done with consultation with peers and/or supervisors. Discussions and consultations about the potential benefits and harms that could occur in such a relationship should be documented and placed into the counselor's records. If the potential benefits can be thoughtfully established, then actions such as attending an important function that is culturally valued and expected can be done. Counselors must always behave in a manner that protects the integrity of the counseling relationship.
- All professional codes address the importance of cultural issues. Counselors must work with clients from diverse cultures and backgrounds in an aware, knowledgeable, competent, and respectful way. Cultural meanings and the worldview of the client must be incorporated into all areas of practice.
- All professional codes address the necessity of using a systematic process of ethical decision making when encountering ethical dilemmas (Cormier & Hackney, 2012, pp. 180–185).

Ethical Decision Making

Principle-Based Ethics and Ethical Decision Making

Ethical principles are general norms that provide a rationale for standards in the ethical codes of most health professions. They are obligations that are always considered in ethical decision making (Meara, Schmidt, & Day, 1996). Kitchener and Anderson (2011) have identified foundational ethical principles, which are norms which provide the foundation for behavior in the helping professions, particularly in the United States and Canada. These foundational principles are:

- *Nonmaleficence:* This refers to the duty to do no harm or to not engage in actions that risk harm to others. Harm means that the interests or well-being of another has been reduced in a substantial way. The ACA's *Code of Ethics* (2014) requires that counselors must minimize or remedy unavoidable or unanticipated harm. The risk of harm must also be balanced with other ethical principles.

- *Beneficence:* This means doing good or benefitting others. This principle has two aspects (Beauchamp & Childress, 2001). First, one must provide benefits to others by acting in ways that increase their general well-being. The second obligates the counselor or psychologist to balance the potential benefit of an action against the potential harm.

- *Respect for a person's autonomy:* This imposes the moral requirement that we respect others, including their choices and desires, regardless of their personality type or characteristics. This includes freedom of action and freedom of choice. One can do what one wants to do with one's own life as long as it doesn't interfere with similar actions of others. Freedom of choice means making one's own judgments.

- *Fidelity:* This is at the core of the relationship between the counselor or psychologist and the client. This includes the qualities of truthfulness and loyalty as well as honesty and trustworthiness—core components of human trust.

- *Justice:* Justice involves treating equals equally and unequals unequally but in proportion to their relative differences (Beauchamp & Childress, 2001). Justice implies that the judgment of relevant and irrelevant characteristics in a particular case should be done impartially. Professionals in the helping professions are forbidden to unfairly discriminate on the basis of age, gender, race, ethnicity, national origin, religion, sexual orientation, socioeconomic status, and so on. Psychologists and counselors ought to have a commitment to being fair where they agree to promote the worth and dignity of each individual and work to ensure that people have access to a minimum of goods and services such as education and health care. Practitioners often contribute a portion of their work to help those with limited resources (Kitchener & Anderson, 2011, pp. 25–37).

In ethical decision making, the question arises about how decisions are made when ethical principles conflict. Kitchener and Kitchener (2008) support the process of using a balancing approach. This suggests that all principles are valuable and, in a particular situation, must be balanced to get the best overall combination.

The American Psychological Association (APA) identifies the principles of beneficence and nonmaleficence, fidelity and responsibility, integrity, justice, and respect for people's rights and dignity in its code of ethics (2002). The Canadian Counselling and Psychotherapy Association's (CCPA) *Code of Ethics* (2007) identifies the principles of beneficence, fidelity, nonmaleficence, autonomy, justice, and responsibility to society. The Canadian Psychological Association (2002) organizes the values and standards in its *Code of Ethics* based on the principles of respect for the dignity of persons, responsible caring, integrity in relationships, and responsibility to society. The American Counseling Association's *Code of Ethics* (2014), identifies the principles of autonomy, nonmaleficence, beneficence, justice, fidelity, and veracity. A great deal of similarity exists for the principles underlying these codes of ethics.

Should ethical codes not be specific or thorough enough to answer a question you encounter in your practice, you should employ ethical principles in evaluating the situation. Ethical principles are used to make decisions about moral issues inherent in a particular dilemma. An ethical dilemma is a situation in which one must make a choice between competing and contradictory ethical mandates. Pope and Vasquez (2011), in their discussion about ethical dilemmas, state that "ethical awareness is a continuous, active process that involves constant questioning and personal responsibility" (p. 2) and that "we often encounter ethical dilemmas without clear and easy answers" (p. 5). Ethical codes do not and cannot always provide solutions to the dilemmas we encounter.

Ethical behavior begins with the counselor's familiarity with the professional codes of ethics. These are the first source for standards regarding appropriate behaviors and responsibilities inherent in the counseling profession. Developing sensitivity to the ethical principles in the code enables the counselor to feel more secure when faced with situations that are ethically problematic. Ethical decision making is rarely an easy task for the counselor. Ethical decision making involves the application of the code of ethics coupled with one's own values and morals and one's own interpretation of what is in the best interest of the client.

Corey (1996) suggested that developing a sense of professional and ethical responsibility is never-ending. It demands that the professional must periodically review a number of ethical issues. According to Corey these issues are as follows:

1. Counselors need to be aware of what their own needs are, what they are getting from their work, and how their needs and behaviors influence their clients. It is essential that the therapist's own needs not be met at the client's expense.
2. Counselors should have the training and experience necessary for the assessments they make and the interventions they attempt.
3. Counselors need to become aware of the boundaries of their competence, and they should seek qualified supervision or refer clients to other professionals when they recognize that they have reached their limit with a given client. They should make themselves familiar with the resources in the community so that they can make appropriate referrals.
4. Although practitioners know the ethical standards of their professional organizations, they also must be aware that they must exercise their own judgment in applying these principles to particular cases. They realize that many problems have no clear-cut answers, and they accept the responsibility of searching for appropriate solutions.
5. It is important for counselors to have some theoretical framework of behavior change to guide them in their practice.
6. Counselors need to recognize the importance of finding ways to update their knowledge and skills through various forms of continuing education.
7. Counselors should avoid any relationships with clients that are clearly a threat to therapy.
8. It is the counselor's responsibility to inform clients of any circumstances that are likely to affect the confidentiality of their relationship and other matters that are likely to negatively influence the relationship.
9. It is imperative that counselors be aware of their own values and attitudes, recognize the role that their belief system plays in their relationships with clients, and avoid imposing these beliefs, either subtly or directly.
10. It is important for counselors to inform their clients about matters such as the goals of counseling, techniques and procedures that will be employed, possible risks associated with

entering the relationship, and any other factors that are likely to affect the client's decision to begin therapy.

11. Counselors must realize that they teach their clients through a modeling process. Thus, they should attempt to practice in their own lives what they encourage in their clients.

12. Counseling takes place in the context of the interaction of cultural backgrounds. Counselors bring their culture to the counseling relationship, and clients' cultural values also operate in the process.

13. Counselors need to learn a process of thinking about and dealing with ethical dilemmas, realizing that most ethical issues are complex and defy simple solutions. The willingness to seek consultation is a sign of professional maturity (Corey, 1996, pp. 79–80).

Ethical codes provide general broad guidelines for ethical conduct. However, each client's situation is unique and does not always fit exactly into the guidelines. The American Counseling Association *Code of Ethics* (2014) states that "when counselors are faced with ethical dilemmas that are difficult to resolve, they are expected to engage in a carefully considered ethical decision-making process" (p. 3). Resolving ethical issues is described in the code as a process which considers professional values, professional ethical principles, and ethical standards. An ethical counselor recognizes an ethical challenge and accepts the responsibility to make an ethical decision and takes the considered action. The counselor then assumes the responsibility for the consequences.

Kitchener and Anderson (2011) have identified an ethical decision-making model (Reasoning about Doing Good Well) which includes steps which highlight a critical evaluative level of moral reasoning. The following steps are identified:

1. Pause and think about your response. Include how your beliefs and values influence your response.

2. Review the available information including the client diagnosis, presenting problem, and contextual information.

3. Identify possible options. Consult with colleagues to generate other possible options.

4. Consult the ethics code. If no single option emerges, continue with your evaluation.

5. Assess the foundational ethical issues. Assess the ethical questions and balance the principles involved in each option. Identify the option which is most justifiable from a moral point of view.

6. Identify legal concerns and agency policy.

7. Reassess options and identify a plan. Have you found an action which balances value over disvalue that respects individual rights?

8. Implement the plan and document the process. This may involve talking to the people involved (pp. 47–49).

Virtue-Based Ethics and Ethical Decision Making

Virtue ethics starts with the assumption that professional ethics involve more than moral actions: they also involve traits of character or virtue (Remley & Herlihy, 2014). This perspective asks you to look at who you are rather than what you do. Principle ethics alone can't account for why some people know the right thing to do but fail to do it. Principle- and rule-bound ethics fail to address questions of moral character (Beauchamp & Childress, 2001; Fowers, 2005). Jorden and Meara (1990) argue that character is critical and you can't teach someone of poor moral character to be ethical. Virtue ethics presumes that counselors and psychologists with good character will be better able to understand the moral dilemmas they face and make good decisions about them. Virtue ethics involves questions about "what a 'good person' would do in real life situations" (Pence, 1991, p. 249).

According to Kitchener and Anderson (2011), the virtues that have been identified as essential to counseling and psychology are as follows:

- *Practical wisdom or prudence.* Prudence refers to the ability to reason well about moral matters and apply that reasoning to real-world problems in a firm but flexible manner (Annas, 1993). Fowers (2005) uses the term *practical wisdom*, which involves the components of moral perception of what is at stake, deliberation about what is possible, and reasoning among choices about what is the best course of action.
- *Integrity.* This is a "firm adherence to a code of, especially, moral or artistic values" (*Webster's Ninth New Collegiate Dictionary*, 1988). To have integrity means we uphold standards even when upholding them might not be popular and may be difficult for other reasons.
- *Respectfulness.* This implies that one considers others' wants or points of view. It involves giving moral recognition to some aspect of a person, such as racial background, gender, or disability, or even the law or social institutions.
- *Trustworthiness.* To trust someone means that we can rely on his/her character, truthfulness, and ability to get things done. We can count on him/her.
- *Care or compassion.* This is defined as a deep concern and empathy for another's welfare and sympathy or uneasiness with another's misfortune or suffering (Beauchamp & Childress, 1994).

A virtue-based approach assumes there are certain ideals toward which one should strive. Virtues are character traits that enable one to be and act in ways that develop one's highest potential (Velasquez, Andre, Shanks, & Meyer, 1996). When practicing virtue-based ethical decision making, one asks the following kinds of questions:

- How can my values best show caring for my client in this situation? (CCPA, 2007).
- What decision would best define me as a person? (CCPA, 2007).
- What emotions and intuitions am I aware of when considering this decision? (CCPA, 2007).
- What course of action develops moral values? (Velasquez, Andre, Shanks, & Meyer, 1996).
- What will develop character in myself and my community? (Velasquez, Andre, Shanks, & Meyer, 1996).
- What course of action honors the trust my client has toward me?

Remley and Herlihy (2014) have reviewed a variety of ethical decision-making models and derived an ethical decision-making process that describes steps that many of the models have in common. The steps proposed are:

- Identify and define the problem. Take time to reflect and gather information. Examine the problem from several perspectives.
- Consider the principles and virtues. How do the moral principles apply? Rank them in the order of their priority in this situation. Consider the virtue ethics and the effect of your actions on your sense of moral self.

- Tune in to your feelings. How do your feelings impact your possible actions?
- Consult with colleagues or experts.
- Involve your client in the decision-making process.
- Identify desired outcomes. Brainstorm to generate new options.
- Consider possible actions. Think about the implications and consequences of each action for all concerned.
- Choose and act on your choice (pp. 15–16).

Pope and Vasquez (2011) have proposed a 17-step ethical decision-making process. There is overlap with the above process. Possible additions which you can consider incorporating are:

- Assess your areas of competence. Are you a good fit for the situation?
- Consider whether personal feeling, bias, or self-interest might affect your judgment.

Self-Tests After Resolving an Ethical Dilemma

After you have progressed through a systematic ethical decision-making process and come to an action plan, several self-tests may be considered.

> The Test of Justice: Ask yourself if you would treat others the same way in this situation (CCPA, 2007).
>
> The Test of Universality: Would you be willing to recommend this course of action to other counselors (CCPA, 2007)?
>
> The Test of Publicity: Would you be willing to have this action headlined in the news (CCPA, 2007)?
>
> The Test of Reversibility: Would you make this same choice if you were in the client's shoes (Remley & Herlihy, 2014)?
>
> The Mentor Test: Consider someone you respect and trust and ask how they might solve the same ethical dilemma (Strom-Gottfried, 2008).
>
> The Moral Traces Test: Are there lingering feelings of doubt or discomfort (Remley & Herlihy, 2014)?

Other sources for your reference are *A Practitioner's Guide to Ethical Decision-Making* (counselors can contact the ACA for a free copy of this document) and *Counselling Ethics: Issues and Cases* (counsellors can contact the CCPA's national office).

The Use of Technology in Counseling

The use of technology in counseling covers a broad range of practices. We are providing you with suggested guidelines regarding (a) the use of telephone and technologies related to telephone use, (b) the use of electronic mail, (c) the practice of technology-assisted distance counseling, (d) the use of social media, and (e) the use of Web-based discussion groups for mental health professionals.

Telephones and technologies related to telephone use (such as answering machines, answering services, cell phones, pagers, and facsimile machines): These are used widely and often not thought of as technology. All professional codes hold the counselor responsible for safeguarding the privacy and confidentiality of the client and client information. Actions taken to safeguard confidentiality when using telephones and related devices include making certain that only the counselor hears or has access to phone messages. Turn off the audio portion of answering machines when not in the office and ensure that access codes to voice mail or answering services are not disclosed to unauthorized persons. Any notes taken from phone messages should be treated as confidential and handled carefully. When contacting the client, check first with the client about how, where, when, if, and with whom they prefer messages to be left. When calling, identify yourself and state the message so that third persons won't hear anything clients would not want them to hear. Text messaging should be avoided because it could be accessed by unauthorized persons. Get a release from the client for fax transmissions, and do not send sensitive personal information by fax.

Electronic mail: The use of electronic mail (e-mail) is becoming a preferred method of communication. Usually there is a time lapse between messages, but it is possible to send and receive messages instantly. Although this may seem secure because a secret password must be used by both parties, it is easy to make errors and send messages to the wrong person or many persons. The main problem with e-mail is that it creates a record that is vulnerable to exposure. If you use e-mail, be extremely cautious about disclosing confidential information and warn clients about risks to confidentiality. Include guidelines for e-mail communications in your written statement to indicate when you check e-mails and the time frame when they will be answered. Be clear that e-mail is to be used only for changing appointments or for notifying about an unexpected cancellation (Remley & Herlihy, 2014, pp. 154–158). Wheeler and Bertram (2008) reported that counselors have had complaints filed "based on an e-mail being sent to the wrong person, voice mail being inappropriately overheard, and computerized records landing in the wrong place" (p. 76).

Technology-assisted distance counseling: Most professional codes of ethics address technology-assisted distance counseling (Web counseling). When providing these services, counselors must provide extensive information to clients prior to initiating counseling regarding risks and benefits, confidentiality, local back-up in an emergency, and access to computer applications. Counselors who use these services must first determine if the client is capable of using these applications and whether this appropriately meets the client's needs (Cormier & Hackney, 2012). Web counseling services can be provided by e-mail only; by e-mail along with chat, telephone, or video services; or by video only. Web counseling presents many potential risks to client confidentiality. The client must be informed of the potential risks. Pope and Vasquez (2011) have identified a series of questions to assess your use of digital media. The questions related to how you safeguard confidentiality are:

- Where is your computer? Who can see it or hear it? Is it secure from unauthorized access or theft?
- Is the computer protected from hackers? From malicious codes? From viruses?
- Is the computer password protected? Is confidential information encrypted?
- How are your confidential files deleted? How are computer disks discarded?
- How do you make sure only the intended recipient receives confidential information?

It is important in Web counseling that the counselor can verify the identity of the client. Examples of verification include the use of code words or phrases. An additional consideration when providing Web counseling is that you must comply with the laws in the state or province in which the client resides. Several states (Maryland, New Mexico, Tennessee, and Virginia) specifically state that they do not support electronic communication under scope of practice for professionals (Kaplan, Wade, Conteh, & Martz, 2011). When practicing Web counseling, be certain to practice according to a set of professional standards for the practice of Web counseling. The

National Board of Certified Counselors has a recently revised *Policy Regarding the Provision of Distance Professional Services* (2012). Guidelines by the International Society of Mental Health Online can be accessed at www.ismho.org.

The American Mental Health Counselors Association (2010) has devoted a specific section of their most recent code of ethics to the practice of technology-assisted counseling. We are reproducing that section here:

American Mental Health Counselors Association *Code of Ethics**

Section 6.
   Technology-Assisted Counseling
   Technology-assisted counseling includes but is not limited to computer, telephone, internet and other communication devices.
   Mental health counselors take reasonable steps to protect patients, clients, students, research participants and others from harm.

Mental health counselors performing technology-assisted counseling comply with all other provisions of this Ethics Code.

Mental health counselors:

   a. Establish methods to ascertain the client's identity and obtain alternative methods of contacting the client in an emergency.
   b. Electronically transfer client information to authorized third party recipients only when both the mental health counselor and the authorized recipient have secure transfer and acceptance capabilities as state and federal laws regulate.
   c. Ensure that clients are intellectually, emotionally and physically capable of using technology-assisted counseling services, and of understanding the potential risks and/or limitations of such services.
   d. Provide technology-assisted services only in practice areas within their expertise. Mental health counselors do not provide services to clients in states where doing so would violate local licensure laws.
   e. Confirm that the provision of counseling services are [sic] not prohibited by or otherwise violate any applicable state or local statutes, rules, regulations or ordinances, codes of professional membership organizations and certifying boards, and/or codes of state licensing boards.

*American Mental Health Counselors Association, 2010, *Code of ethics*, Alexandria, VA: Author, pp. 6–7. Reprinted with permission.

Social media (such as Facebook, LinkedIn, Google, MySpace, Twitter, blogs, texting, instant messaging): Social media are used widely by millennials, and the range of options is increasing rapidly. Professional organizations are struggling to update ethical guidelines for their use. The use of social media in exchanging information with clients has been addressed in the recently published *Policy Regarding the Provision of Distance Professional Services*. Standard 13 states, "NCC's shall avoid the use of public social media (e.g. tweets, blogs, etc.) to provide confidential information. To facilitate the secure provision of information, NCC's shall provide in writing the appropriate ways to contact them." (p. 3). Standard 16 states, "NCC's shall limit use of information obtained through social media sources (e.g., Facebook, LinkedIn, Twitter, etc.) in accordance with established practice procedures provided to the recipient at the initiation of services" (National Board of Certified Counselors, 2012, p. 3). Kaplan et al. (2011) have provided a list of suggestions for the counselor who uses social media in professional interactions. They recommend that you:

- Create separate professional social media accounts and always use these accounts when interacting with clients professionally.
- Reserve your professional name (i.e., Dr. Jane Smith) for social media messages sent through this account.
- Use high-level privacy settings on your personal accounts.
- Be selective about what you post on your private accounts. Avoid potentially embarrassing names, pictures, or statements.
- If you choose to use instant messaging and Twitter with clients, provide them with a written policy about specific hours and anticipated response time to messages.
- Avoid searching for or making unsolicited visits to a client's social media pages.
- Check whether your agency, school, or institution has a policy on social media use and do not violate these rules (p. 6).

When using social media to facilitate the exchange of information, a counselor must clearly define how he/she uses social media in professional interactions. In general, we advise that you do not accept clients as "friends" and that you do not accept current or former friends as clients. Students have been disciplined or dismissed from field sites due to inappropriate or unprofessional content on such internet sites or due to having clients as "friends" on these sites (Cormier & Hackney, 2012).

Web-based professional discussion groups: Counselors often use listservs or Web-based professional discussion groups to exchange ideas about professional practice or as a resource for consultation. Safeguarding client confidentiality remains a priority in these consultations. It is not sufficient to change only a client name when discussing such matters. You must ensure that any client data you share are fully disguised. If this is not possible, you must have a signed release from the client for that purpose (Remley & Herlihy, 2014).

Summary

Knowledge of the ethical issues presented by the authors in this chapter is critical for the establishment and maintenance of the counseling relationship. Knowledge of the ethical codes for counselors and psychologists ensures that the practitioner is well aware of the standards for conducting proper therapeutic activities. It is our hope that students will take the time to become familiar with the codes of their specific professional organizations before meeting with clients at their practicum and internship sites. This will ensure that their counseling practices will comply with the appropriate professional standards. We have, in particular, provided material regarding ethical decision making and the use of technology in counseling as applied areas to which the practicum/internship student must pay thoughtful attention.

Suggested Readings

Davis, T. (1996). *A Practitioners guide to ethical decision-making*. Alexandria, VA: American Counseling Association.

Schulz, W., Sheppard, G., Lehr, R., & Shepard, B. (2006). *Counselling ethics: Issues and cases*. Ottawa, ON: Canadian Counselling and Psychotherapy Association.

References

American Counseling Association (2014). *Code of ethics*. Alexandria, VA: Author.

American Mental Health Counselors Association. (2010). *Code of ethics*. Retrieved from www.amhca.org/assets/content/CodeofEthics1.pdf.

American Psychological Association. (2002). *Ethical principles of psychologists and code of conduct with the 2010 amendments*. Retrieved from www.apa.org/ethics/code/index.aspx.

Annas, J. (1993). *The morality of happiness*. Oxford, England: Oxford University Press.

Beauchamp, T. L., & Childress, J. P. (1994). *Principles of biomedical ethics* (4th ed.). Oxford, England: Oxford University Press.

Beauchamp, T. L., & Childress, J. P. (2001). *Principles of biomedical ethics* (5th ed.). Oxford, England: Oxford University Press.

Canadian Counselling and Psychotherapy Association (CCPA). (2007). *Code of ethics*. Retrieved from www.ccpa-accp.ca/_documents?CodeofEthics_en_new.pdf/.

Canadian Psychological Association. (2002). *Canadian code of ethics for psychologists* (3rd ed.). Ottawa, ON: Author.

Corey, G. (1996). *Theory and practice of counseling and psychotherapy* (5th ed.). Pacific Grove, CA: Brooks/Cole.

Corey, G., Corey, M. S., & Callahan, P. (2011). *Issues and ethics in the helping professions* (8th ed.). Belmont, CA: Brooks/Cole, Cengage.

Cormier, S., & Hackney, H. (2012). *Counseling strategies and interventions* (8th ed.). Upper Saddle River, NJ: Pearson.

Fowers, B. J. (2005). *Virtue and psychology: Pursuing excellence in ordinary practice*. Washington, DC: American Psychological Association.

Gert, B. (2012). The definition of morality. In Edward N. Zalta (ed.), *The Stanford encyclopedia of philosophy*. Retrieved from http://plato.stanford.edu/archives/fall2012/entries/morality-definition/.

Herlihy, B., & Remley, T. P. (1995). Unified ethical standards: A challenge of professionals. *Journal of Counseling and Development, 74*(2), 130–138.

Huber, C. H., & Baruth, L. G. (1987). *Ethical, legal, and professional issues in the practice of marriage and family therapy*. Columbus, OH: Merrill.

Jorden, A. E., & Meara, N. M. (1990). Ethics and the professional practice of psychologists. *Professional Psychology: Research and Practice, 21*, 107–114.

Kaplan, D. M., Wade, M. E., Conteh, J. A., & Martz, E. (2011). Legal and ethical issues surrounding the use of social media in counseling. *Counseling and Human Development, 43*(8), 1–10. Retrieved September 25, 2013, from www.counseling.org/docs/ethics/title.

Kitchener, K. S., & Anderson, S. K. (2011). *Foundations of ethical practice, research, and teaching in psychology and counseling* (2nd ed.). New York: Routledge/Taylor & Francis.

Kitchener, K. S., & Kitchener, R. F. (2008). Social science research ethics: Historical and philosophical issues. In D. M. Mertens & P. E. Ginsberg (Eds.), *Handbook of social science research ethics* (pp. 5–22). Thousand Oaks, CA: Sage.

Meara, N. M., Schmidt, L. D., & Day, J. D. (1996). Principles and virtues: A foundation for ethical decisions, policies, and character. *Counseling Psychologist, 24*(1), 4–77.

National Board of Certified Counselors. (2012). *Policy regarding the provision of distance professional services.* Retrieved from www.nbcc.org/Assets/Ethics/NBCCPolicyRegardingPracticeDistanceCounselingBoard.pdf.

Pence, G. E. (1991). Virtue theory. In P. Singer (Ed.), *A companion to ethics* (pp. 249–258). Oxford, England: Blackwell.

Pope, K. S., & Vasquez, M. J. T. (2011). *Ethics in psychotherapy and counseling: A practical guide* (4th ed.). Hoboken, NJ: Wiley.

Remley, T. P., Jr., & Herlihy, B. (2014). *Ethical, legal, and professional issues in counseling* (4th ed.). Upper Saddle River, NJ: Pearson.

Seligman, L. (2004). *Diagnosis and treatment planning in counseling* (3rd ed.). New York: Springer.

Strom-Gottfried, K. (2008). *The ethics of practice with minors: High stakes, hard choices.* Chicago, IL: Lyceum Books.

Velasquez, M., Andre, C., Shanks, T., S. J. & Meyer, M. J. (1996). Thinking morally: A framework, for moral decision making. *Issues in ethics, 7*(1). Retrieved from www.scu.edu/ethics/practicing/decision/thinking.html.

Webster's Ninth New Collegiate Dictionary. (1988). Springfield, MA: Merriam-Webster.

Welfel, E. R. (2010). *Ethics in counseling and psychotherapy: Standards, research and emerging issues* (4th ed.). Pacific Grove, CA: Brooks/Cole.

Wheeler, A. M., & Bertram, B. (2008). *The counselor and the law* (5th ed.). Alexandria, VA: American Counseling Association.

CHAPTER 9

SELECTED TOPICS ON LEGAL ISSUES IN COUNSELING

The law, as arbitrated through the court system, is society's attempt to ensure predictability, consistency, and fairness. Its purpose is to offer an alternative to private action in settling disputes. Legal issues are an important part of the day-to-day functioning of professional counselors. Almost all areas of counselor practice are affected by the law (Remley & Herlihy, 2014). Areas such as informed consent or disclosure statements; privacy, confidentiality, and privilege; handling of records; statutes regarding harm to self or others and the protection of minors and vulnerable others; and malpractice are all affected by the law. As Swenson (1997) noted, "The question is not whether mental health professionals will interact with laws and legal professionals; it is *how* they will interact both now and in the future" (p. 32). Therefore, it is imperative that mental health professionals understand the legal system. In this chapter we will review information on the law as it relates to mental health professionals. Elements of malpractice; privacy, confidentiality, and privilege; risk management; times when counselors must breach confidentiality; and client record keeping are topics covered.

The Law

The law should be viewed as dynamic, not as static. It is not an entity that rigidly adheres to historically derived rules, but neither does it deny their relevance to current disputes. Legal principles derive from social interactions. At the same time, the law places a great deal of importance on precedence. As enforced through the legal system, the law can be seen as an instrument of concern by the state for the social well-being of the people. Its primary concerns are predictability, stability, and fairness; at the same time, the system must be sensitive to expansion and readaptation. "Laws are the agreed upon rules of a society that set forth the basic principles for living together as a group" (Remley & Herlihy, 2014, p. 4).

Classifications of the Law

Laws are classified as constitutional laws, statutes passed by legislatures, regulations, or case laws. The distinctions between these four classifications are explained in the following descriptions:

- *Constitutional laws* are those found in the US Constitution and in state constitutions.
- *Statutory laws* are those written by legislatures.
- *Statutory laws* may have enabling clauses that permit administrators to write *regulations* to clarify them. Once written, these regulations become laws. An important aspect of statuary

laws is that the laws vary from state to state. Professional counselors have the responsibility to be informed of the state laws that relate to their scope of practice, just as they have the responsibility to be informed about the ethical codes and standards of practice that have been established for their profession.

- Finally, decisions by appeals courts create *case laws* for the people who reside in their jurisdictions. If a legal problem manifests itself and parties differ on how to solve it, they may go to a trial court. The decision made in the trial court is not published and does not become law. However, if lawyers do not believe the trial court (the lower court) interpreted the law correctly, they may bring their case to an appeals court (a higher court). The function of the appeals court is to determine whether the trial court applied the law correctly. The members of the appeals court publish the decision, and the majority decision becomes the law for that jurisdiction. The appeals court is then said to have set a precedent for that jurisdiction. *Case law* is the set of existing rulings which have made new interpretations of law and therefore can be cited as precedent. In the United States, all states (except Louisiana, which has adapted the French legal tradition) follow the English common law tradition. In the common law tradition, courts decide the law applicable to a case by interpreting statutes and applying precedents which record how and why prior cases have been decided.

Types of Laws

Functionally, we can define three types of law: civil law, criminal law, and mental health law (Swenson, 1997), as described in the following:

- *Civil law* is applicable, for the most part, to disputes between or among people. Losing the lawsuit usually means losing money. If a person fails to obey the stipulations made as an analogue to a civil lawsuit, he/she may be subject to a criminal charge called *contempt of court*. An example would be a mother or father who does not pay child support. *Tort law* is a body of rights, obligations, and remedies that is applied by courts in civil proceedings to provide relief to persons who have suffered from the wrongful acts of others (*Free Dictionary*, n.d.). Each state has its own legislation (statuary laws) and accumulated case laws that can serve as the basis for malpractice suits against therapists and counselors (Pope & Vasquez, 2011).
- *Criminal law* is applicable to disputes between the state and people. Losing defendants often face a loss of liberty. The standard of proof is higher in a criminal case than in a civil case. Each state has its own set of criminal laws, usually set forth in the penal code.
- *Mental health law* regulates how the state may act regarding people with mental illnesses. These laws enact a permission from the state to protect people from serious harm to themselves or others. They allow the state to act as a guardian for those with mental disorders and to institutionalize them if necessary. Most experts believe mental health law is part of civil law.

The Steps in a Lawsuit

Laws are enacted to settle disputes that occur in society. They arise out of social interactions as members of society develop values that are necessary to the maintenance of order and justice. They come into being based on the common thoughts and experiences of people. They are antecedents to judgments regarding right and wrong. The person who claims to have been wronged is called the *plaintiff;* the person accused of committing the wrong is the *defendant.* The dispute is known as *a lawsuit.*

A lawsuit proceeds through standard steps. Each step has serious legal consequences and rules that must be followed. It is important to remember that most lawsuits do not go to trial; instead, they are settled at an earlier stage.

First, the plaintiff files a complaint through a lawyer with a court in the appropriate jurisdiction. *Jurisdiction* is determined by geographical and substantive factors. Filing this complaint initiates the legal proceeding.

Once the complaint is filed, the plaintiff must make a judicial effort to inform the defendant of his/her intentions (legal notice). This proceeding is called *due process.* The reason for this procedure is to allow the defendant to rebut the accusation.

Once valid due process is accomplished, a *discovery process* is in order. At this point the lawyers involved investigate the facts of the case.

To obtain the facts, the lawyers may use a *subpoena.* The subpoena demands access to the facts and to the presence of witnesses at court hearings. On the basis of this information, the two sides may settle the dispute, or they may proceed to litigation.

If the attorneys and clients decide to proceed with the lawsuit, the next step is to have *pretrial hearings.* At this step the judge determines how the laws apply to the facts. The lawsuit may be settled at this point. "The general policy of most courts is to promote settlements and, in fact, disputants settle about 90% of all cases" (Swenson, 1997, p. 46).

In the *trial phase,* each side presents evidence and attempts to discredit the evidence of the opponent.

Ultimately, the lawsuit is decided by a judge or jury. If either party is dissatisfied with the verdict, he/she may claim that the law was not correctly applied and appeal to a higher court (Swenson, 1997).

Elements of Malpractice

As a legal term, *malpractice* describes complaints in which a professional is accused of negligence within a special relationship. The law of malpractice refers to torts. A *tort* is a wrongful act, injury, or damage (not including a breach of contract) for which a civil action can be brought. Malpractice involves professional misconduct and has been defined as

> Failure of one rendering professional services to exercise that degree of skill and learning commonly applied under all circumstances in the community by the average prudent reputable member of the profession with the result of injury, loss or damage to the recipient of those services or to those entitled to rely on them. (Black, 2004, p. 959)

The role of incompetency must be established in a malpractice lawsuit. It is not easy to prove that the counselor did not follow established practices. Although malpractice lawsuits have increased over the last decade, the total number of lawsuits is relatively small. Clients come to counseling with a reasonable expectation that the counselor has a legal obligation not to harm them. If clients believe they have been harmed by their counselor, they can file a malpractice lawsuit. The counselor is then obligated to defend himself/herself against the lawsuit before a judge or jury (Remley & Herlihy, 2014).

Prosser, Wade, Schwartz, Kelly, and Partlett (2005) identified the following elements that must be proven in order for the plaintiff to win a tort or malpractice claim:

- The counselor had a duty to the client to use reasonable care in providing counseling services.
- The counselor failed to conform to the required duty of care.
- The client was injured.
- There was a reasonably close causal connection between the conduct of the counselor and the resulting injury.
- The client suffered an actual loss or was damaged.

Why Clients Sue

We live in a litigious society. Mental health professionals do therapy with clients who are emotionally distraught. Good relationships with clients reduce the likelihood of lawsuits. Counselors should thus use their skills to create positive feelings between themselves and the clients they serve. People do not want to sue someone they like or someone who is acting in their best interests.

Counselors are sued most often for sexual misconduct with clients. Counselor incompetence is the second most reported area of ethical complaints (after dual relationships with clients), according to one survey of state licensure boards (Neukrug, Milliken, & Walden, 2001). Many lawsuits brought by clients alleging that they were harmed as clients focus on competence. The next reason revolves around situations where clients attempt or complete suicide (Remley & Herlihy, 2014). Because blaming and anger are nearly universal reactions by family survivors, the mental health professional is particularly vulnerable. Other reasons for lawsuits include inappropriate dual relationships, ineffective treatment, improper diagnosis, custody disputes, and breach of confidentiality (Pope & Vasquez, 2011).

Other reasons to sue involve the breaking of a contract and libel or slander. Breaking a contract is essentially the same as breaking a promise. The counselor's spoken and written word is another aspect of a duty to use reasonable care in providing counseling services. If the breach in spoken or written word causes damage or injury, the law may provide a monetary remedy. A client who is angry does not have to show negligence on the part of the mental health professional, only that the therapy did not achieve the purpose it was intended to achieve (Schwitzgebel & Schwitzgebel, 1980). Damages typically involve at least the cost of the therapy.

Injury to a person's reputation may occur when derogatory words or written statements are made to a third party about the person. Such injurious statements are called *defamation* of character; *slander* is spoken defamation, and *libel* is written defamation. In a recent unpublished case, a trade school counselor made a public remark to the effect that a student had missed classes because she had a venereal disease contracted while working as a prostitute. In fact, the disease was the result of a rape. Because of stress related to gossip, the girl quit school, went into therapy, and sued the school district. The school settled the case, paying $50,000 in damages for the injury. The school also fired the counselor (Swenson, 1997).

Mental health professionals should be extremely careful about information given in letters of recommendation, notes on educational records, or any other oral comments to students. Communication of an opinion, when it can be said to imply a false and damaging statement, could be judged as slanderous or libelous (*Milkovich v. Loraine Journal Inc.*, 1990).

Risk Management and the Counselor

Counseling, like many other professions, has some inherent risk of liability. Recognizing liability can be an asset that enables the counselor to examine carefully the level of risk in his/her decision-making processes in therapy. Risk management is an action practitioners can take that will reduce the risk of liability in the form of a lawsuit for malpractice and disciplinary action before the review board of an institution or an ethics challenge before a state licensing board or professional organization. According to Hackney (2000, pp. 133–136), a number of counselor actions can be helpful in minimizing liability risks. Hackney grouped these actions according to the following themes, and we have added other references as appropriate:

1. Competence: This is awareness on the part of the counselor of the limits of his/her training and not practicing outside the boundaries of his/her competence (Corey, Williams, & Moline, 1995). That is, taking on a client whose treatment and needs are beyond the counselor's skill level is both unethical and a major liability risk.
2. Communication and attention: Communicating and paying attention to the therapeutic relationship with clients help the counselor to minimize the risk of mistakes and misunderstanding in the counseling process. Particularly important is the ongoing process of informed consent, which helps with the avoidance of client misunderstandings about therapy and with clients who have unrealistic expectations for treatment or who may be generally dissatisfied with the counseling received. The counselor must remain open to discussing these issues openly and honestly throughout the therapy process.
3. Supervision and consultation: Feedback from colleagues, supervisors, and consultants is invaluable in gaining insight into clinical problems of a legal or ethical nature. Establishing relationships with other mental health professionals before the need to consult arises is an important consideration. Active involvement in professional organizations can also be an excellent source of information on legal and ethical matters. According to Knapp and VandeCreek (2006), the very best step a counselor can take when faced with a difficult ethical decision or a legal question is to consult.
4. Record keeping: Record keeping is an axiom of practitioners of risk management; that is, if it isn't written down, it didn't occur. In an action against a mental health practitioner, accurate, contemporaneous records enhance the practitioner's testimony in a deposition or at trial (Woody, 2013). The pitfalls of overdocumentation and underdocumentation should be understood by the counselor. Overdocumentation includes irrelevant or sensitive material or observations that are disparaging of the client or others. Underdocumentation is the failure to document phone calls, significant events, decisions, and disclosures for informed consent and failure to obtain and review prior records. Documenting decisions or actions in your clinical case notes protects you in the case that such decisions or actions are questioned later by anyone else (Mitchell, 2007).
5. Insurance: It goes without saying that obtaining liability insurance is an absolute practice essential. Counselors also need to understand their insurance policies, especially regarding exclusions, limits of liability, requirements to report claims, or circumstances that may give rise to a claim.
6. Knowledge of ethics and relevant laws: Familiarity with ethical and legal guidelines aids in the avoidance of liability claims and problems. The websites of the American Counseling Association (ACA), American Psychological Association (APA), Canadian Counselling

and Psychotherapy Association (CCPA), and Canadian Psychological Association (CPA) frequently contain information about ethics, the law, and ethical decision making.

7. Practitioner self-care: The stress and tension generated by situations that present a potential for counselor liability necessitate that counselors address their own health and emotional well-being, which can help to ensure that they can maintain perspective and balance (Hackney, 2000).

Liability Insurance

All mental health professionals should purchase liability insurance before they begin practice. An occurrence-based policy covers incidents no matter when the claim is made, as long as the policy was in force during the year of the alleged incident. Thus, if a therapist is accused today of an infraction alleged to have occurred 2 years ago (when the policy was in effect), he/she is covered, even if the policy is not in force at present. A claims-made policy covers only claims made while the policy is in force. However, if a counselor previously had a claims-made policy, he/she may purchase tail-coverage insurance, which covers him/her if an alleged incident occurring during the period the policy was in effect is reported after the policy has expired.

Privacy, Confidentiality, and Privileged Communication

The client entering the counseling relationship has the expectation that thoughts, feelings, and information shared with the counselor will not be disclosed to others. The nondisclosure in the counseling relationship can be viewed from the vantage point of three separate concepts: privacy, confidentiality, and privilege. These three concepts are interrelated and are sometimes used interchangeably.

Privacy: Privacy is the broad concept that refers to the societal belief that individuals have a right to privacy. Although this right is not specifically stated in the US Constitution, it is derived from interpretations of the Fourth Amendment in the Bill of Rights. Individuals have the right to decide what information about them will be shared with or withheld from others (Remley & Herlihy, 2014). Privacy, when used in the context of counseling, is the "freedom or right of clients to choose the time, circumstances and information others may know about them" (Corey et al., 1995, p. 163).

Confidentiality: Confidentiality applies to the relationship between counselors and clients. Confidentiality is an ethical responsibility and affirmative legal duty on the part of the counselor not to disclose client information without the client's prior consent. According to Welfel (2010), "confidentiality refers to an ethical duty to keep client identity and disclosures secret" (p. 116). The counselor's confidentiality pledge is the cornerstone of the trust that clients need in order to openly tell their stories and share their feelings. Any limitations to this promise of confidentiality must be identified at the outset before counseling begins. Remley and Herlihy (2014) provide a list of exceptions to confidentiality and privileged communication:

- when sharing information with subordinates or fellow professionals, when consulting with experts, when working under supervision, when coordinating client care, when using clerical assistance;
- when protecting someone who is in danger, when suspecting abuse or neglect of children or others with limited ability for self-care, when client poses a danger to others, when the client

is suicidal, when the client has a fatal communicable disease and the client's behavior puts others at risk;

- when counseling multiple clients such as group counseling or couples and family counseling;
- when counseling minors; and
- when mandated by law.

Privilege: Privilege is a common law and statutory concept that protects confidential communication made within certain special relationships from disclosure in legal proceedings (Hackney, 2000). Privilege applies to the relationship between counselors and clients. Wigmore (1961) identified the requirements for a relationship to be privileged under the law.

1. The communication originates in a confidence that it will not be disclosed.
2. The element of confidentiality is essential to the relationship between the parties.
3. The relationship is one that, in the opinion of the community, ought to be fostered.
4. The injury to the relationship that would occur with disclosure of communication would be greater than the benefit gained for the correct disposal of the litigation.

Privileged communication is a legal concept. Privileged communication laws protect clients from having their confidential communication disclosed in a court of law without their consent (Shuman & Weiner, 1982). Privileged communication is conferred by enacting a statute that grants privilege to a category of professionals and to those they serve. When a competent client presents for therapy, any disclosure he/she makes may be protected from legal disclosure. Such communication is considered privileged. The issue at hand is the conflict between the individual's right to privacy and the need of the public to know certain information. The client is considered the holder of the privilege, and he/she is the only one who can waive that right. Privileged communication is established by statutory law enacted by legislators. Client communication with a specified group of mental health professionals may be privileged in some states but not in others. Also, statutes may specify a wide range of exceptions to privileged communication. For instance, privileged communication laws are abrogated, in all states, by an initial report of child abuse.

Privileged communication is not absolute, and a wide range of exceptions to privilege exist (Glosoff, Herlihy, & Spence, 2000). In their research, these authors studied the statutory codes in all 50 states and the District of Columbia and determined that exceptions to these concepts are numerous and varied across jurisdictions. However, they concluded that several categories of exceptions were found in 15% of the jurisdictions (see Glosoff et al., 2000), for a state-by-state listing). In addition, it is important to note that statutes and rules regulating privileged communication and its exceptions must be interpreted with caution because in some codes the rules are not readily apparent and existing statutes are continually modified. With these facts in mind, Glosoff et al. (2000) found the following nine categories of exceptions:

1. *When there is a dispute between client and counselor:* This is the most frequent exception, found in 30 jurisdictions wherein clients filed complaints either in court or with licensing boards. In 30 jurisdictions, clients can be considered to have waived their privilege when they bring complaints of malpractice against their counselor(s).
2. *When the client raises the issue of mental condition in a court proceeding:* This was found in 21 jurisdictions, with two primary circumstances: (a) the individual raises the insanity

defense in response to a criminal charge, and (b) the individual claims in court that he/she has been emotionally damaged and the damage required him/her to seek mental health treatment.

3. *When the client's condition poses a danger to self or others:* This was found in 20 jurisdictions. Counselors who work with clients who pose a danger to self or others cannot rely solely on knowledge of statutory law. Case law may affect the status of their duty to warn and the requirement to breach confidentiality.

4. *Child abuse or neglect:* This was found in 20 jurisdictions. All states and US jurisdictions have mandatory child abuse and neglect reporting statutes of some type. Counselors must know the exact language of the statutes in their state because the laws vary significantly.

5. *Knowledge that a client is contemplating commission of a crime:* 17 jurisdictions waive privilege when the counselor knows that the client is contemplating the commission of a crime.

6. *Court-ordered examinations:* This was found in 15 jurisdictions. Communication made during ordered examinations is specifically exempted from privilege.

7. *Involuntary hospitalization:* 13 jurisdictions waive privilege when counselors participate in seeking the commitment of a client to a hospital.

8. *Knowledge that a client has been a victim of a crime:* 8 states waive privilege.

9. *Harm to vulnerable adults:* 8 jurisdictions waive privilege when the counselor suspects abuse or neglect of older people, adults with disabilities, residents of institutions, or other adults who are presumed to have limited ability to protect themselves (Glosoff et al., 2000, pp. 454–462).

It is crucial that you have knowledge of your state statutes to protect yourself and your client from breaches of privilege and confidentiality.

Release of Information

The essence of a counseling relationship is trust. Mental health professionals must protect the information they receive from clients. They must keep confidential communications secret unless a well-defined exception applies. Confidential information may be disclosed if the client (or the client's parent or legal representative) agrees and signs a consent form for such a disclosure. A consent to a waiver does not always have to be in writing, but it is best if it is. The client should be informed of any and all implications of the waiver.

When the Counselor Must Breach Confidentiality

As stated in the previous section on confidentiality, there are circumstances when a counselor is required, by law, to breach confidentiality. We have included the following information concerning the most frequently encountered circumstances when the counselor must make this difficult decision.

The Law and the Duty to Protect: The Suicidal Client

Counselors have an ethical duty to protect clients from harm to self. You must be prepared to take measures to prevent suicide attempts. Prevention measures begin with a risk assessment, and then, based on the level of danger, one must take action by involving a family member or significant other, by working with the client to arrange for voluntary hospitalization, or by initiating a process of involuntary commitment (Remley & Herlihy, 2014). Any of these actions involve a waiver of confidentiality and result in life disruption to the client. Counselors can be accused of malpractice for neglecting to take action to prevent harm, and they can be accused of malpractice for taking actions when there is no basis for doing so (Remley, Hermann, & Huey, 2003). The law requires the counselor to make risk assessments from an informed position and to take action in a manner comparable to what other reasonable counselors operating in a similar situation would do (Sommers-Flanagan, Sommers-Flanagan, & Lynch, 2001). The practicum/internship student should review again the literature regarding suicide risk assessment. We have included a section on harm to self in Chapter 10 of this text for your review and reference. Most practicum/internship sites already have in place guidelines for how to manage potentially suicidal clients. Speak with your field site supervisor to become informed of guidelines at your site, and follow them in consultation with your supervisor. No matter where you work as a counselor, you are likely to come into contact with individuals who might express suicidal thoughts. In situations where you must assess the potential risk of suicide, it is important that you document carefully. Counselors must know how to assess the risk for suicide, and they must be able to defend their decision at a later time. Remley and Herlihy (2014) have identified essential items to include in your documentation notes:

- what caused your concern (a referral from another person or something the client said);
- what you asked the client and his/her response;
- who you consulted, what you said, and how they responded; and
- what interactions you had with any other person regarding the situation, from when you became concerned until you completed your work regarding the situation.

The Law and the Duty to Warn: The Potentially Dangerous Client

Counselors are sometimes presented with a situation where they must decide whether a client has the potential to harm another person. If you determine that there is foreseeable danger that a client may harm someone or someone's property, then you must take the necessary action to prevent harm (Hermann & Finn, 2002). Ethical guidelines state that confidentiality doesn't apply when you must protect clients or identified others from serious and foreseeable harm (ACA, 2014). However, predicting with certainty whether a person is going to harm someone else is not possible. The burden of deciding whether to breach confidentiality places the counselor in a complicated situation which requires informed assessment practices and documented consultation with other mental health professionals. You have both a legal requirement and an ethical duty to assess the potential danger and to take action when you decide that violence is imminent. Is the client just venting out of anger and frustration, or is he/she likely to act out in violence? Once you assess that a client is dangerous and might harm someone, the law requires that you take action to prevent harm and that the steps you take are the least disruptive ones possible (Rice, 1993). In addition to the requirement to take steps to prevent harm, in most states you are also required to warn an identifiable or foreseeable victim of a dangerous client. This duty to warn arose out of the *Tarasoff* court case in California where the precedent was established that the therapist (in cases where serious danger to another was determined) "incurred an obligation to use reasonable care to protect the foreseeable victim from such danger" (McClarren, 1987, p. 273). Decisions after the *Tarasoff* case throughout the United States have interpreted the holding of the case in a variety of different ways. The only state that has rejected the *Tarasoff* duty to warn is Texas (Remley & Herlihy, 2014).

When taking action to prevent harm, the counselor has a range of choices from the least to the most intrusive. The least intrusive action would be to have the client promise not to harm anyone. Other actions would be to notify family members to have them take responsibility to keep the client under control; persuade the client to voluntarily commit to residential care; call the police; or call the client periodically (Remley & Herlihy, 2014). In addition, you would need to decide whether to warn intended victims, the police, or both. The steps identified for assessment, consultation, and documentation in managing potentially suicidal clients would also be appropriate to managing the potentially dangerous client. We have included a section on the potentially dangerous client in Chapter 10, where we review guidelines for assessing danger to others.

Mandatory Reporting: Suspected Child Abuse and Neglect

All states and US jurisdictions now have mandatory reporting statutes of some type regarding child abuse and neglect. The statutes require that these situations be reported to the appropriate governmental agency. In cases of child neglect, the statutes conclude that absolute confidentiality in counseling must be broken out of the need to protect children. The statutes vary in their wording from state to state, so it is necessary for counselors to check the exact language in the statute that requires them to make reports. The United States Department of Health and Human Services (n.d.) provides information regarding mandatory child abuse reporting statutes for each state and US jurisdictions (www.childwelfare.gov/systemwide/laws_policies/state). The laws have clauses that protect counselors who make reports in "good faith" so they can be protected from lawsuits by people who have been reported.

As in other situations where confidentiality is breached, counselors must exercise their professional judgment with several goals in mind. These include

a. maintaining, if possible, any counseling relationship with those involved;
b. expressing concern about the alleged victim before and after a report is made;
c. helping those involved deal with the process that follows the report; and
d. fulfilling their legal obligations (Remley & Herlihy, 2014, p. 237).

Although reporting suspected abuse is a legal requirement, counselors must use their clinical judgment when they suspect that abuse is occurring. Perhaps the counselor has observed marks on the child, has observed behavior that indicates abuse, or has noticed something the child has said in the counseling session. Counselors must also consider the credibility of the alleged victim, the prevailing standards for discipline in the community, and information that is known about the alleged victim and the alleged perpetrator. Consult immediately with your supervisor when you have a suspicion that abuse is occurring. We have included a section in Chapter 10 that provides information about the definitions of abuse and guidelines for recognizing signs of child physical abuse, neglect, sexual abuse, and emotional maltreatment. Before a report is filed, consult with your supervisor and colleagues and inform the appropriate administrator. Follow any procedures that are in place at the field site. Anytime a report is made, document the date and time that an oral report is made, the name of the person who took the report, and a written summary of what was said when the report was made.

Mandatory Reporting: Suspected Harm to Vulnerable Adults

Counselors have both an ethical and a legal duty to intervene when they suspect that a vulnerable adult is being harmed in some way. They have a duty to intervene to prevent the harm from continuing and to promote client welfare. Adults who might be considered vulnerable include developmentally disabled, severely mentally ill, elderly, and physically disabled persons. The elderly are the largest group of adults who are vulnerable to neglect and abuse. Types of elder abuse include physical abuse, sexual abuse, emotional abuse, financial exploitation, neglect, abandonment, and self-neglect (National Center on Elder Abuse, 2005). Neglect can be self-inflicted when elderly patients fail to take medication, skip meals, use alcohol to self-medicate for depression, and fail to maintain personal hygiene. Many states now have laws requiring reports of suspected abuse or neglect of vulnerable adults. All states have some form of legislation aimed at reducing elder maltreatment. In some ways these statutes are similar to those regarding child abuse. However, not every state mandates that professionals report suspected abuse to authorities. Elder abuse reporting statutes usually allow older adults to refuse protective services if they don't want them (Welfel, Danzinger, & Santoro, 2000). Stetson University School of Law Center for Excellence in Elder Law (2014) provides information about specific laws regarding mandatory reporting of older and vulnerable adult abuse.

If, after careful analysis, you believe you must make a report, you must try to do this in a way that will not damage the counseling relationship. Consult your supervisor. Welfel et al. (2000) recommend that you involve the client in the reporting process, report only essential information to protect confidentiality to the extent possible, and follow up to make sure that needed services are being provided.

The Law and the Practice of Counsellor–Client Confidentiality in Canada

Canadian students are referred to an article by Bryce and Mahaffy (2007). Topics covered include confidentiality, times when a counsellor must breach confidentiality, counsellor–client privilege, and Canada's private sector privacy legislation.

Managed Care and the Counselor

Managed mental health care rules and regulations have a significant impact on how counselors provide counseling services and often determine whether the services provided are reimbursable. Considerable debate has arisen over the effectiveness of mental health care. Managed care means that people are not given all the health care services that people want or that their providers want for them. Instead, health plan members are given the services that the health care plan company has determined are appropriate and necessary. The idea of managed care was that this would lead to lower costs to the company for health care by managing the care provided. However, as costs in health care have increased, so have the number of restrictions placed by insurers on reimbursement for mental health services (Cooper & Gottlieb, 2004). Most managed care companies require that mental health professional assign a diagnosis from the *Diagnostic and Statistical Manual of Mental Disorders (DSM)* in order to qualify for reimbursement for services. The *DSM* contains a variety of diagnostic codes that are not reimbursable. Most companies limit in some way the diagnoses for which they will pay benefits. Some companies will not reimburse for V-code conditions, typical developmental transitions, adjustment disorders, or family or couples counseling

(Remley & Herlihy, 2014). As a result, counselors struggle to meet the mental health needs of clients while at the same time recognizing the demands of managed care. The denial of services based on the *DSM* codes is widespread. As a result of these rules and regulations, many counselors are tempted to, and in some cases do, misdiagnose to get reimbursement. Their misguided efforts are an attempt to provide services for those clients who, without insurance reimbursement, would otherwise terminate therapy and, unfortunately, in some cases, to enhance the number of clients seen in therapy. Braun and Cox (2005), in an article titled "Managed Mental Healthcare: Intentional Misdiagnosis of Mental Disorders," discussed the ethics and legal status of the consequences of intentional misdiagnosis of mental disorders. These authors suggested that many counselors believe that it is in the client's best interest when they agree to intentionally misdiagnose mental status to receive reimbursement. They further stated that by intentionally misdiagnosing clients' mental statuses, they abuse their position of power and break client trust because intentional misdiagnosis involves deceptive behavior. A review of the ACA, American Mental Health Counselors Association (AMHCA), and APA codes of ethics points to the fact that misdiagnosis is a violation of moral and legal standards and may also violate state and federal statutes. The misdiagnosis of a client's mental status for reimbursement is an ethical violation as well as a violation of legal statutes. Intentional misdiagnosis of mental disorders for reimbursement is considered health care fraud (Infanti, 2000). The provisions of the 1986 False Claims Act, embodied in the US Code 31, chapter 37, subsection III, allow the government to investigate individuals (i.e., counselors) with the requisite knowledge who (a) submit false claims, (b) "cause" such claims to be submitted, (c) make or use false statements to get false claims paid (i.e., intentional misdiagnosing of mental disorders), or (d) "cause" false statements to be made or used (Slade, 2000, cited in Braun & Cox, 2005, p. 430). Remember: The dilemma of attempting to counsel a client who otherwise could not afford treatment without reimbursement simply does not justify insurance fraud and the violation of professional ethics. DON'T BE TEMPTED.

In addition to the problem of misdiagnosis, a variety of other significant issues need the counselor's thoughtful consideration when confronted with legal and moral issues. Braun and Cox (2005) suggested that counselors grapple with ethical and legal challenges involving the following:

1. *Informed consent:* Clients in the world of managed care may not know and understand their mental health benefits.
2. *Confidentiality:* Clients may be unaware that counselors can no longer ensure privacy of disclosure because managed care organizations may require client information for determining treatment and insurance reimbursement (Cooper & Gottlieb, 2000; Danzinger & Welfel, 2001).
3. *Client autonomy:* Under managed care, providers and types of treatment are oftentimes determined by policies and utilization reviews (Weinburgh, 1998).
4. *Competence:* Managed care organizations emphasize brief therapy models. When counselors have not received adequate training in brief therapy techniques and interventions, they may not be able to effectively provide services when a managed care organization limits counseling to only five sessions (Cooper & Gottlieb, 2000).
5. *Treatment plans:* The first task of mental health psychotherapy is to accommodate the treatment parameters of the benefit package.
6. *Termination:* The termination of counseling services may be imposed by managed care limitations (Cooper & Gottlieb, 2000).

As noted above, managed care often limits treatment options and the number of sessions allowed. Counselors must discuss this with clients in the beginning session as part of informed consent (Daniels, 2001). Counselors must also let clients know what information the managed care company requires the counselor to disclose and any implications of the diagnosis assigned. A particularly troublesome aspect of limiting the number of sessions is the issue of abandonment. Counselors have ethical obligations not to abandon or neglect clients, and to assist in helping clients make appropriate arrangements to continue treatment when necessary (ACA, 2014, Standard A.12). Remley and Herlihy (2014) recommend several actions to protect counselors from legal liability:

- If needed services are denied, request additional services on behalf of the client. If the request is denied, file a written complaint.
- Instruct the client regarding the right to appeal to receive additional services.
- If patient is in crisis and can't afford to pay you, continue services until care can be transferred to another facility that can provide care.

Client Records

Naturally, mental health professionals should keep records for each client. Records provide an excellent inventory of information for assisting the mental health professional in managing client cases. They also serve as documentation of a therapist's judgments, type of treatment, recommendations, and treatment outcomes. Therapists must also keep financial records. Financial records are necessary to obtain third-party reimbursement for the counselor or the client. The content of records may be defined by agency policy, state licensing laws, statutory laws, or regulation laws. Records may be read in open court; as a result, derogatory comments about clients should never be included.

In most jurisdictions, the paper belongs to the agency, but the information on the paper belongs to the client. Clients can request copies of their records. Some jurisdictions limit access to records if such access is considered to be harmful to a client's mental health.

The evolving standard of practice is to keep records for 7 years, although some suggest they should be kept forever. The appropriate regulatory agencies in one's jurisdiction should be consulted regarding record retention and disposition. The following lists some types of information that should be kept in client records:

1. basic identifying information, such as the client's name, address, and telephone number; also, if the client is a minor, the names of parents or legal guardians;
2. signed informed consent for treatment;
3. history of the client, both medical and psychiatric, if relevant;
4. dates and types of services offered;
5. signature and title of the person who rendered the therapy;
6. a description of the presenting problem;
7. a description of assessment techniques and results;
8. progress notes for each date of service documenting the implementation of the treatment plan and changes in the treatment plan;
9. documentation of sensitive or dangerous issues, alternatives considered, and actions taken;
10. a treatment plan with explicit goals;

11. consultations with other professionals, consultations with people in the client's life, clinical supervision received, and peer consultation;
12. release of confidential information forms signed by the client; and
13. fees assessed and collected.

The keeping of clinical case notes is the record of most concern for clients because these notes often contain specific details the clients have disclosed about their concerns, as well as the counselor's clinical impressions. This is very sensitive and personal information about clients. Counselors must be aware of how often these notes are reviewed by clients, agencies, and the law. Counselors never know whether others will read their clinical notes. Therefore, counselors must assume that notes they write will become public information at some later time. There are two basic reasons to keep clinical case notes: to provide quality counseling services to clients and to document decisions you make regarding your actions as a counselor (Remley & Herlihy, 2014). The important decisions to document are when you take action to prevent harm (when you assess that a client is a danger to self or others), when you consult with other professionals regarding a client's situation, or when you make decisions a client may not like. If you decide to terminate counseling over a client's objection, advise a client to take some action he/she is reluctant to take, or limit a client's interactions with you outside of sessions, it is wise to document how and why you did this and the client's reactions. When you document such actions or decisions in case notes, you are doing this to protect yourself in case such decisions are later questioned by anyone else (Mitchell, 2007). Some situations where clear documentation is called for are if someone accuses the counselor of unethical or illegal behavior, a counselor reports suspected child abuse or determines a client is a danger to self or others, or a client who is being counseled is involved in legal proceedings. Questions about counselor action or inaction could be reviewed by an ethics panel, licensure board, or administrator, or within a legal proceeding.

Summary

The legal issues addressed in this chapter were aimed at the major considerations necessary to ensure that counselors are able to protect both themselves and their clients from legal liability. It is important that all counselors and therapists have a complete understanding of the meaning of privacy, confidentiality, and privileged communication and the rights and responsibilities of helping professionals in legal situations. In addition, mental health professionals should be familiar with the steps in a lawsuit, the issue of negligence, and the elements of malpractice in an effort to avoid the liability that results from such claims. Important considerations that relate to the legal obligation to breach confidentiality in cases of harm to self or others, or suspected abuse of children and/or vulnerable adults, were detailed. Before beginning the practicum and internship experience, students will want to again familiarize themselves with the critical issues reviewed in this chapter.

References

American Counseling Association (2014). *Code of ethics.* Alexandria, VA: Author.
Black, H. C. (2004). *Black's law dictionary* (8th ed.). St. Paul, MN: West.
Braun, S., & Cox, J. (2005). Managed mental healthcare: Intentional misdiagnosis of mental disorders. *Journal of Counseling and Development, 83,* 425–443.

Bryce, G. K., & A. Mahaffy. (2007). *How private is private: A review of the law and practice of counsellor-client confidentiality in Canada and its exceptions.* Paper presented at Connecting With Our Clients: Counseling in the 21st Century, the Canadian Counselling Association National Conference, Vancouver, BC. Retrieved from www.acadiau.ca/~rlehr/How20%Private20%is20%Private_pdf.

Cooper, C. C., & Gottlieb, M. C. (2000). Ethical issues with managed care: Challenges facing counseling psychology. *Counseling Psychologist, 28,* 179–236.

Corey, G., Williams, G. T., & Moline, M. E. (1995). Ethical and legal issues in group counseling. *Ethics and Behavior, 5*(2), 161–183.

Daniels, J. A. (2001). Managed care, ethics and counseling. *Journal of Counseling and Development, 79,* 119–122.

Danzinger, P. R., & Welfel, E. R. (2001). The impact of managed care on mental health counselors: A survey of perceptions, practices, and compliance with ethical standards. *Journal of Mental Health Counseling, 23,* 137–151.

Free Dictionary. (n.d.). Retrieved December 28, 2013, from http://legal-dictionary.thefreedictionary.com/Tort+law.

Glosoff, H. L., Herlihy, B., & Spence, E. B. (2000). Privileged communication and the counselor–client relationship. *Journal of Counseling and Development, 78*(4), 450–462.

Hackney, H. (2000). *Practice issues for beginning counselors.* Boston: Allyn & Bacon.

Hermann, M. A., & Finn, A. (2002). An ethical and legal perspective on the role of counselors in preventing violence in schools. *Professional School Counseling, 6,* 46–54.

Infanti, M. C. (2000). Malpractice may not be your biggest risk. *RN, 63*(7), 67–71.

Knapp, S., & VandeCreek, L. (2006). The ethics of advertising, billing and finances in psychotherapy. *Journal of Clinical Psychology: In Session, 64,* 613–625.

McClarren, G. M. (1987). The psychiatric duty to warn: Walking a tightrope of uncertainty. *University of Cincinnati Law Review, 56,* 269–293.

Milkovich v. Loraine Journal Inc., 497 US 1 (1990).

Mitchell, R. W. (2007). *Documentation in counseling records: An overview of ethical, legal, and clinical issues* (3rd ed.). Alexandria, VA: American Counseling Association.

National Center on Elder Abuse. (2005). *Fact sheet: Elder abuse prevalence and incidence.* Retrieved December 28, 2013, from www.ncea.aoa.gov/Resources/Publication/docs/FinalStatistics050331.pdf.

Neukrug, E., Milliken, T., & Walden, S. (2001). Ethical complaints made against credentialed counselors: An updated survey of state licensing boards. *Counselor Education and Supervision, 41,* 57–70.

Pope, K. S., & Vasquez, M. J. T. (2011). *Ethics in psychotherapy and counseling* (4th ed.). Hoboken, NJ: Wiley.

Prosser, W. I., Wade, J. W., Schwartz, V. E., Kelly, K., & Partlett, D. F. (2005). *Cases and materials on torts* (11th ed.). Westbury, NY: Foundation Press.

Remley, T. P., Jr., & Herlihy, B. (2014). *Ethical, legal, and professional issues in counseling* (4th ed.). Upper Saddle River, NJ: Pearson.

Remley, T. P., Jr., Hermann, M. A., & Huey, W. C. (Eds.). (2003). *Ethical and legal issues in school counseling* (2nd ed.). Alexandria, VA: American School Counselors Association.

Rice, P. R. (1993). *Attorney-client privilege in the United States.* Rochester, NY: Lawyers Cooperative.

Schwitzgebel, R. L., & Schwitzgebel, R. K. (1980). *Law and psychological practice.* New York: Wiley.

Shuman, D. W., & Weiner, M. F. (1982). *The psychotherapist-patient privilege: A critical examination.* Springfield, IL: Charles C. Thomas.

Slade, S. R. (2000). Health care fraud: How far does the Fake Claims Act reach? Quackwatch. Retrieved from www.Quackwatch.org/02consumerprotection/fac.html.

Sommers-Flanagan, R., Sommers-Flanagan, J., & Lynch, K. L. (2001). Counseling interventions with suicidal clients. In E. R. Welfel & R. E. Ingersoll (Eds.), *The mental health desk reference* (pp. 264–270). New York: Wiley.

Stetson University School of Law Center for Excellence in Elder Law (2014), *Guide to U.S. state and mandatory reporting status and statutes*. Retrieved June 15, 2014 from www.stetson.edu/law/academics/elder/ecpp/statutory-updates.php.

Swenson, L. C. (1997). *Psychology and law for the helping professions*. Pacific Grove, CA: Brooks/Cole.

Tarasoff v. Regents of the University of California, 13 Cal. 3d 177, 529 P.2d 533, vacated, 17 Cal. 3d 425, 551 P.2d 334 (1976).

United States Department of Health and Human Services. (n.d.). *The child welfare information gateway*. Retrieved June 15, 2014 from www.childwelfare.gov/systemwide/laws_policies/state.

Weinburgh, M. (1998). Ethics, managed care and outpatient psychotherapy. *Clinical Social Work Journal, 26*(4), 433–443.

Welfel, E. R. (2010). *Ethics in counseling and psychotherapy: Standards, research and emerging issues* (4th ed.). Pacific Grove, CA: Brooks/Cole.

Welfel, E. R., Danzinger, P. R., & Santoro, S. (2000). Mandated reporting of abuse/maltreatment or older adults: A primer for counselors. *Journal of Counseling and Development, 78*, 284–293.

Wigmore, J. H. (1961). *Evidence in trials of common law* (vol. 8). Reviewed by John McNaughton. Boston: Little Brown.

Woody, R. (2013). *Legal self-defense for mental health practitioners: Quality care and risk management strategy*. New York: Springer.

CHAPTER 10

WORKING WITH CLIENTS IN CRISIS AND OTHER SPECIAL POPULATIONS

This chapter is designed to provide the student with information critical to working with the special populations they will encounter most frequently in their work. The populations discussed include clients who are harmful to themselves, clients who are a threat to others, abused children, sexual abuse victims, and substance-abusing clients. The chapter begins first with a review of basic crisis intervention information. Forms for use with these client populations are included for the student's reference and use.

Understanding Crisis and Trauma

James and Gilliland (2013) defined crisis as a perception of an event or situation as an intolerable difficulty that exceeds a person's resources and coping mechanisms. Unless a person obtains relief, the crisis has the potential to cause severe affective, cognitive, and behavioral malfunctioning. However, with support, most people do have the capacity to bounce back after a crisis-causing event.

Crises can unfold in various ways. Myer and Cogdal (2007) outlined four types of crisis-causing events, including developmental crises, existential crises, situational crises, and systemic crises. Developmental crises tend to emerge at marker moments or transitional periods in the life span and disrupt the typical flow of life events. For instance, a person who is just completing college or who is at the point of retirement may experience a crisis related to not knowing how to proceed next in life. Existential crises emerge with a person's reflection on his/her life; they have to do with how one puts meaning to life and how one evaluates his/her self-worth. An existential crisis can surface for people when they realize they have not fulfilled their dreams or desires in the realm of work and career, or they can experience a crisis when people realize they always wanted a family and are not capable of having children. Situational crises refer to the unforeseen circumstances that happen outside of the typical sequence of life events and overwhelm a person's coping mechanisms. These include such things as having a child diagnosed with a life-threatening medical condition, being in a serious car accident, or finding out that one is being laid off from work. Finally, systemic crises are large-scale events that not only have an impact on the individuals most directly affected by the crisis but also have a ripple effect that touches the local and even global community (Myer & Moore, 2006). Examples of systemic crises include the 9/11 terrorist attacks, hurricanes, school shootings, tornados, and the like.

A trauma tends to differ from a crisis in regard to the severity of the impact on human growth and functioning. Trauma is often characterized as a situation (one-time or continuous) that causes a person to feel an overwhelming sense of helplessness in the face of real physical or psychological threat, and it has the potential to upset a person's normal pathway to human development (Murray, Cohen, & Mannarino, 2013; Myer & Cogdal, 2007). Trauma victims can experience persistent alterations in their beliefs about the world (e.g., that most situations, even neutral ones, are fraught with danger), damage with regard to the ability to form healthy interpersonal relationships, altered neurological pathways, flashbacks and nightmares, and difficulty in processing and regulating complex emotions (Curtois & Ford, 2013; Lawson, Davis, & Brandon, 2013; Murray et al., 2013). Trauma victims also may be prone to developing other psychological problems such as addictive or self-injurious behaviors. Though we do not have the space to expand beyond this cursory definition of trauma here, students are highly recommended to review the current literature on trauma in order to broaden their knowledge in this area. There is a large and expanding body of research related to evidence-based practices when working with trauma survivors from a multitude of circumstances such as abusive family dynamics, exposure to community violence, and wartime violence. Interventions include helping clients to repair early, insecure attachment styles that have persisted into adulthood and that were harmed due to abuse and maltreatment; motivating clients to stay in counseling (Lawson et al., 2013); applying cognitive-behavioral methods to help transform belief systems that the world is always (or nearly always) a dangerous place (Murray et al., 2013); and helping clients create concrete and specific safety plans when they feel threatened (Murray et al., 2013).

The following sections review two models of crisis intervention that highlight some of the critical stages and tasks in crisis intervention. The first model was proposed by Kanel (2010), while the second was developed by James and Gilliland (2013). Both are useful for counselors who work in community-based settings.

The Kanel Model of Crisis Intervention

The ABC model of crisis intervention (Kanel, 2010) is a method of conducting very brief mental health interviews with clients whose functioning level has decreased following a psychosocial stressor. It is a problem-focused approach and is effectively applied within 4 to 6 weeks of the stressor. Kanel's (2010) model is designed around three specific stages: (a) developing and maintaining contact, (b) identifying the problem, and (c) developing coping strategies for the client. The following is a summary of the key points of the ABC model:

A. *Developing and maintaining contact:* Essential to the establishment of crisis intervention strategies is the development of rapport with the client. Thus, counselors need to be effective at employing basic attending skills learned early in their training programs. These skills include eye contact, body posture, vocal style, warmth, empathy, and genuineness. Skill in the use of open and closed questions and the skills of clarifying, reflecting, and summarizing are all used to develop and maintain contact with the person in crisis.

B. *Identifying the problem and therapeutic intervention:* By identifying the precipitating event, the counselor can gain information regarding the trigger(s) of the client's crisis. The actual cause of the crisis can vary from a recent event to an event that occurred several weeks or even months ago. The time of the event is important to determine. Kanel uses the following diagram to illustrate the process of crisis formulation:

Precipitating Event—Perception—Subjective Distress—Lowered Functioning

■ *Perception of the event:* This suggests that how an individual views the stressful situation contributes to the development of a crisis. The meaning and assumptions the person makes about the crisis event serve to color and magnify the meaning for the client. Careful perception checking of the client's view of the precipitating event must be thoroughly considered.

■ *Subjective distress:* This refers to the level of distress experienced by the client. Symptoms can affect academic, behavioral, occupational, social, and family functioning. Discussing the affected functional area(s) and the degree to which the crisis event impacts them is crucial (Kanel, 2010).

■ *Lowered functioning:* It is essential that pre- and postlevels of functioning are understood so that the counselor can ascertain the client's realistic level of coping and the severity of the crisis to the person.

C. *Developing coping strategies for the client:* The counselor assesses the past, present, and future coping behaviors of the client. Included in such an assessment are the client's unsuccessful coping strategies so that alternate coping strategies can be developed. Clients are encouraged to propose their own coping strategies in addition to learning the new or alternative strategies proposed by the counselor.

The James and Gilliland Model of Crisis Intervention

The following is a summary of the seven-task model of crisis intervention developed by James and Gilliland (2013):

1. *Engaging and initiating contact:* The counselor needs to develop an understanding of the events that precipitated the crisis and the meaning that it has for the client. It is therefore essential that a helping relationship be established. The use of basic attending skills coupled with the counselor's calm and direct approach can help the client see that something is being done to alleviate the problem.

2. *Exploring the problem and defining the crisis:* Assessing how dangerous the client is to himself/ herself or to others is one of the first concerns in crisis intervention (Aguilera, 1998). The myriad reasons why the client comes for counseling need to be explored. Suicidal ideation, homicidal ideation, danger from a third party, and fear of being harmed are potential reasons that pose a serious risk to a client's physical or psychological safety (Myer, Lewis, & James, 2013). It is essential that direct questioning focus on these possible motivators. Assuring safety involves determining the client's risk for harm or recent exposure to harm so that the counselor can then, if needed, involve others, seek the support of family and friends, recommend hospitalization, or protect intended victims. In conducting an assessment, the counselor inquires as to the event that precipitated the crisis, the meaning it has for the client, the support systems available to the client, and the level of functioning prior to the crisis (Aguilera, 1998). Aguilera further suggested that the assessment process begins with a direct question that elicits the client's reasons for coming to counseling, such as "What happened today?" and "Why today?" The counselor needs to determine what may have been the "last straw" for the client. Proceeding with the techniques of concreteness, leading, structuring, and questioning, the counselor can narrow the focus to the precipitating event. Determining what the client is feeling (rage, confusion, anger, hopelessness) gives the counselor an

understanding of the meaning that the crisis event had for the client. Once the meaning is understood, it is necessary, according to Roberts (2005), to listen for and to note cognitive distortions, overgeneralizations, misconceptions, and irrational beliefs. Attention should focus on the client's physical appearance, behavior, mood, and any signs of distress. In addition, the counselor must assess the client's coping mechanisms, decision-making skills, and stress management skills.

3. *Providing support:* It is essential to assess the client's support systems. The client who has inadequate resources needs support from someone who cares about him/her, including the counselor. Counselors first and foremost can offer psychological support to people in crisis by expressing empathy and concern over their current situation. In addition, counselors can offer logistical and social support to clients by helping to meet their physical and social needs.

4. *Examining alternatives:* The counselor helps the client explore a variety of available options, especially because the client may feel as though there are no available options. It is not necessary to provide the client with a multitude of options; rather, it is more effective to discuss options that are reasonable, appropriate, and realistic.

5. *Planning in order to reestablish control:* In this practical step, the counselor must tenaciously hold the client's attention on one problem whose moderation will begin to restore equilibrium. The counselor attempts to get the client to look at possible alternatives or solutions. It is also helpful to elicit from the client pre-crisis coping strategies that can then be modified. Specifically, the counselor helps the client identify concrete resources (e.g., people, organizations, etc.) that can be of assistance in relieving the crisis, and he/she provides some coping mechanisms, which may take the form of psychoeducation about what to expect during a crisis. Before ending the session, the counselor must assess the degree to which the client understands and can describe the action plan that has been developed. It is important to remember that client ownership of the plan is crucial.

6. *Obtaining commitment:* The counselor demonstrates the need to carry out the action plan. Commitment should go well if the previous steps have been carried out successfully. Follow-up contact or telephone contact with the client will aid the counselor in determining the client's status, whether or not the action plan has been implemented, and the degree to which the client has progressed toward a resolution.

7. *Following up:* Finally, counselors who do crisis intervention follow up with clients about their action plans and their coping skills in the short term. Follow-up happens in the hours or days after the crisis and indicates to the client that the counselor is in touch with the gravity of the crisis event.

By reviewing just these two models, it may be clear that Kanel (2010) and James and Gilliland (2013) both include similar tasks that must be undertaken by counselors in the process of crisis response. Indeed, Myer et al. (2013) reviewed nine different models of crisis intervention in order to identify areas of similarity and difference in the various approaches to crisis counseling. They concluded that nearly all of the models recommended counselors to engage in three continuous activities: (a) assessing the crisis situation in order to gain a sense of how to tailor the response intervention, (b) ensuring safety, and (c) providing support. Likewise, all models described at least four focused tasks that include (a) creating an alliance with the client, (b) defining the problem at hand (e.g., What is the crux of the crisis?), (c) helping the client to regain a sense of control, and (d) following up after the intervention has been enacted. In line with the James and Gilliland model

(2013), Myer and colleagues (2013) also noted that crisis intervention is best conceptualized as a group of clinical tasks that can unfold concurrently and repeatedly (especially those that are seen as continuous tasks) rather than as static stages. With this in mind, counselors do well to conceptualize crisis response more as a dynamic and fluid process than as a checklist of stages.

Crisis Intervention in Schools

In this section, we look at crisis response in the school setting in order to address how school counselors prevent and intervene in the case of various types of crisis and violence. A later section will propose more specific response suggestions related to suicide prevention and intervention in schools. The tasks described above in the Kanel (2010) and James and Gilliland (2013) models can certainly be applied by school counselors. However, because of their unique position in schools and because school counselors do not necessarily have one-to-one counseling relationships with all students (operating instead on behalf of the good of a student body), the focus and role of school counselors with respect to crisis response are somewhat different than for mental health counselors.

Riley and McDaniel (2000) recommended a set of tasks and roles for school counselors in the face of crises. These tasks involve counselors in interacting directly with students, as well as with parents, teachers, and school districts. Citing best practices from the Idaho School Counselor Association, Riley and McDaniel (2000) noted that when working with students relative to crisis response, school counselors can intervene individually with students at risk (e.g., students who are the target of bullying) or with groups of students. When operating at the group level, school counselors can engage in crisis prevention and/or intervention by creating classroom lessons and school programs that encourage mentoring and that discourage school violence; they also might lead counseling groups that help students to deal effectively with anger and emotions related to school-based crises. With regard to parents, school counselors can provide information or training on appropriate parenting and disciplining techniques, as well as act as a referral source for children who are struggling to be successful in the classroom and with peers. At the systemic level, counselors can assist teachers, staff, and administration in handling students' discipline problems as well as participate in the school district's crisis response team (Riley & McDaniel, 2000).

In addition to pointing out the above-mentioned specific tasks, Riley and McDaniel (2000) also discussed how school counselors can act as prevention, intervention, and crisis response specialists. Although counselors wear many hats in the schools in which they work, they are usually viewed as helpful prevention specialists when it comes to crisis work. Counselors who work toward the goal of decreasing the likelihood of crisis and violence in their schools aim to create an environment that is supportive and cohesive. To some extent, this means that they forge individual relationships with students, especially those who appear to be at high risk for becoming either a perpetrator or a victim of violence. School counselors can also partner with local law enforcement to have officers assigned to the school premises. These officers can be attentive to potential crisis and violence situations, as well as act as resources to school personnel. Finally, school counselors can petition to be on the school's or school district's crisis response team. Being familiar with district-wide response plans enables counselors to be an advocate for their own schools, students, and teachers.

Riley and McDaniel (2000) also described the school counselor as the interventionalist with regard to crises. They noted that intervention is most effective when it is early—prior to the unfolding of a crisis or emergency. Counselors therefore may be called on to help assess the needs or risk levels of students who are identified by teachers as exhibiting early warning signs for violence or other types of crises. Thus, counselors themselves have to be familiar with the signs that precede violence among youths. Working with parents and teachers to educate them about children's social and emotional needs, as well as their risk factors for committing violence, is a key part of intervening to reduce violence.

Finally, Riley and McDaniel (2000) pointed out that counselors have a central role to play on crisis response teams. Especially because of the increase in natural and manmade disasters, such as shootings and suicides that are occurring in and around schools, it is imperative that schools have plans in place to aid teachers, counselors, and all personnel in knowing what to do in the event of a crisis. Some responsibilities that fall to counselors on crisis teams include the following: organizing and providing counseling services to students in need, connecting and communicating with teachers and administrators, contacting parents and providing them with social support, cancelling activities if needed, making connections with a feeder school in the event of crises, and coordinating follow-up care after a crisis. Sometimes this involves making sure additional counselors are available to students on the school premises following a crisis event (Riley & McDaniel, 2000).

School Counselors as Prevention Consultants for Crises

As noted above, school counselors play both a preventive and responsive role in crisis intervention. Some of the prevention-related tasks that fall to counselors involve training and consultation with regard to crisis intervention. Training related to crisis response is especially important to and beneficial for teachers and other school personnel who spend nearly their whole day with students and who are in a unique position to gather information and note danger symptoms of children who are prone to commit or be victims of violence. School counselors thus should ally themselves with teachers and other school personnel in working to reduce school violence. Callahan (1998) outlined a helpful crisis response model for teachers that we believe to be applicable for any school personnel. More important, the response model can be a useful resource for counselors who are compiling crisis intervention trainings for their schools. The highlights of Callahan's model are presented here as an aid for school counselors who are looking to put together crisis-related education sessions for teachers and school personnel.

Suggestions for a School-Based Training on Crisis Response

Callahan (1998) noted that when teachers or school personnel gather information about impending crises, they should pass these on to other teachers, counselors, and administrators who may be able to observe and take the necessary action when violence is about to erupt. Accordingly, school personnel need to understand how to manage aggressive behavior. Similarly, the teacher and other school personnel must know that when a student hits a state of disequilibrium (lack of judgment and control) and his/her body is in a defensive state of readiness to attack or flee. Normal processes, such as the ability to hear, think logically, and react normally, may be limited, and the more upset an individual is, the less likely it is that the individual will be able to respond to others. When a person in crisis becomes alarmed and moves into a resistance stage, the person is closer to acting out; thus, it is important to conduct an immediate assessment of the student and the situation. Greenstone and Leviton (as cited in Callahan, 1998) suggested the following points for assessing students in crisis:

1. School personnel begin by engaging the student in conversation about what is going on, and especially what is precipitating the crisis at the moment. Remaining as calm and controlled as possible is important.
2. The adult should determine the most immediate need from the student's perspective and should not belittle any problems presented by the student in crisis.
3. The adult should outline problems that can be quickly managed and determine variables that might hinder the crisis management process.
4. The adult should prioritize actions that can effectively and quickly diffuse the crisis situation.
5. The adult should look for similarities between the present situation and previous incidents of stress.

Callahan (1998) suggested further that if a crisis is occurring outside the classroom, adults in the school should follow safety guidelines, including the following:

1. Intervene with a partner, especially if there is more than one person involved in the crisis.
2. Approach the crisis situation slowly and judiciously.
3. Be careful not to turn one's back on the student in crisis.
4. Visually determine if there is any weapon available.
5. Note any objects that could be used as a weapon.
6. Be prepared for unexpected behavior.
7. Note entrances and exits in the area so that if the situation turns violent, the adult can help other students to safety.
8. Remove audiences from escalating situations when possible.
9. Know where to find assistance (Callahan, 1998, pp. 226–227).

In addition to preparing school personnel and faculty for how to attend to the signs of crisis and to any acts of violence, counselors are well positioned to advocate on behalf of students who need assistance in dealing with the crisis. The American Academy of Experts in Traumatic Stress (2003) made the following recommendations for responding to students during a crisis event that occurs within or near the school setting:

- Gather facts about the crisis, and after getting the consent of the principal, explain the crisis event to students in a manner they can understand.
- Appropriately model expression of feelings so that students know they are also allowed to react emotionally to the crisis.
- Become aware of when the crisis is personally overwhelming and hinders one's ability to attend to children's needs.
- Explain the normal range of emotional reactions to students and validate their responses in a nonjudgmental and noncritical fashion.
- Be aware that children usually reorient themselves within 6 weeks of experiencing a crisis, though longer-term responses can occur and should be dealt with sensitively.
- Be attentive to students who seem to have a more difficult time reorienting after a crisis and refer them to trained professionals such as counselors and psychologists.

- Provide opportunities for students to share their reactions as a group.
- Create nonverbal means through which students can process the crisis event (e.g., through art, drawing, and writing, etc.).
- Develop lessons meant to help students address their feelings about the crisis.
- Be aware that crisis intervention is ongoing and that some students may need ongoing or individualized attention.

The last point noted above recommends that counselors be attentive to students who may not bounce back from a crisis as readily as their peers. In those instances, counselors or other persons in the school might notice that these children and teens appear emotionally elevated, depressed, or withdrawn when their peers seem to have regained homeostasis; they may flounder in their academic performance; older students may show signs of suicidal or homicidal ideation or use of alcohol or drugs; and students may not attend to their hygiene. Students who have ongoing difficulty in dealing with a crisis and who show some of these behavioral changes may benefit from an outside referral for individualized attention and counseling. Other signs of post-crisis response in children are noted next.

Post-Crisis: Understanding Children's Responses

The American Academy of Experts in Traumatic Stress (2003) provided information about how crises affect children specifically and what counselors can do when they know or suspect that a student(s) has been exposed to a traumatic event. The following is a summary of the behavioral responses a school counselor might observe in children or learn about secondhand from parents during and after a crisis.

- *Regression in behavior:* Children may behave in ways more akin to those younger than themselves (e.g., sucking their thumb even if they have not used this form of comfort for some time, wetting the bed, or becoming clingy with trusted adults and parents).
- *Increase in fears and anxiety:* Children may respond to a crisis by appearing excessively afraid or worried about situations that do not normally cause anxiety, such as going to school alone or going to bed alone or in the dark.
- *Decreased academic performance and poor concentration:* Children may not be able to concentrate on or complete schoolwork as usual, especially if they are preoccupied with the crisis event or the fear caused by the event.
- *Increased aggression and oppositional behavior and decreased frustration tolerance:* Some children may show a disproportionate increase in aggressive behavior or, in adolescents, oppositional or defiant behaviors.
- *Increased irritability, emotional lability, and depressive feelings:* Children can show signs of depressed mood, lack of interest in the activities that previously were entertaining, and overall irritability.
- *Denial:* Children may deny or act as if a crisis or traumatic event such as a death of a parent, a beloved teacher, or a friend has not occurred. Although denial responses are as common in children as in adults, children may need help coming to terms with the reality of the crisis in gentle yet direct ways.

It is important to keep in mind that the reactions described above are typical responses to crises for children and adolescents and thus ought not be seen primarily as signs of psychological illness. Rather, they ought to be evaluated within the context of the crisis that occurred for the child or teenager.

The High-Risk Client: Understanding and Assessing Harm to Self

One of the most stressful experiences for mental health professionals in training involves helping people who pose a risk to their own safety and well-being. A question often asked by trainees is: What do I do when I have a client who wants to commit suicide? Meichenbaum (2005) noted that it is not unusual for counselors to work with suicidal clients over the course of their careers. Similarly, intern students who are placed in settings with highly stressed, chronically depressed, and under-resourced clients, as well as in placements such as inpatient hospitals, may be more likely than not to work with suicide-prone persons. The first part of this section introduces basic information about suicide, the suicidal client, and risk assessment with clients who pose a threat to their own lives.

Defining Suicide and Debunking Common Myths

We begin with a brief definition of suicide. Beauchamp (1985) talked about suicide this way:

- the person intentionally brings about his/her own death,
- the person is not coerced by others to take the action, and
- death is caused by conditions arranged by the person for the specific purpose of bringing about his/her own death.

Possibly because suicide is counter to natural instincts to persevere through even the most difficult of human situations (Joiner, 2010), there are many misconceptions about the act of suicide itself, as well as about people who commit suicide. Being aware of some of these myths is helpful for counselors so that they are better able to tailor their discussions with clients who are suicidal. Conversely, it is important for mental health professionals not to structure their clinical interventions around common misunderstandings about suicide in order to be of maximal benefit to clients and to ensure that they are not acting negligently with regard to their professional obligations. According to Fujimura, Weis, and Cochran (1985) and Joiner (2010) the following is a sample of some of those myths.

- Discussing suicide will cause the client to move toward doing it.
- Clients who threaten suicide don't do it.
- Suicide is an irrational and a selfish act.
- Persons who commit suicide are insane.
- Suicide runs in families—it is an inherited tendency.
- Once suicidal always suicidal.
- When a person has attempted suicide and pulls out of it, the danger is over.
- A suicidal person who begins to show generosity and share personal possessions is showing signs of renewal and recovery.
- Suicide is always an impulsive act.
- Suicide is an act of aggression or anger toward oneself.

Greene (1994) identified five additional myths surrounding childhood suicide:

- Children under the age of 6 do not commit suicide.
- Suicide in the latency years is extremely rare.

■ Psychodynamically and developmentally, true depression is not possible in childhood.
■ Children are cognitively and physically incapable of implementing a suicide plot successfully.

In the face of these many myths, it is important to keep in mind that most suicide attempts are expressions of extreme distress, not bids for attention (Captain, 2006; Joiner, 2010). Thus, Captain (2006) rightly noted that counselors should not be afraid to ask clients about suicidal thoughts. Most clients who are suicidal are relieved to talk about their feelings and to be assured that they are not out of the ordinary for thinking this way. Indeed, about a third of the population of people not in therapy has had suicidal thoughts (Meichenbaum, 2005).

Risk Factors for Suicide*

Working effectively with clients who are at high risk for suicide entails the intern gathering a body of knowledge about the signs and characteristics that commonly surface for people who commit suicide. Knowing risk factors aids directly in being able to conduct an assessment about a client's level of lethality and to structure the most appropriate clinical response. Risk factors for suicide are characteristics or conditions that increase the chance that a person may try to take his/her life. Suicide risk tends to be highest when someone has several risk factors at the same time.

The most frequently cited risk factors for suicide are:

■ Mental disorders, in particular:
  • Depression or bipolar (manic-depressive) disorder
  • Alcohol or substance abuse or dependence
  • Schizophrenia
  • Borderline or antisocial personality disorder
  • Conduct disorder (in youth)
  • Psychotic disorders; psychotic symptoms in the context of any disorder
  • Anxiety disorders
  • Impulsivity and aggression, especially in the context of the above mental disorders
■ Previous suicide attempt
■ Family history of attempted or completed suicide
■ Serious medical condition and/or pain

It is important to bear in mind that the large majority of people with mental disorders or other suicide risk factors do not engage in suicidal behavior.

Environmental Factors That Increase Suicide Risk

Some people who have one or more of the major risk factors above can become suicidal in the face of factors in their environment, such as:

■ A highly stressful life event, such as losing someone close, financial loss, or trouble with the law
■ Prolonged stress due to adversities such as unemployment, serious relationship conflict, harassment, or bullying

- Exposure to another person's suicide or to graphic or sensationalized accounts of suicide (contagion)
- Access to lethal methods of suicide during a time of increased risk

Again, though, it is important to remember that these factors do not usually increase suicide risk for people who are not already vulnerable because of a preexisting mental disorder or other major risk factors. Exposure to extreme or prolonged environmental stress, however, can lead to depression, anxiety, and other disorders that, in turn, can increase risk for suicide.

Protective Factors for Suicide

Protective factors for suicide are characteristics or conditions that may help to decrease a person's suicide risk. While these factors do not eliminate the possibility of suicide, especially in someone with risk factors, they may help to reduce that risk. Protective factors for suicide have not been studied as thoroughly as risk factors, so less is known about them.

Protective factors for suicide include:

- Receiving effective mental health care
- Positive connections to family, peers, community, and social institutions such as marriage and religion that foster resilience
- The skills and ability to solve problems

Protective factors may reduce suicide risk by helping people cope with negative life events, even when those events continue over a period of time. The ability to cope with or solve problems reduces the chance that a person will become overwhelmed, depressed, or anxious. Protective factors do not entirely remove risk, however, especially when there is a personal or family history of depression or other mental disorders.

Warning Signs for Suicide

In contrast to longer-term risk and protective factors, warning signs are indicators of more acute suicide risk. Thinking about heart disease helps to make this clear. Risk factors for heart disease include smoking, obesity, and high cholesterol. Having these factors does not mean that someone is having a heart attack right now but rather that there is an increased chance that they will have heart attack at some time. Warning signs of a heart attack are chest pain, shortness of breath, and nausea. These signs mean that the person may be having a heart attack right now and needs immediate help. As with heart attacks, people who die by suicide usually show some indication of immediate risk before their deaths. Recognizing the warning signs for suicide can help us to intervene to save a life. A person who is thinking about suicide may say so directly: "I'm going to kill myself." More commonly, they may say something more indirect: "I just want the pain to end," or "I can't see any way out." Most of the time, people who kill themselves show one or more of these warning signs before they take action:

- Talking about wanting to kill themselves or saying they wish they were dead
- Looking for a way to kill themselves, such as hoarding medicine or buying a gun
- Talking about a specific suicide plan
- Feeling hopeless or having no reason to live
- Feeling trapped, desperate, or needing to escape from an intolerable situation

- Having the feeling of being a burden to others
- Feeling humiliated
- Having intense anxiety and/or panic attacks
- Losing interest in things or losing the ability to experience pleasure
- Experiencing insomnia
- Becoming socially isolated and withdrawn from friends, family, and others
- Acting irritable or agitated
- Showing rage or talking about seeking revenge for being victimized or rejected, whether or not the situations the person describes seem real

*Permission to use this material has been granted by the American Foundation for Suicide Prevention.

Risk Assessment for Suicide

Unfortunately, suicide assessment can tend to be impressionistic and fail to consider pertinent information regarding a person's lethality. To guard against impressionistic evaluations of suicidal risk, it is helpful to review the research and the clinical data about suicide that outline the factors counselors ought to assess when they encounter a high-risk client. Joiner et al. (2007) noted that suicide can reliably be understood as involving (a) the desire to die, (b) the capacity to commit suicide, (c) the intent to harm oneself, and (d) buffers against self-harm. An effective suicide assessment addresses each of these areas.

Assessment Point 1: Desire to Die

The desire to die refers to a client's sense that life is simply not worth living and that he/she would be better off not alive. There is a strong psychological component to this factor that involves clients perceiving that they are a burden to others, as well as feeling hopeless and helpless with regard to their life situation. In assessing a client's desire to die, a counselor should inquire about the following (Joiner et al., 2007):

- the client's stated desire to die,
- the client's perceptions about being a burden to others in his/her life,
- the client's sense of hopelessness and helplessness (a depression screening can be helpful here),
- the client's feelings of being deeply alone, and
- the client's sense of being trapped by life circumstances with no way out.

Joiner et al. (2007) noted that while the desire to die is always present in those who are suicidal, in itself this factor is not the most critical in determining whether or not a client is at high risk to die. The authors point out that many people have a wish to die but not every person is actually capable of committing the act. Thus, in the global assessment of risk, clients who desire to die but who do not have the capacity or intent to die are not at as high a risk as those with the latter two factors in place.

Assessment Point 2: Capacity to Commit Suicide

The second area that counselors want to assess for suicide relates to a person's actual ability to go through with the suicidal act (Joiner, 2005; Joiner et al., 2007; Rudd et al., 2006). To take one's life is not an easy task, and it involves both courage and desensitization to death and dying (Joiner, 2005). Joiner (2005) noted that the courage to commit suicide is not meant to be emulated or held up on a pedestal; rather, he noted that it speaks to the difficulty of actually overcoming the natural, inborn instinct to live. Overcoming the instinct to live can get eroded in repeated exposures to violence and death (including those that are experienced personally and those witnessed in others). To assess a person's capacity to die, Joiner et al. (2007) recommended asking clients about the following:

- the client's history of suicide attempts,
- the client's exposure to others' suicide attempts,
- the client's history or current participation in violence to others,
- the available means to kill oneself,
- the client's current substance use or current level of intoxication,
- the client's level of active symptoms of mental illness, and
- the client's expression of anger, rage, or agitation.

The presence of any or all of the above factors increases a person's capacity for suicide.

Assessment Point 3: Suicidal Intent

One of the most critical areas to assess with regard to suicide is a person's intent to commit the act (McGlothlin, Rainey, & Kindsvatter, 2005). Clients may have both a desire not to live and the ability to commit suicide, but if they do not have the intent or a specific plan to die, they are less likely to pursue their own deaths (Joiner et al., 2007). When counselors are assessing for a client's suicidal intent, they should consider the following points:

- The client is in the midst of an attempt to die or has a clear plan for how and when to die.
- The client has an identified means of taking his/her own life.
- The client has left important possessions to others.
- The client expresses the intention to die.

Assessment Point 4: Buffers Against Suicide

A suicide assessment should include not only the points of vulnerability that make a person desirous, capable, and intending of dying; it should also include an evaluation of the factors that mitigate against the suicide attempt. Buffers against suicide are the elements that protect people against death, provide points of hope, and indicate a will to continue living. When people can be reconnected to reasons to live, they will be less likely to follow through on suicidal intent, though it may not always directly decrease the risk level for suicide. Buffers for which counselors should assess include the following, as noted by Joiner et al. (2007):

- The client perceives he/she has immediate support available (e.g., in the person of the counselor, family, or friends).
- The client can identify a reason(s) to continue living and has a plan for the future.
- The client has core values that are strong.
- The client has a sense of purpose for life.
- The client is able to engage in the dialogue of the counseling session.

Evaluating Suicide Risk: Putting It All Together

The risk assessment model outlined by Joiner et al. (2007) and described above uses three levels of evaluation: high risk, moderate to high risk, and moderate to low risk.

■ *High risk:* A client who is considered high risk has elements of the first three assessment points present; that is, the person has a desire to die, is capable of committing the suicidal act, and has the intent and/or a plan to die. In this instance, even the presence of buffers tends not to decrease risk, and a client with this presentation of factors should be aided in seeking immediate safety.

■ *Moderate to high risk:* A client who is at moderate to high risk has a desire to die and also has either the capacity or the intent to die. In this case, the presence of buffers for safety can reduce the overall level of risk, and, conversely, the absence of any buffers can increase the risk level. When buffers against suicide are in place, a counselor may not need to recommend immediate action for the protection of a client's safety but likely will want to follow up and regularly monitor a client's risk and overall well-being. If buffers are not in place, immediate action to ensure a client's safety still may be needed.

■ *Moderate to low risk:* A client has any of the three core elements of risk present, and the level of risk can be lessened by the presence of buffers for safety or elevated in the absence of such buffers.

Conducting a thorough risk assessment for suicide is part of competent clinical practice. However, Granello (2010) wisely pointed out that suicide assessment is as much about the process of conducting the risk assessment as it is about knowing the specific warning signs and risk factors for suicide. She identified numerous principles that guide the implementation of a suicide assessment. Specifically, she encouraged clinicians to keep in mind that assessment is unique to each person; an ongoing, collaborative, and complex process; responsive to warning signs; sensitive to cultural issues; reliant on clinical judgment; documented; errant on the side of caution; inclusive of tough questions; and a form of treatment itself.

Suicide Risk Assessment Instruments

The use of empirical evaluation can help ground suicide risk assessments. Suicide scales, checklists, and other psychological instruments can be helpful in determining suicidal risk (Granello, 2010; Klott, 2012). Empirical instruments are excellent resources for those who may be inexperienced in dealing with suicide. In addition, consultation and discussions with a more experienced supervisor, therapist, or treatment team help promote a multifaceted approach and decrease the probability of suicide resulting from flawed treatment interventions (Granello, 2010).

The Substance Abuse and Mental Health Services Administration recommended a five-step process in assessing suicide known as the Suicide Assessment Five Step Evaluation and Triage (SAFE-T) model (a free copy of the model can be downloaded or ordered from: http://store.samhsa. gov/product/Suicide-Assessment-Five-Step-Evaluation-and-Triage-SAFE-T-/SMA09-4432). SAFE-T is based on best practice guidelines established by the American Psychiatric Association (2003) for assessing and treating suicide. Using this assessment tool, counselors first identify current risk factors for suicide; these can include a history of abuse, history of suicide attempts, diagnostic risk factors, history of family suicide attempts, and high level of impulsivity. Second, clinicians investigate with the client any potential protective factors that would mitigate against suicidal behavior, such as religious beliefs, positive relationships, and responsibility for children. Third, counselors inquire into suicidal thoughts, plans, behaviors, and overall intent. Fourth, clinicians must use their knowledge and experience in conjunction with the clinical interview to determine the level of risk that the client is facing with regard to suicide and, together with the client, make treatment decisions. Finally, all clinicians should document the details of the interview, the characteristics of risk, and interventions used to address risk. Fowler (2012) recommended that clinicians who use this or other assessment tools align themselves with the client and make a concerted effort to approach the process with concern and an attitude of curiosity (rather than authority). A collaborative style can help clients feel more at ease during the assessment and ultimately be more upfront about suicidal plans and intent.

Intervention and Planning

Listed below are some techniques generally recognized by therapists to facilitate the counseling process for suicidal clients:

- Listen intelligently, sensitively, and carefully to the client.
- Accept and understand the client's suicidal thoughts.
- Don't give false assurances such as "Everything is going to be all right."
- Be supportive.
- Assure the client of your availability.
- Be firm and caring at the same time.
- Don't use euphemisms. Ask direct questions such as "Would you like to kill yourself?" rather than using vague expressions.
- Bring out any ambivalence the client has. Try to increase his/her choices.
- If the client is in crisis, don't leave him/her alone.
- Intervene to dispose of any weapons the client has.
- Tell others, especially those who would be concerned and can help. (You have already informed the client of the limits of confidentiality.)
- Help the client identify and develop support systems, especially when in crisis.
- Trust your own judgment.
- Know the suicide hotline numbers.
- Be aware of commitment procedures in your area.

The above suggested actions are helpful to counselors in putting together an overall safety plan for clients who are suicidal. Students who are interested in reviewing a more comprehensive list of possible questions and active interventions are referred to Meichenbaum (2005).

Finally, students may have questions about the role and use of suicide contracts in the process of working with suicidal clients. Though many clinicians used to be in the habit of developing suicide contracts with their clients (that both suicidal clients and counselors would sign, acknowledging the client's agreement not to self-harm), these contracts are not strongly encouraged today (Rudd et al., 2006). Instead, counselors are urged to put together commitments to treatment (Rudd et al., 2006) or safety plans (Klott, 2012) that include a list of clients' and counselors' responsibilities and preferred actions in the event that clients are tempted to act on suicidal intentions. A safety plan can encourage clients to contact family members, walk away from stress-inducing circumstances, and utilize means of emotional regulation (Klott, 2012). However, even with the best-prepared plan for safety, some clients still may desire to act on suicidal intentions and will neither comply with the plan nor consent to hospitalization. In serious cases, counselors may be in the position to consider involuntary commitment to a treatment center. The procedures for commitment, whether voluntary or involuntary, vary a great deal from area to area, and laws on commitment procedures are different from state to state. Mental health professionals should be familiar with the legal aspects of commitment in their areas. A copy of a Suicide Consultation Form (Form 10.1) is included in the Forms section at the end of this book; students may use this form, in consultation with their supervisors, to facilitate their counseling of clients who are potentially harmful to themselves.

Ethical and Legal Mandates Relating to Danger to Self

Working with people who are suicidal has ethical and legal implications for counselors. All codes of ethics from well-established mental health professional associations clearly address the welfare of clients as paramount in the clinical process. The following excerpts highlight the types of responses that are expected of professional clinical counselors and school counselors in the case of clients who pose harm to themselves.

Professional School Counselors

a. Inform parents/guardians and/or appropriate authorities when a student poses a danger to self or others. This is to be done after careful deliberation and consultation with other counseling professionals.
b. Report risk assessments to parents when they underscore the need to act on behalf of a child at risk; never negate a risk of harm as students sometimes deceive in order to avoid further scrutiny and/or parental notification.
c. Understand the legal and ethical liability for releasing a student who is a danger to self or others without proper and necessary support for that student (American School Counselors Association, 2010, Standard A.7.a–c).

Professional Counselors

The general requirement that counselors keep information confidential does not apply when disclosure is required to protect clients or identified others from serious and foreseeable harm or when legal requirements demand that confidential information must be revealed. Counselors consult with other professionals when in doubt as to the validity of an exception. Additional considerations apply when addressing end-of-life issues (American Counseling Association, 2005, B.2.a.).

In addition to ethical responsibilities to do good by the client by protecting his/her bodily welfare in the instance of possible self-harm, the counselor also faces legal responsibilities around client suicidality. The mental health professional's special relationship with the client creates the context for the legal accountability for negligent malpractice with potentially suicidal persons. A therapist is assumed to possess superior knowledge and skills beyond those of the average person and may be considered by the courts to bear responsibility for the suicide of his/her client. The client's reliance on the counselor alone is enough to shift some of the weight of the responsibility for the client's actions to the mental health professional.

This was not always the case. In England, for example, toward the latter part of the 19th century, suicide was considered self-murder, and authorities buried the bodies of those who committed suicide at the side of the road with a stake through the heart (Bednar, Bednar, Lambert, & Waite, 1991). In contrast, today a mental health professional who does not take appropriate action to prevent a suicide can be held liable. At the same time, liability has not been found when apparently cooperative clients suddenly attempt suicide (*Carlino v. State*, 1968; *Dalton v. State*, 1970) or when an aggressive client does not reveal any suicidal symptoms (*Paridies v. Benedictine Hospital*, 1980). In determining liability, courts also must decide whether the recommendations of a mental health professional were followed. In one case, a hospital was found liable when the staff did not follow the psychiatrist's recommendations (*Comiskey v. State of New York*, 1979).

Liability may be imposed if a therapist is determined to be negligent in his/her treatment of a client. Negligence is found when the mental health professional does not perform his/her duties according to the standard of care for that particular profession. As a consequence, mental health professionals should make as accurate an assessment of the danger as possible (based on the client interview, observation of client behavior, and review of the client's history); determine what action is reasonable, which may mean intensifying treatment, referring the client for a medication check, advising voluntary commitment, or authorizing involuntary commitment; and make sure the recommendation is followed.

Suicide Risk Assessment and Prevention in Schools

Suicide among American youths is cause of concern for counselors, who must not discount the possibility that young people can take their own lives. Gould, Shaffer, and Greenberg (2003) point out that 5.8% of deaths among children aged 10–14 are due to suicide. The American Association of Suicidology (2007) reported that for youth aged 15–19 suicide is the third leading cause of death, which accounts for the loss of over 4,100 lives per year. Perhaps of greater concern is that actual cases are considered to be underreported (Barrio, 2007). The American Association of Suicidology (2007) also reported that for every completed suicide, youths make about 100–200 attempts. The tragedy of suicide is further complicated by the strong possibility that it can be prevented (Barrio, 2007). Professionals concur that most potential suicide victims want to be saved and often send out signals for help. Considering the magnitude of this problem, schools have a moral imperative to develop suicide prevention programs (Joe & Bryant, 2007).

Basics of Suicide Prevention Programs in Schools

School counselors have responsibility for the welfare and safety of students in their schools and therefore may be actively involved in creating and updating the school-based suicide prevention plan. Thinking globally about the welfare of students is necessary for counselors who act on behalf of hundreds of students at a time; for this reason, program-based prevention approaches are often the most accessible and effective in the school setting. The literature suggests that to be effective, school-based programs must be comprehensive and systematic and include strategies for suicide prevention, intervention, and postvention following a completed suicide (Miller, Eckert, & Mazza, 2009). Comprehensive and systematic programs also must be ongoing, intact, and continuously updated. Many researchers who have developed models of school-based programs share this position. A review of recent literature (e.g., Doan, LeBlanc, Roggenbaum, & Lazear, 2012) reveals the following components as those most often recommended for school-based adolescent suicide prevention and intervention programs:

- a written formal policy statement for reacting to suicide and suicidal ideation, as well as following up with postvention strategies;
- staff training and orientation for recognizing at-risk students, determining the level of risk, and knowing where to refer the student;
- "booster" trainings for teachers, staff, and personnel every 2–3 years to keep school personnel updated about suicide risk and risk assessment;
- mental health professionals on-site;
- a mental health team;
- information programs and prevention materials for distribution to parents;
- incorporation of suicide curriculum and education for students;
- psychological screening programs to identify at-risk students;
- prevention-focused classroom discussions;
- mental health counseling for at-risk students;
- development of peer support groups for students who are at risk;
- suicide prevention and intervention training for school counselors;
- postvention component in the event of an actual suicide;
- written statement describing specific criteria for counselors to assess the lethality of a potential suicide; and
- a written policy describing how the program will be evaluated.

Learning About and Responding to Potentially Suicidal Students

School-based mental health professionals may encounter suicide-related crisis situations in at least three different ways, each of which requires some specific guidelines. First, the student may attempt suicide on school premises. In this case, the counselor should refer to the school's policy regarding this intervention. Second, the student may disclose suicidal ideation directly to the counselor without having attempting suicide. When this happens, the counselor should assess lethality as the first level of response (steps for assessing risk are outlined in the next section) and consult the school's prevention and intervention plan. Third, peers may inform the counselor of a suicidal student. Seven out of 10 students will tell a peer about suicidal ideation before telling anyone else. It is especially important to take this information seriously, conduct a risk assessment, and inform a student's parents of the concern in order to help the student receive appropriate care and to avoid acting negligently (Pate, 1992). Below are some additional guidelines for action in each of the situations noted above:

1. *If a suicide attempt occurs on the premises*, involve appropriate school personnel, then notify the police and an ambulance service. Also notify the parents (or guardian). Let them know where their child is being taken. If the parents (or guardian) are not available, notify the next closest relative. See to it that the student receives proper medical and psychiatric care.
2. *If the student discloses suicidal ideation to you*, first consult your supervisor or another mental health professional. Go over the assessment of lethality with the student. This process will help you establish the standard of care. Call the parents (or guardian) and tell them to go to the appropriate psychiatric facility. Explain to the parents and the student that an evaluation

or diagnosis does not necessarily mean commitment. If the parents resist this process, you may need to contact your local children and youth services for assistance. Be sure to contact the parents in the presence of the child, to eliminate the "he said–she said" phenomenon.

3. *If a peer tells you about another student's suicidal intent*, confront the student. If the student admits the suicidal ideation, follow the procedure outlined above. If the student denies the ideation, notify the parents (or guardian). Of course, you must inform the student about this disclosure.

Suicide Risk Assessment for Students

One of the elements of a suicide prevention program, as mentioned above, involves determining whether or not a student is at risk for attempting suicide. Appropriate intervention steps cannot be implemented until lethality is determined. The following process suggests actions that school teachers, counselors, and other personnel can take when a student is suspected of being suicidal (Pate, 1992):

1. *Ask directly during a session.* Ask the student, without hesitation, if he/she is thinking about killing himself/herself. If the student claims to have had suicidal ideation, the strength of the intent should be determined. Continue with the questioning.
2. *Ask if he/she has attempted suicide before.* If so, ask how many times attempts were made and when they were made. The more attempts, and the more recent the attempts, the more serious the situation becomes.
3. *Ask how the previous attempts were made.* If the student took aspirin, for example, ask how many. One? Six? Twenty? Then ask about the consequences of the attempts. For example, was there medical intervention?
4. *Ask why.* Why did the student attempt suicide before? Why the suicidal thoughts now?
5. *Does the student have a plan?* Ask about the details. The more detailed the plan is, the more lethal it is. Does the student know when and how the attempt will be made? Assess the lethality of the method. This assessment is critical. Does the student have a weapon or access to one? Using a gun or hanging oneself leaves little time for medical help.
6. *Ask about the student's preoccupation with suicide.* Does he/she think about it only at home or during a particular incident—or does it go beyond all other activities?
7. *Ask about drug use.* Drug use complicates the seriousness of the situation because people tend to be less inhibited when under the influence of drugs. Although the student may deny drug use, try to get as much information as possible.
8. *Observe nonverbal actions.* Is the student agitated, tense, or sad? Is he/she inebriated? Use caution if the student seems to be at peace. This peaceful state may be the result of having organized a suicide plan, with completion being the next step.
9. *Try to gauge the level of depression.* A student may not be depressed because he/she is anxious about completing the plan.

Using the points outlined in this process will help in determining the level of suicide risk for a student. A low-risk student may have thoughts about suicide but has never attempted suicide in the past, does not have a plan, is not taking drugs, and is not preoccupied with the ideation. Most students at low risk will agree to the therapist's contacting their parents, which should be done. The statements must be monitored closely, however, as a low-risk student can quickly become a high-risk student.

A high-risk student has a plan but may or may not have attempted suicide in the past. Of course, a previous attempt is an important factor in assessing lethality, especially if the attempt was recent (Joiner, 2005). But counselors should remember that many first-time attempts are successful. The current situation must never be minimized. The plan of a high-risk student is usually detailed, and the ideation frequent. At this point, other people need to become involved, including the counselor's supervisor, principal, and school nurse.

Ideally, the school will have some type of suicide intervention policy. The goal in a high-risk situation is to have the student undergo a psychiatric evaluation as soon as possible, whether by voluntary or involuntary commitment. The student's parents must be notified; confidentiality is not an issue if the limits of confidentiality were explained previously via informed consent. Although confidentiality laws vary from state to state, a counselor usually is not bound if the client intends to harm himself/herself or someone else (Moyer & Sullivan, 2008). It is absolutely imperative, however, that school counselors discuss confidentiality limits at the beginning of every client intake session.

The High-Risk Client: Potential Harm to Others

Working with clients who pose harm to others, like working with potentially suicidal clients, is an anxiety-provoking experience for seasoned counselors and for those in training. Mental health professionals become acutely aware of their own liability in such situations and thus must be prepared with regard to knowing about their professional obligations, being able to identify persons who pose a threat to others, and developing competence around assessing risk and determining an action plan for potentially dangerous clients. In this section we look first at the issue of professional obligation (through the lens of the *Tarasoff* case) and then at the issues surrounding risk assessment.

The *Tarasoff* Case: The Events

Prosenjit Poddar was a graduate student at the University of California, Berkeley. In 1968 Poddar attended dancing classes at the International House in Berkeley, where he met a woman named Tatiana (Tanya) Tarasoff. This meeting quickly led to an obsessive, one-sided love affair. Poddar began harassing Ms. Tarasoff, calling and pestering her continually. He was consistently and repeatedly rebuffed by the young woman. In the summer of 1969, Tarasoff went to Brazil. When she returned, Poddar went to her home and again was rebuffed. Poddar drew a pellet gun and shot at her. Desperate, the young woman ran from the house, only to be chased down and caught by Poddar, who fatally stabbed her with a kitchen knife. This tragic chain of events unleashed some unforeseen and shocking consequences for mental health professionals. While Tarasoff was in Brazil, Poddar had sought help for depression at Cowell Memorial Hospital, an affiliate of the University of California, Berkeley. His intake interview was conducted by Dr. Stuart Gold, a psychiatrist, and his therapy was conducted by a psychologist, Dr. Lawrence Moore. In August 1969, Poddar told Dr. Moore he was going to kill Tarasoff when she returned from Brazil. Moore immediately consulted his supervisor, and they agreed that Poddar should be involuntarily committed. Dr. Moore called the police, who detained Poddar, but after questioning the man, police officials decided he was rational and released him. His freedom led directly to Tarasoff's death.

Implications of the Tarasoff *Case*

In late 1974 the California Supreme Court ruled there was cause for action for negligence against the therapist, the university, and the police for the failure to warn (*Tarasoff v. Regents of the University of California*, 1974). This case is commonly known as *Tarasoff I*. The court, apparently under pressure from various professional groups, agreed to a rehearing in 1976 (*Tarasoff v. Regents of the University of California*, 1976). This case is commonly known as *Tarasoff II*.

Whenever we mention the *Tarasoff* case throughout this book, we are citing *Tarasoff II*. In the court's final decision, presented in *Tarasoff II* on July 1, 1976, it set a new standard for therapists. The mandate was clear: *"Therapists who know or should know of patients' dangerousness to identifiable third persons have an obligation to take all reasonable steps necessary to protect the potential victims* [italics added]" (Appelbaum, 1985, p. 425).

Various writers on the subject of *Tarasoff* have defined the term *therapist* to include psychologists; counselors; child, marriage, and family therapists; and community mental health counselors. As Stone (cited in Waldo & Malley, 1992) noted,

> Many mental health professionals and paraprofessionals, including social workers, psychiatric social workers, psychiatric nurses, occupational therapists, pastoral counselors, and guidance counselors, provide some form of therapy. . . . How many of these millions of therapist–patient contacts each year are intended to be covered by the court's decision is unclear. (p. 59)

What Tarasoff *Did Not Require*

Researchers have looked extensively at what the *Tarasoff* ruling requires and does not require of mental health professionals. VandeCreek and Knapp (1993) addressed this issue head on:

> Because the *Tarasoff* decision has been subject to so many misinterpretations, it is important to know what the *Tarasoff* court did *not* say. The court did not require psychotherapists to issue a warning every time a patient talks about an urge or fantasy to harm someone. On the contrary, the court stated that "a therapist should not be encouraged routinely to reveal such threats . . . unless such disclosure is necessary to avert danger to others" (*Tarasoff*, p. 347). Finally, the court did not specify that warning the intended victim was the only required response when danger arises; on the contrary, the court stated that the discharge of such duty may require the therapist to take one or more of various steps. (p. 6)

*Post-*Tarasoff

Since the *Tarasoff* trial, other courts have ruled that liability should not be imposed on the therapist if a victim was not identified (*Thompson v. County of Alameda*, 1980). However, other courts have ruled that the potential victim need only be foreseeably identifiable (*Jablonski v. United States*, 1983) or that the danger need only be foreseeable (*Hedlund v. Superior Court of Orange County*, 1983; *Lipari v. Sears Roebuck*, 1980). Mental health professionals have been found liable for not using prior patient records to predict violence (*Jablonski v. United States*, 1983) and for keeping inadequate records (*Peck v. The Counseling Service of Addison County*, 1985). A Florida appellate court ruled that *Tarasoff* should not be imposed because the relationship of trust and confidence, necessary for the therapeutic process, would be harmed if mental health professionals were required to warn potential victims (*Boynton v. Burglass*, 1991). According to Walcott, Cerundolo, and Beck (2001), the general movement of the courts in recent years has been to limit rather than expand *Tarasoff*.

Risk Assessment for Potentially Dangerous Clients

Walcott and his colleagues (2001) provided two basic guidelines for assessing danger in clients that would prompt the counselor to dispatch the duty to warn and protect others. First, counselors should determine if the client has a specific individual whom they wish to do harm, and, second, counselors need to assess the client's history of violence. If both a specific person is named and a history of violence is present, counselors would seem to have greater responsibility to warn and protect. Appelbaum (1985) also presented a model for fulfilling the *Tarasoff* obligation, urging that clinicians treating potentially dangerous patients undertake a three-stage process of risk assessment and action.

1. The first task, *assessment* of the client, has two components:
   a. First, the therapist must gather the data to evaluate the level of danger.
   b. Second, he/she must make a determination of dangerousness on the basis of that data.
2. The second tasks involves the clinician in *choosing a course of action* to protect potential victims when he/she has determined that a client is likely to be dangerous.
3. The third task entails the therapist implementing his/her decisions appropriately. This task has two components:
   a. First, the therapist must take action to protect potential victims.
   b. Second, he/she must monitor the situation on a continuing basis to assess the success or failure of the initial response, the likelihood that the patient will be violent, and the need for further measures (Appelbaum, 1985, p. 426).

Task I: Risk Assessment

Information needed to assess the level of danger can be found in the client's past and current history of behaviors, demographic factors, psychological diagnoses, and various other risk areas shown to increase the likelihood of violence. A thorough risk assessment should be gathered in the clinical counseling interview. Otto (2000) pointed out that there are various means of risk assessment, including structured and clinical interviews, as well as assessment tools. Webster, Douglas, Eaves, and Hart (1997) authored the HCR-20, a tool for conducting a structured interview when evaluating violent behavior in clients. The HCR-20 aids the counselor in assessing historical factors, clinical factors, and risk-related factors that increase a client's likelihood for violence. Otto (2000) provided an excellent overview of areas to which counselors should attend when conducting a clinical risk assessment. He noted that there are demographic factors that increase likelihood of violence; for instance, people in their late teens to early 40s are more prone to commit violence than those younger or older. In addition, men tend to have a higher prevalence toward violent crimes and acts than do women. Otto (2000) also recommended that counselors assess the following areas, as they form a constellation of factors that increase risk:

■ history of past violent or criminal behavior (this is one of the most reliable predictors of future violence) and start of violent behavior at an early age;

- history of and current use of substances;
- history of child abuse, maltreatment, or neglect;
- presence of a mental illness and presence of hallucinations in which the client hears a command to commit a violent act;
- perception that one is being threatened by others or outside forces;
- difficulty in dealing with life stressors;
- a disposition to be impulsive or respond angrily to stressors without thinking about options;
- presence of significant life stressors, such as financial stressors, unemployment, relationship difficulties, etc.; and
- lack of personal support systems.

The following questions and guidelines, based on the above-mentioned areas that increase risk of harm to others, can be used by counselors to help determine the potential for violent behavior:

1. Does the client have a history of violent behavior? Past violence is the best predictor of future violence.
2. Does the client have a history of violent conduct with a previous assessment or diagnosis of mental illness?
3. Does the client have a history of arrests for violent conduct?
4. Does the client have a history of threats associated with violent conflict?
5. Has the client ever been diagnosed with a mental disorder for which violence is a common symptom?
6. Has the client had at least one inpatient hospitalization associated with dangerous conduct, whether voluntary or involuntary?
7. Does the client have any history of dangerous conduct, apparently unprovoked and not stress related?
8. If the client has a history of dangerous conduct, how long ago was the incident? The more recent the dangerous behavior, the more likely it is that the behavior will be repeated.
9. If the client appears dangerous to someone else, document any threats, including clinical observations related to danger, and notify the person who might be harmed. Those acts that have a high degree of intent or intensity are most likely to recur.
10. Determine if any serious threats, attempts, or acts harmful to others have been related to drug or alcohol intoxication.
11. Ask the client direct and focused questions, such as "What is the most violent thing you have ever done?" and "How close have you come to becoming violent?" (Monahan, 1993, p. 244).
12. Use the reports of significant others. Often family members can provide valuable information about a client's potential for violence. Again, ask direct questions, such as "Are you worried that your loved one is going to hurt someone?" (Monahan, 1993, p. 244).
13. Has the client threatened others?
14. Does the client have access to weapons?
15. What is the client's relationship to the intended victim(s)?
16. Does the client belong to a social support group that condones violence?

Task II: Selecting a Course of Action

Once the mental health professional has assessed the danger a client poses to others, he/she must decide what to do. Use the following guidelines to help form an action plan:

1. *If the danger does not seem imminent, keep the client in intensified therapy.* Deal with the client's aggression as part of the treatment. However, if the client does not adhere to the treatment plan—that is, if he/she discontinues therapy—the danger level should be considered higher.
2. *Invite the client to participate in the disclosure decision.* This process often makes the client feel more in control. It is also prudent to contact the third party in the presence of the client. This may limit paranoia over what has been communicated.
3. *Attempt environmental manipulations.* Medication may be initiated, changed, or increased. Have the client get rid of any lethal weapons.
4. *Keep careful records.* When recording information relevant to risk, note the source of the information (e.g., the name of the spouse), the content (e.g., the character of the threat and the circumstances under which it was disclosed), and the date on which the information was disclosed. Finally, include your rationale for any decisions you make.
5. *If warning a third party is unavoidable, disclose only the minimum amount necessary to protect the victim or the public.* State the specific threat, but reserve any opinions or predictions.
6. *Consult with your supervisor.* Agencies or schools should have a contingency plan for such problems that is derived in consultation with an informed attorney, an area psychiatric facility, and local police (Bernes & Bardick, 2007).

Task III: Monitoring the Situation

Counselors should constantly monitor any course of action to ensure that the objectives of the initial implementation are satisfied. Follow-up procedures should be scrupulously adhered to and well documented. The Harm to Others Form (Form 10.2), which can be used in the facilitation of the assessment and monitoring process, is included in the Forms section at the end of the book.

Clients' Past Criminal Acts

There is a substantial body of literature that addresses what counselors and mental health professionals should do when working with a client who has the potential to act on criminal intent. However, a less addressed issue relates to what to do in the case of a client revealing involvement in past crimes against others. Appelbaum and Meisel (1986) reported that therapists' legal obligations to report past criminal acts differ under state and federal laws. Under federal law, therapist obligations fall under a statute of "misprision of a felony." Appelbaum and Meisel (1986) noted these conditions as necessary to establish guilt for a misprision of a felony:

1. The principal committed and completed the felony alleged.
2. The defendant had full knowledge of the fact.
3. The defendant failed to notify authorities.
4. The defendant took an affirmative step to conceal the crime.

The mere failure to report the crime does not appear to meet the criteria of affirmative concealment. If the mental health professional is questioned by law enforcement officials, he/she must respond truthfully but is not obligated to break confidentiality; it does not appear that the mental health professional has an obligation to say anything at all. Few states have statutes addressing misprision of a felony. Most do require the reporting of gunshot wounds, child abuse, or other specified evidence of certain crimes. Walfish, Barnett, Marlyere, and Zielke (2010) examined the incidence of clients reporting past crimes to their therapists and found that it was not infrequent, which provides good reason for counselors to be familiar with their state laws regarding disclosure of past and unprosecuted crimes.

The Client Who Is Being Abused: Responding, Reporting, and Intervening

People who are victims of abuse can be of any age, race, ethnicity, educational level, and socio-economic status. Intervening on behalf of persons who are being abused is critical in all instances. However, intervening on behalf of children who are being neglected, maltreated, or abused is critical because of the known deleterious effects of childhood maltreatment on normal human development. This section highlights the signs and symptoms of childhood abuse, recommends a course of action for reporting child abuse, and also provides a list of suggested therapeutic approaches for working with adult survivors of childhood abuse.

According to the Children's Bureau, an affiliate of the United States Department of Health and Human Services (DHHS), approximately 3.4 million cases of child abuse were reported to child protective agencies in the United States during the year 2011 (US Department of Health and Human Services, 2011). In addition, it can be conservatively estimated that at least five students have been or will be reported as being possible victims of abuse in a typical teacher's classroom per year in the United States. Sadly, the Children's Bureau also reported that in 2011 an estimated 1,570 children died from abuse and maltreatment.

Child abuse is "an act of omission or commission causing intentional harm or endangerment to the child under age 18" (Bryant & Milsom, 2005, p. 63). Abuse is understood to include sexual, physical, and emotional harm, as well as neglect. Examples of abuse to which counselors must be alert include adults using children for their own sexual gratification, intentionally inflicting physical harm, or threatening or terrorizing a child in such a way that it harms the child's self-esteem. Neglect can be defined to include the failure to provide necessary food, care, clothing, shelter, supervision, or medical attention for a child (i.e., malnourished, ill-clad, dirty, without proper shelter or sleeping arrangements, lacking appropriate health care, unattended, lacking adequate supervision, ill and lacking essential medical attention; irregular or illegal absences from school; exploited, overworked, lacking essential psychological nurturing; abandonment).

Recognizing Child Abuse*

The Child

You should consider the possibility of abuse when the child

- shows sudden changes in behavior or school performance;
- has not received help for physical or medical problems brought to the parents' attention;
- has learning problems that cannot be attributed to specific physical or psychological causes;
- is always watchful as though preparing for something to happen;
- lacks adult supervision;

- is overly compliant, an overachiever, or too responsible; or
- comes to school early, stays late, and does not want to go home.

The Parent

You should consider the possibility of abuse when the parent

- shows little concern for the child, rarely responding to the school's request for information, for conferences, or for home visits;
- denies the existence of or blames the child for the child's problems in school or at home;
- asks the classroom teacher to use harsh physical discipline if the child misbehaves;
- sees the child as entirely bad, worthless, or burdensome;
- demands perfection or a level of physical or academic performance the child cannot achieve; or
- looks primarily to the child for care, attention, and satisfaction of emotional needs.

The Parent and Child

You should consider the possibility of abuse when the parent and child

- rarely touch or look to each other,
- consider their relationship entirely negative, or
- state that they do not like each other.

None of these signs proves that child abuse is present in a family. Any of them may be found in any parent or child at one time or another, but when these signs appear repeatedly or in combination, they should cause the counselor to take a closer look at the situation and to consider the possibility of child abuse. That second look may reveal further signs of abuse or signs of a particular kind of child abuse.

Signs of Physical Abuse

Consider the possibility of physical abuse when the child

- has unexplained burns, bites, bruises, broken bones, or black eyes;
- has fading bruises or other marks noticeable after an absence from school;
- seems frightened of the parents and protests or cries when it is time to go home from school;
- shrinks at the approach of an adult; or
- reports injury by a parent or another adult caregiver.

Consider the possibility of physical abuse when the parent or other adult caregiver

- offers conflicting, unconvincing, or no explanation for the child's injury;
- describes the child as "evil" or in some other very negative way;
- uses harsh physical discipline with the child; or
- has a history of abuse as a child.

Signs of Neglect

You should consider the possibility of neglect when the child

- is frequently absent from school;
- begs or steals food or money from classmates;

- lacks needed medical or dental care, immunizations, or glasses;
- is constantly dirty or has severe body odor;
- lacks sufficient clothing for the weather;
- abuses alcohol or other drugs; or
- states that there is no one at home to provide care.

You should consider the possibility of neglect when the parent or caregiver

- appears to be indifferent to the child,
- seems apathetic or depressed,
- behaves irrationally or in a bizarre manner, or
- is abusing alcohol or other drugs.

Signs of Sexual Abuse

You should consider the possibility of sexual abuse when the child

- has difficulty sitting or walking;
- suddenly refuses to change for gym or to participate in physical activities;
- demonstrates bizarre, sophisticated, or unusual sexual knowledge or behavior;
- becomes pregnant or contracts a venereal disease, particularly if younger than 14 years of age;
- runs away; or
- reports sexual abuse by a parent or another adult caregiver.

You should consider the possibility of sexual abuse when the parent or caregiver

- is unduly protective of the child and severely limits the child's contact with other children, especially of the opposite sex,
- is secretive and isolated, or
- describes marital difficulties involving family power struggles or sexual relations.

Signs of Emotional Maltreatment

Consider the possibility of emotional maltreatment when the child

- shows extremes in behavior, such as overly compliant or demanding behavior, extreme passivity, or aggressiveness;
- is either inappropriately adult (e.g., parenting other children) or inappropriately infantile (e.g., frequently rocking or head banging);
- is delayed in physical or emotional development;
- has attempted suicide; or
- reports a lack of attachment to the parent.

Consider the possibility of emotional maltreatment when the parent or other adult caregiver

- constantly blames, belittles, or berates the child;
- is unconcerned about the child and refuses to consider offers of help for the child's school problems; or
- overly rejects the child.

*Copyright 2013. Permission to reprint granted by Prevent Child Abuse America.

Legal Issues Related to Reporting Child Abuse

Mandated reporters usually are professionals who interact with children in the course of their work. The federal Child Abuse Prevention and Treatment Act (US Department of Health and Human Services, 2003) requires that sexual, physical, and psychological exploitation of children be reported. *Any circumstance that indicates serious harm or threat to a child's welfare must be reported.* Confidentiality and privileged communication are not legal reasons for failing to report abuse. The laws against child abuse supersede the laws of privilege and the ethical mandates of confidentiality (Lambie, 2005). Thus, it is critical that counselors are familiar with the laws in their state that govern their responses to child abuse. State laws can vary with regard to the threshold required to trigger a report to child protective services agencies (Marshall, 2012). For example, some states require that counselors make a report if they suspect that abuse has occurred, while other states have laws that oblige a report if the clinician suspects abuse has occurred or *is likely to occur* (Marshall, 2012). In addition, states have varying definitions of what constitutes abuse, and definitions differ with regard to the specificity of how abuse is delimited. For example, the states of Georgia and Washington are the only ones that do not include psychological abuse in their statutes on child abuse (US Department of Health and Human Services, 2009). It is helpful to keep in mind that if the abuse is reported in good faith, most states do not allow retribution; that is, the mental health professional cannot be sued for defamation of character even if the abuse report is unfounded. Most states do not have a statute of limitations on child abuse cases, unless the abuse was reported previously and the charges were dismissed. This suggests that mental health professionals must report abuse that occurred many years ago. Counselors may be liable in civil lawsuits for failure to report suspected abuse, though no criminal cases have come against counselors in this regard (Lambie, 2005).

Making a Report Related to Child Abuse

Therapists who decide to file a child abuse report typically do so by calling the appropriate social service agency. They must file a written report subsequent to the call. A caseworker will be assigned to the case by the child protective services agency. If the caseworker finds probable evidence that neglect or abuse has occurred, he/she refers the case to a law enforcement agency. At that point, the state either begins a criminal prosecution or takes civil action. If someone other than a parent or caretaker accuses a parent of sexually abusing a child, authorities may initiate both criminal and civil proceedings simultaneously (Bryant & Milsom, 2005). It should be noted that one difficulty in making a report of suspected child abuse is that clinicians may be obliged even if the child does not want the report made and even if the mental health professional does not feel it is in the best interest of the child to do so (Sikes, Remley, & Hays, 2010). Marshall (2012) pointed out that the decision-making process around reporting can be tricky and demands nuanced development of clinical skills. For example, she noted that clinicians will have to determine, in the instance of emotional abuse, the level of abuse that is occurring and consider that evaluation in deciding whether or not to make a report. A clinician will have to assess if the actions on the part of a parent or caregiver are the result of poor, underdeveloped, but nonmalicious parenting skills that can be addressed therapeutically or if the style of interaction with the child is consistently harmful and pernicious enough to constitute abuse. A Child Abuse Reporting Form (Form 10.3) is included in the Forms section. This asks the therapist to record basic information required to make an initial call to the authorities and to file a formal written report. The Child Abuse Reporting Form shows the required information a counselor needs to have prior to filing a report of child abuse.

Interviewing Children Who May Have Been Sexually Abused

Therapists working with young children on possible sexual abuse must be aware that the language, cognition, and logic systems of children are different from those of adults; in other words, children are not miniature adults. A child's vocabulary is much more limited, which means that children understand much more than they can say. Counselors must learn specific interviewing techniques and clinical skills to work with young children (Mart, 2010). For instance, the use of pronouns, double negatives, and compound sentences should not be employed in the interview. Instead, the counselor should focus on familiar events; for example, "Did this take place after your birthday or before your birthday?"

Children remember what happened, but their causal connections are not the same as those of adults. If they have been sexually abused, they may think (indeed, they most often do) that they caused the abuse. Thus, counselors should carefully assess the developmental level and capabilities of their young clients before interviewing them. For example, Berliner and Lieb (2001) suggested assessing younger children's cognitive ability to distinguish between the truth and a falsehood by using concrete examples and questions. In addition, children often are afraid they will no longer be loved; are guilty, ashamed, and afraid they will get into trouble; and may even fear harm or death (their own or others') if the sexual abuse is disclosed.

Before the Interview

It is not possible to predetermine how long the interview should be. The ideal time is one that allows the truth of the matter to purge itself. The therapist should have information pertinent to the history of the case before starting the interview. Information such as the child's name, nicknames, family members' names, and when and where the disclosure was made will contribute to the counselor's efficacy before and during the interview.

Interviewing the Child

The main ingredient for veracity in an interview is the introduction of support and rapport (Mart, 2010). Berliner and Lieb (2001) suggested that a clinical interview of a child who may be a victim of abuse should begin with a good deal of relationship building. The counselor should spend some time getting to know the child by asking about his/her hobbies, schoolwork, things a child likes to do, favorite teacher or subject in school, and so on. It is also important that the therapist appear to be on the same level as the child. This requires an atmosphere that is comfortable. The counselor should be able to get down on the floor or on a pillow and make eye contact with the child. Eye contact is essential when communicating to a child that he/she is not at fault and that what happened was hurtful. It is important to remember that the effects of sexual abuse are pervasive and emotionally difficult for the rest of the child's life. After establishing some rapport, the interviewer may want to get a sense of the child's level of development related to episodic memory, or memory for events that have taken place in his/her life. Asking the child to talk about a recent school happening or a holiday, for example, can give the counselor some insight into how developed the child's ability to accurately recall the details of life events is. In the course of the interview, the counselor will want to transition the conversation to the critical issue of abuse at hand. The interviewer can do this by beginning to ask the child to speak about his/her home environment (e.g., who lives at home with the child?) and then asking the child if he/she knows why the interview is taking place. Focused and open-ended questions about the incident(s) of concern eventually must be addressed. For example, the interviewer might say, "I heard that something happened to you. Tell me from the beginning to the end what happened." Supporting a child emotionally and responding to displays of distress is of utmost importance during an interview (Berliner & Lieb, 2001).

The interviewer must not overreact to any statements the child makes. Some interviews may include interested third parties. The third party may even be the perpetrator or someone from whom the child is keeping a secret. Third parties should be directed to go to the side of the room, where they are not directly part of the interview. The therapist should arrange the parties so that eye contact is not possible between the child and adult. Above all, third parties must be instructed that they are not to be part of the interview.

Therapists must be careful not to ask leading questions. Brainer, Reyna, and Brandse (1996) reported how easy it was to implant memories of events that never happened in 5- to 8-year-old children by suggestion alone. What is more, the implanted false memories often were remembered in more detail than real memories. The biggest danger in examinations of potential sexual abuse is the interviewer who asks leading questions. Questions should be specific; most important, they should not suggest an answer. A question such as "Is it true your Uncle John did this to you?" is leading and may put pressure on the child to answer affirmatively. Likewise, if the child says, "Uncle John touched me," an appropriate response would be "Where did Uncle John touch you?" Asking "Did he touch you on your private parts?" is, again, leading the child. Finally, counselors should be careful to remember that what they conceptualize as sexual abuse may not be experienced in that way by a child, and thus questions that assume distress on the part of the child may not fit a child's understanding of sexuality or abuse (Mart, 2010; Freidrich et al., 2001). Interviewing children is a clinical art form; mental health professionals who conduct such interviews should receive considerable supervised training in this area.

Counseling the Sexually Abused

There are many approaches to counseling people who have a history of childhood sexual abuse, and in a meta-analysis conducted by Martsolf and Draucker (2005), no one therapeutic approach was shown to be more effective than another. What seems important is creating a therapeutic environment that is safe and that allows for the disclosure of the abuse events. Advocating for a person-centered approach, Edwards and Lambie (2009) emphasized positive regard, genuineness, and empathy as key components to helping survivors feel comfortable with the counseling process. Other approaches incorporate cognitive behavioral methods as well as trauma assessments. Harrison (2001, pp. 91–92) discussed several general considerations for therapy with sexual abuse survivors:

1. On the basis of statistics, survivors of sexual abuse are probably telling the truth, so the counselor begins treatment with each client by adopting this assumption.
2. It is not the survivor's fault in any way. The responsibility for the assault or abuse rests solely with the perpetrator.
3. The counselor's initial goal is help the survivor regain a sense of personal control. He/she has had personal power taken away in a manner that affected him/her emotionally, physically, and spiritually.
4. Secondary goals of therapy include building self-esteem, moving toward autonomy, and training in coping skills, anger management, and assertive skills aimed at prevention of sexual abuse in the future.

Harrison (2001) further suggested an expansive list of dos and don'ts of therapy. The list was compiled from various sources, including the Minnesota Coalition Against Sexual Assault (1994) and Slavik, Carlson, and Sperry (1993).

1. Do ensure a safe environment and presence in sessions. If it appears that the abuse is ongoing, enlist help from the appropriate social service agencies to remove the client from an abusive environment so that healing may begin.
2. Do return a sense of control by encouraging clients to solve problems, elicit new choices, and then trust their own judgments to arrive at their own decisions. Also distinguish between then, when the client felt helpless during the sexual abuse, and now.
3. Do not minimize the client's experience. A client once said that a previous therapist's reaction had been to say, "Well, at least he didn't beat you up when he raped you."
4. Do listen to, support, acknowledge, and validate feelings.
5. Do not be a caretaker or rescuer.
6. Do not address the myths about sexual abuse and reeducate clients, especially the prevalent myth that victims are at least partially to blame for the sexual abuse.
7. Do trust the healing and support process, and ask a client to do so, reminding him/her that the time frame will vary for each individual.
8. Do model setting boundaries, for example, by starting and stopping sessions on time.
9. Do be aware of your own blind spots and question your assumptions. Don't assume that the perpetrator was of the opposite sex or that the act involved penetration.
10. Don't judge or use a patronizing manner. Many clients who have been sexually abused have later become very sexually active, some involved in group sex, pornography, and prostitution. If you see yourself as on the same plane as your client, then you will not be patronizing. Many clients verbalize that they take little or no enjoyment in sex, even with a caring partner, yet they feel obligated to perform sexual acts. You must be aware that this hypersexual behavior is based not on self-gratification but on mistaken ideas.
11. Do confer with colleagues and practice self-care.
12. Do listen with a calm curiosity about the sexual assault or abuse when the client is ready to discuss it.
13. Do accept unconditionally the client's ambivalent feelings about discussing the abuse.
14. Do not treat the revelation of sexual abuse as a crisis, because it is important that clients see themselves as having survived something that happened in the past and as now being able to move forward toward their goals.
15. Do see clients as capable of new ways of thinking, feeling, and acting and expect them to be competent and creative.
16. Do not see clients as fragile, although they may act as if they are.
17. Do help clients get in touch with unexpressed anger to combat depression, and teach them how to make choices about using their anger constructively rather than destructively.
18. Do help clients to redefine themselves apart from their role relationships and to explore fears about potential role changes.
19. Do encourage clients to nurture themselves, and reframe this self-focus as essential to healing, not as selfish.
20. Do be specific in giving positive feedback. Note any improvement in grounding skills, especially with a client who may experience either dissociative states or flashbacks. Other

examples might include the client's improvement in "discussing goals" and determining an issue on which to work, bodily awareness, interpersonal skills, keeping of social supports, work skills, and parenting skills (Slavek et al., 1993, pp. 113–114).

The Client Who Is Dealing With Addiction

In this final section, we look at the issue of addiction, which is likely to be an issue that nearly every mental health profession will encounter whether or not he/she works in a specifically designated addictions treatment facility. The information provided below relates primarily to recovery from addiction to a substance (e.g., alcohol or drugs). However, there is growing evidence for the existence of process addictions for which the counselor should be prepared, such as gambling addiction, sexual addiction, and the like.

Understanding Addiction

Until recently, conceptualizations of substance abuse generally adhered to the categories of use, abuse, and dependence, which suggested that people either had an addiction or they did not. Abuse was conceptualized as the mild form of addiction, while dependence was conceptualized as the more severe occurrence of addiction (American Psychiatric Association, 2013b). Current conceptualizations of substance addiction are that it occurs along a continuum, a view advocated by the American Psychiatric Association (2013a) in the *Diagnostic and Statistical Manual of Mental Disorders* (5th ed.; *DSM-5*). Not everyone who uses substances is addicted, and, moreover, clinicians are increasingly recognizing the developmental aspects of addiction. People are not necessarily seen as either having an addiction or not, but are viewed as moving along a path toward greater and greater disordered use of substances or behaviors when their use of substances or behaviors has ongoing adverse effects. In addition, alcohol and drug addiction is often conceived of as a disease that over time causes changes in the person's body, mind, and behavior, and the individual is unable to control his/her use of substances despite the harm that it causes. The chronicity and relapsing of the disease means that an addiction may persist or reappear over the course of an individual's life (Breshears, Yeh, & Young, 2004).

Diagnosing Alcohol and Drug Use

The *DSM-5* (American Psychiatric Association, 2013a) recognizes 10 classes of drugs for which qualified practitioners and supervised interns can make the diagnosis of addiction; it also includes criteria for diagnosis of gambling addiction, as there is a growing body of evidence that some of the same behavior patterns and symptoms associated with substance use are similarly associated with excessive gambling. There are two broad categories of diagnosis in the *DSM-5* that deal with substance-related addiction: substance-induced disorders and substance use disorders. Substance-induced disorders emerge as a result of use and include intoxication, withdrawal, and substance-induced mental illness, such as depression, anxiety, psychosis, and sleep disorders. Substance use disorders involve sets of behavioral, cognitive, emotional, social, psychological, and physiological responses to use that are problematic for a user; in addiction, these symptoms tend to persist even though they are negative. The *DSM-5* (American Psychiatric Association, 2013a) describes a person with substance use disorder as having a pathological relationship to his/her substance of choice, and any number of symptoms can be present with this type of relationship. For example, clients may desire to stop using their substance of choice but be incapable of doing so; they may have cravings for their drug of choice and concurrently need more and more of the drug to be satisfied; they may spend an inordinate amount of time thinking about or trying to obtain the substance; they may experience many social consequences such as loss of a job or divorce; and they may engage in risky behaviors in the effort to obtain the substance.

When making a diagnosis, it is important to remember that the *DSM-5* (American Psychiatric Association, 2013a) considers substance use as part of a continuum. Therefore, it has collapsed the two diagnostic categories of substance abuse and dependence (as outlined in former editions of the *DSM*) into a single disorder known as substance use disorder, for which clinicians will indicate a mild or moderate form after conducting a clinical assessment (American Psychiatric Association, 2013b). According to the American Psychiatric Association (2013b) the former categories of abuse and dependence were not always clear to clinicians and clients, and the association stated that the single diagnostic category of substance use disorder is a better reflection of clients' experiences (American Psychiatric Association, 2013b). We recommend that students make a careful review of the diagnostic criteria and categories as outlined in the *DSM-5* and seek supervision before engaging in diagnosis and treatment of substance-related disorders.

What Is Treatment?

A number of alcohol and drug treatment models are used successfully, and treatment can include a variety of services and activities. Levels of treatment can range from outpatient, day treatment, and short- and long-term residential programs to inpatient hospital-based programs. Prior to beginning treatment, some individuals require detoxification and stabilization. Other individuals may need outreach services to help overcome barriers to treatment. Treatment may involve a single service or a combination of therapies and services. The following is a partial list of treatment services:

- assessment and treatment planning;
- prescription of certain drugs, such as Antabuse for alcohol dependence or methadone and buprenephrine for heroin addiction (Arias & Kranzler, 2008);
- crisis intervention;
- case management to coordinate among the treatment providers;
- individual and group counseling and psychotherapy;
- alcohol and drug abuse recovery programs;
- medical assessment and care;
- diet, physical exercise, and other nontraditional programs;
- self-help groups or 12-step programs; or
- trauma-specific services or other mental health services.

The duration of treatment can range from weeks to years. The type, length, and intensity of treatment are determined by the severity of the addiction, type of drugs used, support systems available, personality, and other behavioral, physical, or social problems of the addicted person. It is important to think about treatment as management of a lifelong disease such as diabetes or high blood pressure rather than as crisis intervention such as emergency treatment for a broken leg. The treatment plan should be developed based on information gathered in the substance abuse assessment process (Breshears et al., 2004).

The National Institute on Drug Abuse ([NIDA], 2012) has developed a number of research-based treatment principles that are important to the recovery process:

- No single treatment is appropriate for all individuals. Treatment and services should be matched to the person's problems and needs.
- Treatment needs to be readily available.
- Effective treatment attends to multiple needs of the individual, not just to his/her drug use.
- Medical, psychological, social, vocational, and legal problems must be addressed in addition to substance addiction.
- Remaining in treatment for an adequate period of time is critical for effectiveness.
- Treatment does not need to be voluntary to be effective. Court-ordered treatment, an employment mandate, or family insistence can increase treatment entry, retention, and success.
- Possible drug use during treatment must be monitored continuously. Monitoring can help reduce the desire to use and provide early warning of use if a slip or relapse occurs.
- Recovery from drug addiction can be a long-term process and frequently requires multiple episodes of treatment.

What Is Recovery?

Treatment does not equal recovery. Treatment is an important part of recovery, but recovery is much more than obtaining sobriety. Recovery is a process of making lifestyle changes to support healing and to regain control of one's life. Recovery involves being accountable and accepting responsibility for one's behavior. It is the process of establishing and reestablishing patterns of healthy living. Former addicts talk about being "in recovery" as opposed to having "recovered," because recovery is viewed as an ongoing process.

Stages of Recovery

There are different stages of recovery. A person who has been drug free for a week and one who has been drug free for a year experience different issues. Recovery is complicated. It may be helpful to view recovery as a developmental process. The developmental model of recovery describes stages and tasks as part of recovery:

- *Transition:* The person recognizes that his/her attempts to control substance use are not working.
- *Stabilization:* The person goes through physical withdrawal and begins to regain control of his/her thinking and behavior.
- *Early recovery:* The person changes addictive behaviors and develops relationships that support sobriety and recovery.
- *Middle recovery stage:* The person builds a more effective lifestyle and repairs lifestyle damage that occurred during substance use.
- *Last recovery stage:* The person examines his/her childhood, family patterns, and beliefs that supported a dysfunctional lifestyle, and the person learns to grow and recover from childhood and adult trauma.
- *Maintenance stage:* The person learns to cope in a productive and responsible way without reverting to substance use.

Counseling Recommendations for Clients With Addiction

It is important for counselors who work with clients who have a substance use disorder to adopt an objective and factual approach to assessment interviews. As many clients enter treatment for substance-related problems because of external pressures (i.e., family, employers, the legal system), the counselor must convey an impression that he/she is an ally to the client in addressing his/her problems (Burrow-Sanchez, 2006). In asking assessment questions, the counselor should use objective criteria as a guideline and proceed in a nonjudgmental and matter-of-fact way. In addition, it is helpful to work with a client's resistance to counseling, rather than to confront it outright, especially in the beginning of a clinical relationship. Initial interviewing goals include establishing a flow of information and disclosure about the client's level of motivation for treatment and obtaining the necessary information to formulate an objective impression. The counselor should relay the results of the assessment interview to the client in the same objective fashion and emphasize that the assessment is based on the information the client provided and on data from assessment instruments. This process may help the client work though treatment resistance as well as reinforce the therapeutic alliance. Below are some general guidelines for working with substance-abusing clients:

1. *Understand the emotional role the substance of choice plays for the client.* A central challenge for the counselor is to identify the client's rationale for using a mood-altering substance. Almost invariably that rationale has an affective base (i.e., substance use to avoid or escape negative situations or to acquire a desired affective state). Once the affective motivation is established, the counselor can undertake treatment to develop adaptive coping responses. Therapists should be cautious in immediately addressing traumatic issues if the client has had only a brief period of abstinence or if affect tolerance or modulation appears tenuous.

2. *Identify the internal and external triggering events for substance cravings and impulses.* Substance-using impulses are often precipitated by events that may or may not be evident to the client. The counselor needs to detect the internal (i.e., thoughts, feelings, memories, attitudes) and external (i.e., interpersonal conflicts, social isolation, interpersonal/existential losses) antecedents for the client's substance use impulses and cravings. Helping the client identify these triggers when they occur allows him/her to implement substance-avoidance behaviors. Once substance triggers are identified, specific plans for coping with them can be constructed.

3. *Confront internal versus external locus of control regarding substance-using behaviors.* Many substance-abusing clients rationalize their substance use by either relinquishing responsibility for control ("I can't help it") or externalizing control over their behavior ("My boss makes me use—he's so demanding"). The counselor must confront the client by reflecting that he/she ultimately chooses to use a substance regardless of the circumstances. Once clients accept this reality, controlling the impulses to use becomes a treatment focus.

4. *Challenge substance dependence–reinforcing cognitions (i.e., beliefs and thinking styles).* Many substance-abusing clients present belief systems that reinforce chemical dependency ("Without my crack, I can't deal with life" or "I need a drink to control myself"). The counselor should challenge such maladaptive cognitions.

5. *Help the client learn and apply abstaining behaviors.* Coping with cravings and impulses is a vital therapeutic goal. A useful resistance skill is for the client to focus on previous negative consequences of substance use when he/she experiences cravings or impulses. This technique

shifts the psychological focus from the desired and expected immediate mood-altering effect to the association of the substance with emotionally negative events. This technique of "thinking the craving through" can divert clients from impulsiveness and make them aware of adaptive options. Counselors should review with clients the distinctions between thinking, feeling, and doing (physical action).

6. *Practice therapeutic rather than antagonistic confrontation.* As treatment engagement on the part of the client is critical, the counselor must be careful not to confuse confrontation with intolerance. Therapeutic confrontation occurs when the counselor presents the client with concrete examples of clinical material representative of the disorder. Therapeutic confrontation is based on objective data or behavior that the client presents, not on a conflict of personal values. Attempts to impose guilt or shame on the client increase the potential for treatment dropout.

7. *Establish healthy developmental goals.* An important part of counseling substance-abusing clients is addressing the frequent developmental disturbances that accompany maladaptive patterns of substance use (dropping out of school, getting fired from jobs, having family disruptions, etc.). Part of the treatment plan should include a return (perhaps gradually) to normal and productive functioning. Frustration and anxiety tolerance may be a central focus, depending on the severity and duration of psychosocial disturbances.

A Substance Abuse Assessment Form (Form 10.4) is included in the Forms section at the end of the book. This form provides questions for the intern to use when working with substance-abusing clients.

Preventing Relapse

Relapse, or the full-blown use of drugs or alcohol after a period of non-use, is a typical experience in long-term recovery and should be anticipated in the same way that relapse occurs with the management of other chronic diseases or illnesses (Burrow-Sanchez, 2006; NIDA, 2012). Behaviorally, relapse prevention can be seen as one set of operationalized target behaviors implemented and practiced consistently over time that results in another set of targeted undesired behaviors being discontinued. Below are some general framework suggestions for an operationalized psychoactive substance relapse prevention program:

1. *Help the client identify high-risk situations.* High-risk situations may include attending social events where substance use is prominent or spending time at places where substances are readily available. Being aware of high-risk situations alerts the client to consider avoidance or to apply specific behavior plans for increasing controls to maintain abstinence (Witkiewitz & Marlatt, 2004).

2. *Help the client make necessary lifestyle changes and relationship modifications.* The client must gain awareness of specific lifestyle behaviors (theft, prostitution, drug sales, etc.) that are specifically related to the substance-using pattern. Often the client must change those behavior patterns to maximize the prognosis for abstinence. Likewise, specific relationships that reinforce substance use must be confronted, modified, or even discontinued until the client has gained sufficient behavioral and impulse controls to withstand the influence of others who advocate substance use.

3. *Reduce access to psychoactive substances.* A strategic component of relapse prevention is reducing access to psychoactive substances. This may occur by removing psychoactive

substances from the client's residence, eliminating routine purchases of substances (alcohol), or identifying specific places (high-risk situations) where substances are readily available or promoted.

4. *Address any underlying psychopathology.* Untreated psychiatric disorders (or psychopathology) constitute one of the most common reasons for psychoactive substance relapse (NIDA, 2012). Mood, anxiety, or personality disorders or other forms of psychopathology that persist into the abstinence period should be formally evaluated and treated. Using simultaneous combination treatments (psychotherapy, pharmacotherapy, family therapy, and self-help groups) may be most advantageous.

5. *Help the client rebound from a relapse.* Relapses happen; in specific patient subtypes (i.e., severe personality disorders, untreated mood or anxiety disorders), they may be common. The counselor must be clinically prepared for relapse and assure the client that a relapse should not be viewed fatalistically but rather as a mistake with the current treatment focus. Relapses can be used as restarting points in treatment if therapeutic engagement is maintained.

Summary

This chapter addressed the key issues in dealing with clients who are harmful to themselves or others, abused clients, survivors of sexual abuse, substance-abusing clients, and victims of crisis. These populations are commonly encountered in standard therapeutic settings, and the student will likely work with them throughout the internship. Thus, it is important that interns familiarize themselves with the issues that can arise in therapy and the special considerations that must be made when determining appropriate interventions. The intervention strategies and clinical forms provided were designed to assist the counselor or therapist in the treatment and reporting of critical client data.

References

Aguilera, D. C. (1998). *Crisis intervention: Theory and methodology* (8th ed.). St. Louis, MO: Mosby.

American Academy of Experts in Traumatic Stress. (2003). *Teacher guidelines for crisis response.* Retrieved from www.schoolcrisisresponse.com/teacherguidelines.pdf.

American Association of Suicidology. (2007). *Youth suicide fact sheet.* Retrieved from http://211bigbend.net/PDFs/YouthSuicideFactSheet.pdf.

American Counseling Association. (2005). *Code of ethics.* Alexandria, VA: Author.

American Psychiatric Association. (2003). *American Psychiatric Association Practice Guideline for the assessment and treatment of suicidal behaviors.* Arlington, VA: Author.

American Psychiatric Association. (2013a). *Diagnostic and statistical manual of mental disorders* (5th ed.). Washington, DC: Author.

American Psychiatric Association. (2013b). *Substance-related and addictive disorders.* Washington, DC: Author. Retrieved from www.psychiatry.org/practice/dsm/dsm5.

American School Counselors Association. (2010). *Ethical standards for school counselors.* Alexandria, VA: Author.

Applebaum, P. S. (1985). *Tarasoff* and the clinician: Problems in fulfilling the duty to protect. *American Journal of Psychiatry, 142*(4), 425–429.

Applebaum, P. S., & Meisel, M. A. (1986). Therapists' obligations to report their patients' criminal acts. *Bulletin of the American Academy of Psychiatry and the Law, 14*(3), 221–229.

Arias, A. J., & Kranzler, H. R. (2008). Treatment of co-occurring alcohol and other drug use disorders. *Alcohol Research & Health, 31,* 155–167.

Barrio, C. A. (2007). Assessing suicide risk in children: Guidelines for developmentally appropriate interviewing. *Journal of Mental Health Counseling, 29,* 50–66.

Beauchamp, T. L. (1985). Suicide: Matters of life and death. *Suicide and Life-Threatening Behavior, 24*(2), 190–195.

Bednar, R. L., Bednar, S. C., Lambert, M. J., & Waite, D. R. (1991). *Psychology with high-risk clients: Legal and professional standards.* Pacific Grove, CA: Brooks/Cole.

Berliner, L., & Lieb, R. (2001). *Child sexual abuse investigation: Testing documentation methods.* Olympia, WA: Washington State Institute for Public Policy. Retrieved from www.wsipp.wa.gov/rptfiles/PilotProjects.pdf.

Bernes, K. B., & Bardick, A. D. (2007). Conducting adolescent violence risk assessments: A framework for school counselors. *Professional School Counselor, 10,* 419–427.

Boynton v. Burglass, No. 89-1409, Fla. Ct. App., 3d Dist. (September 24, 1991).

Brainer, C. J., Reyna, C. F., & Brandse, E. (1996). Are children's false memories more persistent than their true memories? *Psychological Science, 6*(6), 359–364.

Breshears, E. M., Yeh, S., & Young, N. K. (2004). *Understanding substance abuse and facilitating recovery: A guide for child welfare workers.* Rockville, MD: US Department of Health and Human Services, Substance Abuse and Mental Health Services Administration.

Bryant, J., & Milsom, A. (2005). Child abuse reporting by school counselors. *Professional School Counselor, 9,* 63–71.

Burrow-Sanchez, J. (2006). Understanding adolescent substance abuse: Prevalence, risk factors, and clinical implications. *Journal of Counseling & Development, 84,* 283–290.

Callahan, C. J. (1998). Crisis intervention model for teachers. *Journal of Instructional Psychology, 25,* 226–235.

Captain, C. (2006). Is your patient a suicide risk. *Nursing, 36*(8), 43–47.

Carlino v. State, 294 N.Y.S.2d 30 (1968).

Comiskey v. State of New York, 418 N.Y.S.2d 233 (1979).

Curtois, C. A., & Ford, J. D. (2013). *Treatment of complex trauma: A sequenced, relationship-based approach.* New York: Guilford.

Dalton v. State, 308 N.Y.S.2d 441 (App. Div. 1970).

Doan, J., LeBlanc, A., Roggenbaum, S., & Lazear, K. A. (2012). *Suicide prevention guidelines: Issue brief 5.* Tampa, FL: University of South Florida, College of Behavioral and Community Sciences, Louis de la Parte Florida Mental Health Institute, Department of Child & Family Studies (FMHI Series Publication #218-5 Rev 2012).

Edwards, N., & Lambie, G. (2009). A person-centered counseling approach as a primary therapeutic support for women with a history of childhood sexual abuse. *Journal of Humanistic Counseling, Education, and Development, 48,* 23–45.

Fowler, J. C. (2012). Suicide risk assessment in clinical practice: Pragmatic guidelines for imperfect assessments. *Psychotherapy, 49,* 81–90.

Freidrich, W. N., Fisher, J. L., Dittner, C. A., Acton, R., Berliner, L., Butler, J., et al. (2001). Child sexual behavior inventory: Normative, psychiatric, and sexual abuse comparisons. *Child Maltreatment, 6,* 37–49.

Fujimura, L. E., Weis, D. M., & Cochran, F. R. (1985). Suicide: Dynamics and implications for counseling. *Journal of Counseling and Development, 63,* 612–615.

Gould, M. S., Shaffer, D., & Greenberg, T. (2003). The epidemiology of youth suicide. In R. King & A. Apter (Eds.), *Suicide in children and adolescents* (pp. 1–40). New York: Cambridge University Press.

Granello, D. H. (2010). The process of suicide risk assessment: Twelve core principles. *Journal of Counseling & Development, 88*, 363–370.

Greene, D. B. (1994). Childhood suicide and myths surrounding it. *Social Work. 39*, 230–233.

Greenstone, J. L. & Leviton, S. C. (1993). Elements of crisis intervention. Pacific Grove, CA: Brooks/ Cole.

Harrison, R. (2001). Application of Adlerian principles in counseling survivors of sexual abuse. *Journal of Individual Psychology, 57*(1), 91–101.

Hedlund v. Superior Court of Orange County, 669 P.2d 41, 191 Cal. Rptr. 805 (1983).

Jablonski v. United States, 712 F.2d 391 (9th Cir. 1983).

James, R. K., & Gilliland, B. E. (2013). *Crisis intervention strategies* (7th ed.). Belmont, CA: Brooks/ Cole.

Joe, S., & Bryant, H. (2007). Evidence-based suicide prevention screening in schools. *Children & Schools, 29*, 219–227.

Joiner, T. E. (2005). *Why people die by suicide.* Cambridge, MA: Harvard University Press.

Joiner, T. E. (2010). *Myths about suicide.* Cambridge, MA: Harvard University Press.

Joiner, T., Kalafat, J., Draper, J., Stokes, H., Knudson, M., Berman, A., et al. (2007). Establishing standards for the assessment of suicide risk among callers to the national suicide prevention lifeline. *Suicide and Life-Threatening Behavior, 37*, 353–365.

Kanel, K. (2010). *A guide to crisis intervention.* Belmont, CA: Brooks/Cole.

Klott, J. (2012). *Suicide and psychological pain: Prevention that works.* Eau Claire, WI: Premier Publication and Media.

Lambie, G. W. (2005). Child abuse and neglect: A practical guide for professional school counselors. *Professional School Counseling, 8*, 249–258.

Lawson, D. M., Davis, D., & Brandon, S. (2013). Treating complex trauma: Critical interventions with adults who experienced ongoing trauma in childhood. *Psychotherapy, 50*, 331–335.

Lipari v. Sears Roebuck, 497 F. Supp. 185 (D. Neb. 1980).

Marshall, N. A. (2012). A clinician's guide to recognizing and reporting parental psychological maltreatment of children. *Professional Psychology: Research and Practice, 43*, 73–79.

Mart, E. G. (2010). Common errors in the assessment of allegations of child abuse. *Journal of Psychiatry and Law, 38*, 325–343.

Martsolf, D. S., & Draucker, C. B. (2005). Psychotherapy approaches for adult survivors of childhood sexual abuse: An integrative review of outcomes research. *Issues in Mental Health Nursing, 26*, 801–825.

McGlothlin, J. M., Rainey, S., & Kindsvatter, A. (2005). Suicidal clients and supervisees: A model for considering supervisor roles. *Counselor Education and Supervision, 45*, 134–146.

Meichenbaum, D. (2005). 35 years of working with suicidal patients: Lessons learned. *Canadian Psychology, 46*, 64–72.

Miller, D. N., Eckert, T. L., & Mazza, J. J. (2009). Suicide prevention programs in the school: A review and public health perspective. *School Psychology Review, 38*, 168–188.

Minnesota Coalition Against Sexual Assault. (1994). *Training manual.* Edina, MN: Author.

Monahan, J. (1993). Limiting therapist exposure to *Tarasoff* liability: Guidelines for risk containment. *American Psychologist, 48*, 242–250.

Moyer, M., & Sullivan, J. (2008). Student risk taking behaviors: When do school counselors break confidentiality? *Professional School Counselor, 11*, 236–245.

Murray, L. K., Cohen, J. A., & Mannarino, A. P. (2013). Trauma-focused cognitive behavioral therapy for youth who experience continuous traumatic exposure. *Peace and Conflict: Journal of Peace Psychology, 19*, 180–195.

Myer, R. A., & Cogdal, P. (2007). Crisis intervention in counseling. In J. Gregoire & C. M. Jungers (Eds.), *The counselor's companion: What every beginning counselor needs to know* (pp. 550–566). Mahwah, NJ: Erlbaum.

Myer, R. A., Lewis, J. S., & James, R. K. (2013). The introduction of a task model for crisis intervention. *Journal of Mental Health Counseling, 35*, 95–107.

Myer, R. A., & Moore, H. B. (2006). Crisis in context theory: An ecological model. *Journal of Counseling & Development, 84*, 139–147.

National Institute on Drug Abuse (NIDA). (2012). *Principles of drug addiction treatment: A research-based guide*. Retrieved from www.drugabuse.gov/sites/default/files/podat_1.pdf.

Otto, R. (2000). Assessing and managing violence risk in outpatient settings. *Journal of Clinical Psychology, 56*, 1239–1262.

Paridies v. Benedictine Hospital, 431 N.Y.S.2d 175 (App. Div. 1980).

Pate, R. H. (1992, Summer). Are you liable? *American Counselor, 10*, 23–26.

Peck v. The Counseling Service of Addison County, 499 A.2d 422 (Vt. 1985).

Riley, P. L., & McDaniel, J. (2000). School violence, prevention, intervention, and crisis response. *Professional School Counselor, 4*, 120–125.

Roberts, A. R. (Ed.). (2005). *Crisis intervention handbook: Assessment, treatment and research*. New York: Oxford University Press.

Rudd, M. D., Berman, A. L., Joiner, T. E., Jr., Nock, M. K., Silverman, M. M., Mandrusiak, M., et al. (2006). Warning signs for suicide: Theory, research, and clinical implications. *Suicide and Life-Threatening Behavior, 36*, 255–262.

Sikes, A., Remley, T. P., & Hays, D. G. (2010). Experiences of school counselors during and after making suspected child abuse reports. *Journal of School Counseling, 8*, 30.

Slavik, S., Carlson, J., & Sperry, L. (1993). An Adlerian treatment of adults with a history of childhood sexual abuse. *Individual Psychology, 49*(2), 111–131.

Stone, A. A. (1976). The Tarasoff decisions: Suing psychotherapists to safeguard society. *Harvard Law Review, 90*, 358–378.

Tarasoff v. Regents of the University of California, 113 Cal. Rptr. 14, 551 P.2d 334 (Cal. 1976).

Tarasoff v. Regents of the University of California, 13 Cal. 3d 177, 529 P.2d 533 (1974), vacated, 17 Cal. 3d 425, 551 P.2d 334 (1976).

Thompson v. County of Alameda, 614 P.2d 728 (Cal. 1980).

US Department of Health and Human Services. (2003). *The child abuse prevention and treatment act*. Retrieved from www.acf.hhs.gov/sites/default/files/cb/capta2003.pdf.

US Department of Health and Human Services, Administration for Children and Families, Administration on Children, Youth and Families, Children's Bureau. (2009). *Definitions of child abuse and neglect: Summary of state laws*. Washington, DC: US Government Printing Office.

US Department of Health and Human Services, Administration for Children and Families, Administration on Children, Youth and Families, Children's Bureau. (2011). *Child maltreatment*. Retrieved from www.acf.hhs.gov/sites/default/files/cb/cm11.pdf#page=69.

VandeCreek, L., & Knapp, S. (1993). *Tarasoff and beyond: Legal considerations in the treatment of life-endangering patients* (rev. ed.). Sarasota, FL: Professional Resource Press.

Walcott, D. M., Cerundolo, P., & Beck, J. C. (2001). Current analysis of the *Tarasoff* duty: An evolution towards the limitation of the duty to protect. *Behavioral Sciences and the Law, 19*, 325–343.

Waldo, S., & Malley, P. B. (1992). *Tarasoff* and its progeny: Implications for school counselors. *School Counselor, 40*, 56–63.

Walfish, S., Barnett, J. E., Marlyere, K., & Zielke, R. (2010). "Doc, there's something I have to tell you": Patient disclosure to their psychotherapist of unprosecuted murder and other violence. *Ethics & Behavior, 20*, 311–323.

Webster, C. D., Douglas, K. S., Eaves, D., & Hart, S. D. (1997). *HCR-20: Assessing risk for violence* (Version 2). Burnaby, BC: Mental Health, Law, and Policy Institute, Simon Fraser University.

Witkiewitz, K., & Marlatt, G. A. (2004). Relapse prevention for alcohol and drug problems: That was Zen this is Tao. *American Psychologist, 59*, 224–235.

CHAPTER 11

CONSULTATION IN THE SCHOOLS AND MENTAL HEALTH AGENCIES
MODELS AND METHODS

Consultation has become one of the most sought-after services rendered by psychologists and counselors in mental health agencies and in schools. The practice was born out of the Mental Health Act of 1962 and Gerald Caplan's (1970) seminal work *The Theory and Practice of Mental Health Consultation*, which provided a solid basis for understanding and implementing mental health consultation. In the school systems, a formal consultation role for counselors arose in the late 1970s as other helping professionals started branching out from one-to-one relationships to work with caretakers, who then worked with clients (Baker, 2000). Consultation is a way counselors can use their skills to influence other professionals to facilitate the emotional, psychological, academic, and career development of clients or students. Given the importance of consultation in the mental health clinician's range of duties, this chapter was included for the purpose of providing students with a basic understanding of consultation in schools and mental health agencies.

Definition of Consultation

With the growth of consultation, a diversity of opinion has developed with regard to the definition of consultation (Gravois, 2012; Gregoire & Slagel, 2007). Caplan (1970), who provided some of the first perspectives on consultation, viewed it as a collaborative process between two professionals who each have their own area of expertise. Ohlsen (1983) defined consultation as an activity in which a professional helps another person in regard to a third person or party. Kirby (1985) defined consultation in terms of four relationship conditions: (a) the relationship is voluntary, (b) the focus of attention is on the problem situation as articulated by the consultee(s), (c) the consultant is not functioning as a part of the structural hierarchy, and (d) the power that resides in the consultant's expertise is sufficient to facilitate change. Referring to consultation with organizations or systems, Moe and Perera-Diltz (2009) stated, "Rather than focusing solely on the behaviors or attitudes of one member or client, the systemic-organizational consultant focuses on the relationships that connect members of the system and that help the members collectively achieve the system's goal(s)" (p. 29). For purposes of clarity, the definition provided by Dougherty (2005) will be used in this chapter:

> [Consultation is] a process in which a human service professional assists a consultee with a work-related (or caretaking-related) problem with a client system, with the goal of helping both the consultee and the client system in some specified way. (p. 11)

In addition to trying to solve the problem of defining consultation, early authors (Alpert, 1977; Caplan, 1970) disagreed as to the focus of consultation and its distinctive qualities. The disagreement centered on consultation as a direct or an indirect service. It is important to remember that counselors and psychologists traditionally were involved in direct service to clients. By the 1980s, however, attention began to be given to how counselors and psychologists could provide preventive approaches to client care (Erchul, 2011; Neukrug, 2012). This more indirect service approach required counselors to assist *other* professionals who had direct responsibility for the welfare of clients or students. Today, it is clear that consultation is viewed as a unique and *indirect* approach to intervention (Crothers, Hughes, & Morine, 2008). One of the most salient implications of consultation being viewed as an indirect approach to intervention is that providers have to ensure that role confusion around counseling and consultation does not hamper service delivery. Consultation differs from therapy in that the consultant typically does not assume the full responsibility for the final outcome of consultation. The consultant's role is to develop and enhance the role of the consultee, which is in contrast to counseling, where the focus is on the personal improvement of the client. The consultant must remember that the relationship established with the consultee is not primarily therapeutic in nature. Rather, the consultant serves in the capacity of collaborator and facilitator to assist the consultee in performing his/her duties in a more productive and effective manner (Sears, Rudisill, & Mason-Sears, 2006).

Types of Mental Health Consultation

Defining mental health consultation and distinguishing it from counseling are helpful to being able to grasp its particular purpose and unique qualities. Caplan (1970), in his book *The Theory and Practice of Mental Health Consultation*, offered other points of consideration related to consultation when the discipline was first emerging. In particular, Caplan (1970) identified four consultation types practiced in mental health settings that are still useful to consultants today:

- *Client-centered case consultation:* A consultee has difficulty in dealing with the mental health aspects of one of his/her clients and calls in a specialist to advise on the nature of the difficulties and on how the consultee's work difficulty relates to the management of a particular case or group of cases. The consultant makes an assessment of the client's problem and recommends a course of action.
- *Program-centered administrative consultation:* The consultant is invited by an administrator to help with a current problem of program development, with some predicament in the organization of an institution, or with planning and implementation of organizational policies, including personnel policies. The consultant is expected to provide feedback to the organization in the form of a written report.
- *Consultee-centered case consultation:* The consultee's work problem relates to the management of a particular client, and he/she invokes the consultant's help to improve handling of the case. The consultant's primary focus is on clarifying and remedying the shortcomings in the consultee's professional functioning that are responsible for the present difficulties with the case about which he/she is seeking help. This type of interaction is distinguished from supervision in that the consultant does not usually have an ongoing, long-term relationship with the consultee in the way that a supervisor might.

■ *Consultee-centered administrative consultation:* The consultant helps the administrative staff of an organization deal with current problems in organizational policies. The focus of attention is the consultee's work difficulties and attempts to help improve his/her problem-solving skills (Caplan, 1970).

Since the 1970s, Caplan's definition of consultee-centered consultation has been adapted and updated by many professionals in the field (e.g., Caplan & Caplan, 1993; Hylander, 2012; Lambert, Hylander, & Sandoval, 2003). Knotek and Sandoval (2003) summarized consultants' understanding of the consultee-centered model as follows:

1. Consultee-centered consultation emphasizes a nonhierarchical helping role relationship between a resource (consultant) and a person or group (consultee) who seeks professional help with a work problem involving a third party (client).
2. The work problem is the topic of concern for the consultee, who has direct responsibility for the learning, development, or productivity of the client.
3. The primary task of the consultant is to help the consultee pinpoint critical information and then consider multiple views about well-being, development, and interpersonal, intrapersonal, and organizational effectiveness appropriate to the consultee's work setting. Ultimately the consultant may reframe his/her prior conceptualization of the work problem.
4. The goal of the consultation process is the joint development of a new way of conceptualizing the work problem, so that the repertoire of the consultee is expanded and the professional relationship between the consultee and the client is restored or improved. As the problem is jointly reconsidered, new ways of approaching the problem may lead to acquiring new means to address the work dilemma (Knotek & Sandoval, 2003).

Characteristics of Mental Health Consultation

Caplan (1970) described what he considered to be the characteristics of mental health consultation. A summary of Caplan's characteristics is presented to give students a clear understanding of the consultation model in mental health settings.

1. Mental health consultation is a method for use between two professionals in respect to a lay client or a program of such clients.
2. The consultee's work problem must relate to (a) a mental disorder or personality idiosyncrasies of the client, (b) the promotion of mental health in the client, or (c) interpersonal aspects of the work situation.
3. The consultant has no administrative responsibility for the consultee's work or professional responsibility for the outcome of the client's case.
4. The consultee is under no compulsion to accept the consultant's ideas or suggestions.
5. The basic relationship between the two is coordinate. No built-in hierarchical authority tension exists.
6. The coordinate relationship is fostered by the consultant's usually being a member of another profession and coming into the consultee's institution from the outside.
7. Consultation is usually given as a short series of interviews which take place in response to the consultee's awareness of a current need for help with the work problem.

8. Consultation is not expected to continue indefinitely.
9. A consultant has not predetermined a body of information that he/she intends to impart to a particular consultee.
10. The twin goals of consultation are to help the consultee improve his/her handling or understanding of the current work difficulty and to increase his/her capacity to master future problems of a similar type.
11. The aim is to improve the consultee's job performance, not his/her well-being.
12. Consultation does not focus overtly on the personal problems and feelings of the consultee.
13. This doesn't mean that the consultant does not pay attention to the feelings of the consultee. The consultant is particularly sensitive to these and to the disturbance of task functioning produced by personal problems.
14. Consultation is usually only one of the professional functions of a specialist, even if he/she is formally titled "consultant."
15. Finally, mental health consultation is a method of communication between a mental health specialist and other professionals (Caplan, 1970).

Dimensions of Internal and External Consultation

A look at the evolution of the Caplan model over the past 40 years reveals how it has transformed with time and implementation. At least two major updates are notable. First, in Caplan's (1970) original conceptualization, the consultant's base of operations was seen as outside of (i.e., external to) the consultee's work setting. However, in practice, mental health consultants are frequently in-house (i.e., internal) employees and staff members who have specialized training that is brought to bear on the issues with which the whole organization grapples (Caplan, Caplan, & Erchul, 1994; Crothers et al., 2008; Erchul, 2011). This is especially true in the case of school counselors, who often may find that they are wearing the consultant hat in their interactions with teachers and administrators looking for better ways to work with students. School counselors also often act as consultants to their own colleagues with regard to specialized issues, such as training and implementation of crisis response and prevention plans and suicide intervention policies. Caplan et al. (1994) suggested that it is difficult for an in-house consultant to act within the hierarchy of a school when he/she has an official status that is superior to that of many potential consultees and when he/she may be at least as knowledgeable about key practices, such as classroom instruction, as are other people in the system. The practice of internal consultation led to a second, related change to Caplan's original model. With the increased use of insider consultants, it became clear that the consultees in those systems were not as free as first thought to reject the advice or recommendations from in-house consultants (Caplan et al., 1994). When consultants are themselves members of the system for which they are consulting and own responsibility for the outcomes of their own recommendations, they may not find it easy to permit the consultee the freedom to reject their "expert views" (Caplan et al., 1994).

Consultation or Collaboration?

Because the use of in-house consultants is not without challenges, especially regarding the consultee's freedom to accept or reject advice from the consultant, Caplan and his colleagues (1994) proposed that in these instances it may be more appropriate to talk not about consultation but about collaboration. In collaboration, the specialist-collaborator and consultee share responsibility for the general outcome of the client, and the specialist-collaborator takes on the primary responsibility for the mental health–related elements of the case. The specialist-collaborator is seen as a fully participating team member acting as a hands-on clinician or advisor and making the best use of his/her specialized diagnostic and remedial skills to improve the mental health outcomes of the case. The consultant is expected to direct consultees' attention to salient aspects of the case in order to lead to positive outcomes. Also, in collaboration, the consultee-collaborator does not have the same freedom to accept or reject advice from the consultant as happens when an outside consultant is being used. Rather, the consultee is obliged to follow the best possible course of action to improve the client's condition (Brown, Pryzwansky, & Schulte, 2011).

Cook and Friend (2010) point out that in school settings the concept of collaborative consultation (or just simply collaboration) began to emerge in the 1980s as a way to empower teachers, especially special education teachers, to advocate for the needs of children with disabilities. These authors point out that collaboration is comparable to consultation, though with much more emphasis on professionals acting as partners who all have the same goal of meeting children's needs. Often, in schools, counselors, psychologists, and social workers can take on the role of consultant working in a nonhierarchical way to help teachers, for example, to better understand the behavioral, academic, and psychological needs of their students and prompt their overall success in the school environment (Crothers et al., 2008).

Assumptions of and Metaphors for Consultation

Types of mental health consultation have already been described, as have some dimensions of the consultation relationship. This brief section highlights some of the metaphors and assumptions on which the practice of consultation is based. Schein (1969, 1990, 1997) focused on the need for the helper or consultant to understand the assumptions he/she brings to the consultation relationship. Rockwood (1993) discussed Schein's consultation models—examining content versus process components of problems and problem solving. The basic components and major assumptions of the Purchase-of-Expertise Model, Doctor–Patient Model, and Process Consultation Model are outlined next.

The Purchase-of-Expertise Model

The Purchase-of-Expertise Model generally suggests that one seeks out a consultant for his/her special expertise or knowledge and is willing to pay for that knowledge through the practice of consultation. It makes the following assumptions:

1. The client has to have made a correct diagnosis of what the real problem is.
2. The client has identified the consultant's capabilities to solve the problem.
3. The client must communicate what the problem is.
4. The client has thought through and accepted all the implications of the help that will take place (Rockwood, 1993).

The Purchase-of-Expertise Model enables clients to remove themselves from the problem, relying on the skills and expertise of the consultant to fix the problem.

The Doctor–Patient Model

The Doctor–Patient Model also focuses on content and assumes that the diagnosis of and prescription for the problem solution rest solely in the hands of the consultant. It is characterized as follows:

1. The client has correctly interpreted the organizational assumptions and knows where the "sickness" is.
2. The client can trust the diagnosis.
3. The person or group defined as such will provide the necessary information to make the diagnosis.
4. The client will understand and accept the diagnosis, implement the prescription, and think through and accept the consequences.
5. The client will be able to remain healthy after the consultant leaves.

The Process Consultation Model

The Process Consultation Model focuses on how problems are solved in a collaborative effort. It can be characterized as follows:

1. The nature of the problem is such that the client not only needs help in making a diagnosis but would also benefit from participating in the making of the diagnosis.
2. The client has constructive intent and some problem-solving abilities.
3. Ultimately, the client is the one who knows what form of intervention or solution will work best in the organization.
4. When the client engages in the diagnosis and then selects and implements interventions, there will be an increase in his/her future problem-solving abilities.

Process consultation is systematic in that it accepts the goals and values of the organization as a whole and attempts to work with the client within those values and goals to jointly find solutions that will fit within the organizational system (Rockwood, 1993). Finally, Schein (1997) recommended eight principles that can guide process consultants in their work with clients, including aiming to make every contact helpful to the client, using every interaction with the client to unearth information about the client and the system, and being honest about what is unknown about the client or system so as to be able to learn about the client more directly and fully.

Cultural Issues in Consultation

Helping professionals of all specialties, including consultation, have become increasingly aware of the impact of cultural diversity on their practices (Kirmayer, Guzder, & Rousseau, 2014). Behring and Ingraham (1998) sent a call to the field of consultation to incorporate cultural awareness and practices into consultation. They defined multicultural consultation as "a culturally sensitive and indirect service in which the consultant adjusts the consultation services to address the needs and cultural values of either the consultee, or client, or both" (Behring & Ingraham, 1998, p. 58). For all types of consultation, Behring and Ingraham recommended that consultants be aware of their own cultural values and biases and how they are different from those of their consultees.

Furthermore, in multicultural consultation, consultants consider how culture can affect the communication style of both themselves and the consultees and, therefore, directly affect the process and outcome of consultation. In the school setting, Olivos, Gallagher, and Aguilar (2010) discussed the impact of cultural and linguistic diversity on consultation and collaboration. They noted that families who are not part of the majority (i.e., white, European, middle-class) culture and who have children with special needs may not have equal access to services as those families who are members of the dominant culture. Olivos et al. (2010) suggested that consultants or collaborators ensure that culturally diverse families (a) have full access to the school and to those (e.g., teachers, administrators, counselors, etc.) who serve students; (b) feel empowered in the collaboration process so that they know how and to whom to express concerns related to their children; (c) know all of the information that is pertinent to decisions being made on behalf of their children and are free to offer their input on the decision-making process; and (d) are familiar with the general education teachers in addition to special education teachers so that parents can consult them about their child's needs. Given the complexities involved in being culturally competent, consultants are encouraged to become knowledgeable about their consultee's cultural background and look for ways to account for cultural differences.

School Consultation

In mental health consultation, the consultation models focus on a work problem and the consulting relationship facilitates a problem-solving process. With regard to consultation in schools, Schmidt (2003) stated, "School counselors use consultation in a broader context that includes educational, information and problem solving relationships" (p. 176). He went on to frame the school consultation process as a triadic relationship between the counselor-consultant, the consultee (student, teachers, parents, etc.), and a situation with a third party or an external situation (prevention, development, remediation). Crothers et al. (2008) similarly noted that consultants who intervene in schools work with professional personnel, such as principals and teachers, to aid them in bettering their skills so that they can serve students and their families in the best possible ways.

When the focus of consultation is helping schools prevent problems, educational or informational consultation is implemented. Counselors often use large group instruction for parents, students, and teachers to give information or teach new skills. This kind of educational consultation does not include evaluation and thus aims instead at asking questions and sharing opinions. These consulting activities differ from direct counseling because the goal is to remedy a situation that is external to the relationships between the consultant and the consultee. Informational consulting situations occur when students, parents, and teachers have a need regarding community and school resources, career and educational materials, or other referrals. In other words, the counselor has contacts in the community and knowledge of the location of resources where the consultee can get information that is needed.

Kurpius and Fuqua (1993) outlined four generic modes of consulting that identify the different roles counselors take on when performing consulting functions in schools. The first role is "expert." In this role, counselors either provide answers to problems by giving expert information to parents, students, and teachers or use direct skills to fix the problem. The second role is the "prescriptive role," in which the counselor collects information, makes a diagnosis, and recommends solutions. The third role is that of "collaborator," where the counselor works in partnership with consultees to define concerns and develop strategies to change or improve an external situation. The consulting role of collaborator assumes an equal relationship among participants to facilitate change. This role is often used when consulting with students, parents, and teachers as well as with administrators and other professionals. The collaborative role can be more broadly defined when it includes the initiation and formation of collegial relationships with a variety of educational, medical, and other professionals who provide auxiliary services to school populations. These alliances benefit all parties concerned as they work to create circumstances that facilitate the healthy development of children. They also ensure the availability of outside services for students, parents, and teachers who interact with school counselors (Schmidt, 2003). The fourth mode in the Kurpius and Fuqua (1993) framework is that of "mediator." As mediator, the counselor facilitates conflict resolution between two or more persons or between persons and an outside situation. The goal is to find common ground and compromise.

Baker (2000) proposed basic consulting competencies for school counselors as proceeding through stages parallel to those proposed in Egan's (2010) three-stage helping paradigm for problem-solving counseling. Egan's paradigm has been restated for consulting stages, and the word *consultee* was used where the word *client* was used in the original counseling model.

Baker (2000) proposed the basic skills of a comprehensive consulting model in the context of the three stages of identification/clarification, goal setting/commitment, and action. In the identification/clarification stage of consulting, an opening interview is held. The skills used in this consulting interview are the same skills counselors use in an initial client interview: strategies that encourage sharing, identifying, and clarifying. Next, the counselor-consultant invites the consultee to share tier-targeted problems while establishing a facilitative working alliance. As the problem is clarified, the consultant determines the mode of consulting that fits the problem: expert, prescriptive, collaborative, or mediator. The consultant clarifies the problem as he/she understands it, explains his/her understanding of the consultee's motives, and negotiates the role the consultant will take.

The second stage of goal setting/commitment follows. Implicit in proceeding to this stage is the decision to consult. Assuming this decision is made, further exploration of the problem issues and possible solutions is undertaken. Basic challenging skills of information sharing, immediacy, and confrontation are brought in at this stage. If consultants are using the collaborative mode, brainstorming of hypotheses and solutions follows. As many hypotheses and solutions as possible are identified without analysis. In the prescriptive mode, consultants explain their treatment plans and then brainstorm who will implement them. When solutions have been identified, alternatives are evaluated using workability, reasonability, and motivation as criteria. Sometimes more information about the problem is needed before final goals can be established. A shift occurs as the consultant encourages and supports the consultee's understanding of and commitment to the goal.

Table 11.1 Brief Stages and Goals of Consultation

Stage	Goal
I	The consultee's problem situation and unused opportunities are identified and clarified.
II	Hopes for the future become realistic goals to which the consultee is committed.
III	Strategies for reaching goals are devised and implemented.

The final stage in this consulting process is action strategies. The consultee may need help with the final decision making. Depending on the mode of consulting, counseling for rational thinking may apply, or competence enhancement regarding child and adolescent development or classroom management skill training may be deemed appropriate. When mediation is the appropriate mode selected, counselors respond directly to requests from two or more parties to facilitate a mutual agreement or reconciliation. Basic counseling skills, challenging skills, and knowledge of interpersonal communication are requisite skills for mediation. Mediation can be between student and parent, student and student, student and teacher, teacher and administrator—any two parties engaged in the educational endeavor. As with any counseling process, reluctance and/or resistance can be handled using the same skills as those used in counseling interactions (Baker, 2000).

Consulting processes also include a closing phase. Consulting goals that have been established provide the criteria for whether the expected results have occurred. Consultees can also give feedback about their satisfaction with the consulting process and, upon reflection, make suggestions about how things could have been more helpful (Baker, 2000).

In addition to the modes of consultation proposed by Kurpius and Fuqua (1993) and Baker (2000), Gravois (2012) suggested that consultation in schools has three primary dimensions: focus, function, and form. The school-based consultant first has to define who the recipient of the consultation services is or, in other words, who is the focus of services. Gravois (2012) noted that in school settings the focus tends to lie primarily on teachers, students, or the school system itself. In defining the function of school-based consultation, Gravois (2012) proposed that consultation can have the aim of primary, secondary, or tertiary prevention and that consultants need to clarify in which area the consultation will be applied. Last, this model considers form to be the means through which consultation services are provided. The form of consultation includes provision of services through individuals, groups, or teams who are capable of having an impact on the identified consultation focus and issues.

In the 21st century, school counselors are faced with ever-increasing responsibilities on the job. At-risk students, reintegration of special students, and the job of coordinating the school and community services are but a few of the added responsibilities of the school counselor. The American School Counselors Association's (2003) national model advocates that the school counseling program be established as an integral component in the academic mission of the school, with academic development, personal development, and career development as the foci. An outline of a comprehensive school counseling program for the state of Alabama (Alabama Department of Education, 2003) identified consultation as a counselor's role in implementing a guidance curriculum in responsive services and in systems support. Other articles propose that the counselor expand the educational consulting role to include peer facilitator training, counselor–teacher consultation to plan and implement a guidance curriculum, the training and coordination of teacher advisory programs, and others (Dahir, Sheldon, & Valiza, 1998; Myrick, 1997). It is not a leap to conclude that the consulting role for school counselors may become equal to the counseling practice role as the American School Counselors Association model is adopted by more school systems.

Consultation Models and Practices in Schools

In this section, we look at models of consultation that have been proposed for use in school settings. The first model (Clemens, 2007) uses developmental counseling and therapy as a conceptual framework and is meant to aid counselors who consult with teachers, parents, and students in the school setting. The second model, developed by Kahn (2000), draws on solution-focused therapy as its backdrop. The third model, from Truscott et al. (2012), is a school-based model that is explicitly consultee centered (i.e., teacher centered) and draws on the theories of positive psychology and self-determination.

Clemens's (2007) model of consultation for school counselors draws on the work of Ivey, Ivey, Myers, and Sweeney (2005), who recommended a developmental approach to counseling that they call developmental counseling and therapy (DCT). DCT uses Piaget's insights into cognitive development in order to help counselors assess the way in which clients perceive and make meaning of their world. The four cognitive modalities identified by DCT are sensorimotor, concrete, formal-operational, and dialectic/systemic. Clients and consultees who operate from a sensorimotor modality tend to focus on the emotional component of their experience as they relay it to the counselor/consultant. Those who are concrete in their thinking style often speak about their experience in a linear fashion, emphasizing cause-and-effect elements of their experiences. Formal-operational thinkers tend to highlight patterns of thinking and behaving in their accounts of their needs. Finally, dialectic/systemic thinkers also talk about patterns, but they focus on the types of interactions between systems and groups that seem typical (Clemens, 2007). Each cognitive modality has its benefits and limitations, and Clemens (2007) suggested that it is the consultant's job to help consultees (such as stressed teachers) expand their use of multiple modalities in thinking about the issue for which they are seeking consultation. Thus, one goal of the consultation process using DCT is to aid the consultee in using more than one cognitive modality so that the consultee can perceive the situation of concern from a different and more helpful point of view. She recommended using the following questions to prompt thinking in the four cognitive styles identified in DCT consultation:

Sensorimotor

- What are you seeing and hearing?
- What does the classroom look like? Describe in detail.
- Who else is present?
- What are they doing?
- Where are you in the room?
- What are you feeling?
- Where are you feeling X in your body? (Clemens, 2007, p. 355)

Concrete

- Can you think of a specific example?
- Tell me what happened just before the student did X.
- What happened just after the student did X?
- What did you do or say?
- How did you feel?
- So when you did Y, then the student did X and you felt Z? (Clemens, 2007, pp. 355–356)

Formal-Operational

- Is this a pattern for the student/teacher?
- Does this happen a lot in your classroom?

- What are the exceptions to these patterns?
- What are you saying to yourself when this type of situation occurs?
- How do you act or respond? (Clemens, 2007, p. 356)

Dialectic/Systemic

- What purpose do you think the student's behavior is serving?
- How do you think the student learned this way of acting in the classroom?
- How did you learn your way of responding to this pattern of behavior?
- What else might be impacting your response to this particular situation?
- What is the rule or the cognition that guides your response?
- What are the limitations of that rule? (Clemens, 2007, p. 356)

In proposing the above questions, Clemens (2007) cautioned that school counselors should clarify whether or not a teacher is seeking consultation for themselves when they approach the counselor with a student issue. She also noted that counselors must be able to accurately assess a teacher's cognitive style in order to be helpful.

A second model of consultation in the schools is Kahn's (2000) solution-focused consultation approach. According to Kahn, a solution-focused model is an appropriate fit for the school environment because the objectives of education, like this consultation approach, tend to be future oriented, positive, and goal directed. Several steps characterize Kahn's (2000) model, all of which are grounded in the assumption that the consultant and consultee are collaborators in trying to resolve the issue at hand. The process begins when the consultant (usually the school counselor) asks the consultee (a teacher, parent, or administrator) to identify strengths he/she brings to the consultation relationship. Directing the consultee to consider strengths and resiliencies reflects the solution-focused consultant's belief that language is formative and helps play a role in coming to a resolution of the problem (Kahn, 2000). After encouraging the consultee to use positive language throughout the process, both parties attend to goal setting, which typically happens early on in the relationship so that little time is spent ruminating about the problem. The consultant helps the consultee to describe the actions he/she wants to see take place (rather than what should not be happening) and also helps to motivate the consultee to participate fully in the process if he/she is somewhat complacent about seeking help.

After establishing goals for the consultation relationship, the consultant and consultee reflect on any prior workable solutions that the consultee has used for the issue needing to be resolved or any exceptions to the problem of which he/she is aware. This focus emphasizes the solution-centered consultant's beliefs that the consultee has the ability to resolve the issue and that the issue can be successfully addressed and managed. Looking at exceptions to the problem helps the consultant and consultee to ready themselves for the next step in the process, which is to decide on a seemingly workable solution to the consultation issue. Kahn (2000) suggested that consultants ask specific and concrete questions such as "Which solution seems most doable given the resources of the student, the student's family, the school, etc.?" and "In the solution, who is doing what and when and where?" Finally, Kahn (2000) proposed that school-based consultants compliment their consultees in order to highlight their dedication and motivation to change.

A third model of school-based consultation was developed by Truscott and his colleagues (2012) and is known as Exceptional Professional Learning (EPL). This model focuses its attention primarily on the consultee, which usually means its focus is on helping teachers. The EPL model assumes that by aiding teachers to create productive learning environments and implement effective learning practices, the consultant is indirectly helping students, who are seen as the recipients of services. The EPL approach is grounded in theories such as positive psychology (Seligman & Csikszentmihalyi, 2000) and self-determination theory (Ryan & Deci, 2000). In brief, some of the goals of EPL consultation are:

- developing social climates that foster strengths,
- shifting teacher . . [focus] . . from fixing unsuccessful students to building knowledge and confidence about improved teaching practices,
- conceptualizing teachers as active decision-makers who can, and should, exercise choice, and
- using the power of authentic social context and construction for sustained applications of teaching and learning (Truscott et al., 2012, p. 68).

In practice, the EPL model takes up the following tasks (Truscott et al., 2012):

- *Gaining entry into the system:* Generally, this means that consultants focus first on developing authentic relationships with consultees in the school system.
- *Selecting and implementing projects:* The consultant and consultees together determine which areas of focus are of greatest need in their ability to do their jobs effectively; in essence, the consultant conducts a needs assessment.
- *Identifying consultee competencies:* The consultant helps the consultees to identify their existing areas of strength and competencies as relevant to the needs that have emerged.
- *Building knowledge:* The consultant helps to build consultee knowledge about the consultation area of focus by leading presentations, implementing new skills, and practicing those with consultees.
- *Assessing and responding:* Consultants and consultees evaluate the effectiveness of the consultation projects and interactions.

General Guidelines for Consultation

The stages of consultation outlined by numerous authors (e.g., Kurpius & Fuqua, 1993) have been adapted here and serve as guidelines for the development of a consultation plan. To some extent, these guidelines are reflected in many consultation models (for example, reflections of these steps are seen in the EPL school consultation approach described briefly above). At the same time, Tindal, Parker, and Hasbrouck (1992) found that stage descriptions of consultation are not necessarily reflective of the practice of consultation in every instance and should be applied flexibly.

Preentry

Preentry is considered part of the consultation process because it enables the consultant to assess the degree to which he/she is the proper fit for the consultation situation. Preentry is the preliminary stage when the consultant forms a conceptual foundation to work from and through the process of self-assessment and is able to articulate to self and others who he/she is and what services he/she can provide (Neukrug, 2012; Truscott et al., 2012). Kurpius and Fuqua (1993) suggested that throughout this self-assessment and reflective process, consultants should understand their beliefs and values, understanding how individuals, families, programs, organizations, or systems cause, solve, or avoid problems. Furthermore, Kurpius and Fuqua (1993) maintained that in the preentry stage it is essential for consultants to conceptualize the meaning and operation of consultation to themselves and be ready to do the same with their consultees or consultee system. To this end, the following questions are often helpful:

- What models, processes, theories, and paradigms do you draw on to conceptualize your model of helping?
- How do you define consultation to the consultee or consultee system?
- Do you see the process of consultation as triadic (consultant, consultee, client) or didactic (consultant and client)?
- When is having a vision, looking into the future, and planning a better intervention than cause-and-effect problem solving?

Entry Into the System

The consultant's entry into the system is a crucial step in determining the success or failure of consultation efforts. Several tasks characterize formal entry into the system. For the external consultant, entry usually begins with the exploration of the match between the organization's needs and the consultant's skills. Discussions between the consultant and members of the organization center around descriptive information about the organization, its needs, and desired outcomes. The consultant's skill, style of consultation, and plan for how consultation efforts can be implemented in the setting are discussed and negotiated. Once the parties have agreed that consultation is indeed needed, the process proceeds to the negotiation of an informal or formal contract. The formulation of a contract follows the consultant's defining of his/her function and role in the system. A clear understanding of the specific duties and functions of the consultant must be presented to personnel involved in the consultation effort (Truscott et al., 2012; Brown et al., 2011). Negotiating a contract with key personnel serves to ensure that the highest level of administrators participate in the consultation process and helps to facilitate a smooth transition into the system. The formal discussion of the contract should include the following:

- goals or intended outcomes of consultation,
- identity of the consultee,
- confidentiality of service and limits of confidentiality,
- time frame (How long will the service be provided to the organization? To the individual consultee?),
- times the consultant will be available and ways to contact him/her,
- procedures for requesting to work with the consultant,
- the possibility of contract renegotiation if change is needed,
- fees (if relevant),
- consultant's access to different sources and types of information within the organization, and
- the person to whom the consultant is responsible (Brown et al., 2011).

Orientation to Consultation

Orientation to consultation requires the consultant to communicate directly with key personnel in the system. Initially, the consultant, in establishing a working relationship, must discuss the roles the consultant and consultees will play in the process. This enables all parties to share in the expression of their needs and preferences and creates an atmosphere of open communication. Typical questions addressed in the orientation include the following:

- What are the consultant's expectations about consultation?
- What roles will the consultant and consultee assume in the consultative effort?
- What are the boundaries of the consultant's interventions?
- What are the ethical concerns of the consultee?
- What are the guidelines of confidentiality?
- How long will the consultation take?
- What are the procedures governing the gathering of data?
- What are the guidelines for the giving and receiving of feedback?
- What are the procedures used in the assessment of the consultation plan?

Problem Identification

Once the consultant and consultee have oriented themselves to the process of consultation, the consultant needs to identify the problem(s) to be addressed (Neukrug, 2012). A first step in problem identification is to meet with the consultee to gather appropriate data. Problem identification begins with establishing goals and objectives to be accomplished in consultation. Specific outcomes to be expected and the format for assessing outcomes are discussed. For example, questions to be considered might include the following:

- What are your general concerns about the problem?
- What needs to be accomplished to overcome your concerns?
- What role will the consultee play in overcoming the problem?
- What aspects of the consultee's problem are most distressing?

Consultation Intervention

Having defined the problem and reviewed the data gathered with the consultee, the consultant proceeds with the development of a specific intervention plan. The plan will include the establishment of objectives, the selection of strategies to be implemented, and the assessment procedures to be followed (Neukrug, 2012). Bergan and Kratochwill (1990) suggested the following four-point outline as part of implementing a consultation plan:

1. *Make sure the consultee and consultant agree on the nature of the problem:* Problem identification during the consultation process is critical to the overall success of consultation and sets the stage for the establishment of the consultant–consultee relationship. During the process, the consultant's main priority is to assist the consultee in identifying and clarifying the main problem that is experienced by the client. According to Baker (2000), the skills and techniques of focusing, paraphrasing, setting goals, and showing empathy and genuineness are particularly valuable at this problem identification stage. These skills assist in the development of a plan based on authenticity and collaborative commitment between the consultant and consultee.

2. *Complete either the setting and intrapersonal analysis or the skills analysis:* One role of the consultant is to help the consultee to accurately estimate the importance of situations, as well as

to develop self-efficacy expectations regarding performance. Once performance of a productive behavior has been completed, self-evaluation based on reasonable standards must occur. These processes can be facilitated through modeling and feedback to the consultee. Often motivation can be enhanced by reminding the consultee about the possible positive outcomes of consultation, helping to set goals that correspond with his/her own standards and developing situations that will build confidence that he/she can perform the skills needed to solve the problem (Brown et al., 2011).

3. *Design a plan to deal with the identified problem:* Once the problem has been identified, the consultant and consultee work to establish realistic goals—the objectives of the consortium effort. Setting realistic expectations for the outcomes of consultation implies communication about and knowledge of environmental consultee constraints. Furthermore, successful consultation requires consultees who are knowledgeable of the consultation process. Without this understanding, discordant expectations between consultant and consultee frequently will lead to resistance (Kilburg, 2010). Unless consultees actively contribute during consultation interactions, they often will be frustrated by recommendations that are inconsistent with their own thinking, will feel little psychological ownership of treatment plans, and will fail to expand their own professional skills. This agreement to and acceptance of the objectives of the consultation plan must be ensured before consultation interventions can be planned.

   The selection of intervention strategies should rest with the consultee (Cook & Friend, 2010). The consultee's involvement in the selection process will raise the client's awareness of the problem and should enhance motivation by engaging clients in goal setting and evaluation. The major issue in selecting intervention strategies is their appropriateness to the setting and the amount of time needed to monitor strategies.

4. *Make arrangements for follow-up sessions with the consultee:* Successful termination of consultation includes the need on the part of the consultant to express an openness to work with the consultee again with other presenting problems. In addition, the collection of data from the consultee on the outcomes of change efforts can document effective consultation and justify its use in professional practice (Neukrug, 2012).

Assessing the Impact of Consultation

The success or failure of consultation interventions is determined by assessing the degree to which the results are congruent with the specific objectives. Data for making this determination come from the observations that began during the entry process and have continued throughout the consultation process. Brown et al. (2011) suggested that steps in the evaluation process are as follows:

1. *Determine the purpose(s) of the evaluation:* The extent to which consultees provide or gather data affects their involvement at this point. The opportunity to make choices that will affect the time that needs to be directed to evaluation as well as the types of information that are collected will contribute to ownership of the evaluation. A major issue to be considered is the confidentiality of the information to be presented.

2. *Agree on measurements to be made:* The consultant and consultee must agree on methods and procedures of measurement. Measures must specifically address the objective and goals of the intervention plan.

3. *Set a data collection schedule:* The consultant and consultee must agree on a formalized calendar of data collection. The method of collection, the tasks assigned to each party, and the method for summarizing and reporting data are discussed.

4. *Develop a dissemination plan:* The dissemination plan, which includes the format in which data are reported, needs to be carefully considered by both parties. Issues surrounding the reporting of data, the individuals to whom data are reported, and the confidentiality of the data are agreed on and follow a predetermined plan of action.

5. *Concluding consultation:* The termination of the consultation process is as important as the initial entry into the system. An imperative step is for the consultant to act in a culturally competent fashion with regard to the disengagement process, as well as to provide the consultee with an open invitation to seek further assistance as the need arises (Dougherty, Tack, Fullam, & Hammer, 1996). Follow-up of consultation activities ensures that the consultant and consultee have the opportunity to measure the effects of the process over time. The degree to which the termination process is perceived as a smooth transition can determine whether consultation services will be sought in the future.

Resistance to Consultation

Resistance in consultative relationships can happen as in any other human relationship. Kilburg (2010) noted that consultants must put concerted effort into developing trust with the consultee in order to have a positive outcome and to help reduce the potential for resistance in the process. Various authors have discussed different manifestations of organizational resistance as noted below:

1. *The desire for systems maintenance:* The entrance of the consultant into the system requires the system to adapt to new input that drains energy and threatens the system (Crothers et al., 2008; Gilman & Gabriel, 2004). To avoid this pitfall, the consultant should be careful not to threaten existing roles or challenge others' jobs or role definitions. The simpler the consultant's entry and the less change in structure, tone, process, or product it entails, the easier it will be for the consultant to avoid resistance based on system maintenance.

2. *The consultant as the outsider:* The consultant is viewed as an alien in the organization and is treated with suspicion. The consultant should become familiar with the institution's history, mission, philosophy, and procedures and increase his/her availability to and contact with the staff to reduce outsider status.

3. *The desire to reject the new as nonnormative:* There is often a desire to maintain the status quo by conforming to existing norms in the organization. The consultant must guard against tampering with time-honored programs, processes, and procedures. Consultant sensitivity to organizational vulnerability is essential.

4. *The desire to protect one's turf or vested interests:* The consultant must recognize that his/her presence is often viewed as an intrusion on the consultee's area of interest or professional responsibility. Involving the consultee in the process tends to lessen the resistance (Crothers et al., 2008).

5. *Being so close to a problem that one loses perspective:* Consultees sometimes can feel as if they have invested so much energy and thought into a client or student that they are hesitant to engage consultation because they cannot see how new approaches will aid the problem or because their view of the client or student is distorted by continuous close contact (Hylander, 2012).

Similarly, some specific variables can increase resistance to consultation. For example, the less time and resources needed to implement interventions, the greater the acceptance. Gonzales, Nelson, Gutkin, and Shwery (2004) proposed that when the costs of consultation and its potential required outcomes outweigh the perceived benefits, consultees (especially teachers) may resist the process. Discordant expectations between consultant and consultees will frequently lead to resistance. Finally, Maital (1996) discussed resistance as emerging when consultees, such as parents who are seeking consultation for their children, lose objectivity and find it difficult to implement a plan of action created by a consultant.

Contracting and the Forces of Change in the Organization

Kurpius and Fuqua (1993) suggested that an understanding of the cycles of change and the forces of change within the organization is helpful in gaining a better understanding of the problems and the culture surrounding the problems in the organization. Stages of change include the following:

1. *Development:* Help is needed at an early stage of a new problem or program.
2. *Maintenance:* Things are becoming stagnant and falling behind, needing help to improve. This stage shows signs of consultee desire and motivation for change.
3. *Decline:* Things are worse, and consultees recognize that they cannot solve the problem. Consultees may want a quick fix and have high expectations for the consultant.
4. *Crisis:* Consultees or consultee system is desperate for help. The consultant may look for dependency first, but it is important that consultees understand that their situation and the investment need to return to a stable state.

The forces of change within the system need to be understood for consultation to proceed. When the system is closed to change and internal forces vary between being for and against change, there is usually little opportunity for change to occur. When the system recognizes that change is needed but forces for and against change are balanced, progress is possible but slow moving. When the forces for change are external to the members who prefer not to change, one can expect a high degree of conflict and slow change. Finally, when the members recognize the need for help and all want help to improve, then the best chance for successful helping occurs (Kurpius & Fuqua, 1993).

These models can serve as a test of the feasibility of the consultant's effort and the type of contract the consultant will implement. The formal discussion of the contract between the consultant and the consultee should include a number of critical questions to be answered before a contract is developed and implemented. According to Remley (1993), consultation contracts should do the following:

1. clearly specify the work to be completed by the consultant,
2. describe in detail any work products expected from the consultant,
3. establish a time frame for the completion of the work,
4. establish lines of authority and the person to whom the consultant is responsible,
5. describe the compensation plan for the consultant and the method of payment, and
6. specify any special agreement or contingency plans agreed on by the parties.

Remley (1993) suggested that some individuals complain that written contracts are too legalistic and signify a distrust between the consultant and the consultee. Consultation is a business arrangement and should be entered into in a businesslike fashion. By reducing to written form agreements that have been reached by the parties, misunderstandings can be identified and resolved before further problems arise.

Summary

Consultation in schools and mental health agencies is a highly sought-after skill, and one with which counseling and psychotherapy interns should become familiar. In this chapter, the models and methods of consultation were presented to provide the student with an overview of the ways to organize and establish consultative relationships. The differences between mental health consultation and school consultation have been discussed, along with critical issues such as resistance. Systems and integrative approaches to consultation were chosen as representative samples of consultation strategies, and guidelines for consulting in the school were presented.

References

Alabama Department of Education. (2003). *The revised comprehensive counseling and guidance model of Alabama public schools.* In D. C. Cobia & D. A. Hendeson, *Handbook of school counseling* (p. 48). Upper Saddle River, NJ: Pearson Education.

Alpert, J. L. (1977). Some guidelines for school consultation. *Journal of School Psychology, 15,* 308–319.

American School Counselors Association. (2003). ASCA national model: A framework for school counseling programs. *Professional School Counseling, 6*(3), 54–58.

Baker, S. B. (2000). *School counseling for the twentieth century* (3rd ed.). Upper Saddle River, NJ: Prentice Hall.

Behring, S. T., & Ingraham, C. L. (1998). Culture as a central component of consultation: A call to the field. *Journal of Educational and Psychological Consultation, 9,* 57–72.

Bergan, J. R., & Kratochwill, T. R. (1990). *Behavior consultation and therapy.* New York: Plenum.

Brown, D., Pryzwansky, W. B., & Schulte, A. C. (2011). *Psychological consultation and collaboration: Introduction to theory and practice.* Upper Saddle River, NJ: Pearson.

Caplan, G. (1970). *The theory and practice of mental health consultation.* New York: Basic Books.

Caplan, G., & Caplan, R. B. (1993). *Mental health consultation and collaboration.* San Francisco: Jossey-Bass.

Caplan, G., Caplan, R., & Erchul, W. P. (1994). Caplanian mental health consultation: Historical background and current status. *Consulting Psychology: Practice and Research, 46,* 2–12.

Clemens, E. (2007). Developmental counseling and therapy as a model for school counselor consultation with teachers. *Professional School Counselor, 10,* 352–359.

Cook, L., & Friend, M. (2010). The state of the art of collaboration on behalf of children with special needs. *Journal of Educational and Psychological Consultation, 20,* 1–8.

Crothers, L. M., Hughes, T. L., & Morine, K. A. (2008). *Theory and cases in school-based consultation: A resource for school psychologists, school counselors, special educators, and other mental health professionals.* New York: Routledge.

Dahir, C. Q., Sheldon, C. B., & Valiza, M. J. (1998). *Vision into action: Implementing the national standards for school counseling program.* Alexandria, VA: American School Counseling Association.

Dougherty, A. M. (2005). *Psychological consultation and collaboration in school and community settings* (4th ed.). Pacific Grove, CA: Brooks/Cole.

Dougherty, A. M., Tack, F. E., Fullam, C. B., & Hammer, L. A. (1996). Disengagement: A neglected aspect of the consultation process. *Journal of Educational and Psychological Consultation, 7,* 259–274.

Egan, G. (2010). *The skilled helper: A problem management approach to helping* (9th ed.). Pacific Grove, CA: Brooks/Cole.

Erchul, W. P. (2011). School consultation and response to intervention: A tale of two literatures. *Journal of Educational and Psychological Consultation, 21,* 191–208.

Gilman, R., & Gabriel, S. (2004). Perceptions of school psychological services by educational professionals: Results from a multi-state survey pilot study. *School Psychology Review, 33,* 271–286.

Gonzales, J. E., Nelson, J. R., Gutkin, T. B., & Shwery, C. (2004). Teacher resistance to school-based consultation with school psychologists: A survey of teacher perceptions. *Journal of Emotional and Behavioral Disorders, 12,* 30–37.

Gravois, T. A. (2012). Consultation services in schools: A can of worms worth opening. *Consulting Psychology Journal: Practice and Research, 64,* 83–87.

Gregoire, J., & Slagel, L. (2007). A look at consultation. In J. Gregoire & C. M. Jungers (Eds.), *The counselor's companion: What every beginning counselor needs to know* (pp. 528–548). Mahwah, NJ: LEA.

Hylander, I. (2012). Conceptual change through consultee-centered consultation: A theoretical model. *Consulting Psychology Journal: Practice and Research, 64,* 29–45.

Ivey, A. E., Ivey, M. B., Myers, J. E., & Sweeney, T. J. (2005). *Developmental counseling and therapy: Promoting wellness over the lifespan.* Boston: Lahaska.

Kahn, B. B. (2000). A model of solution-focused consultation for school counselors. *Professional School Counselor, 3,* 248–254.

Kilburg, R. R. (2010). Executive consulting under pressure: A brief commentary on some timeless issues. *Consulting Psychology Journal: Practice and Research, 62,* 203–206.

Kirby, J. (1985). *Consultation: Practice and practitioner.* Muncie, IN: Accelerated Development.

Kirmayer, L. J., Guzder, J., & Rousseau, C. (Eds.). (2014). *Cultural consultation: Encountering the other in mental health care.* New York: Springer.

Knotek, S. E., & Sandoval, J. (2003). Current research in consultee-centered consultation. *Journal of Education and Psychological Consultation, 14*(3–4), 243–250.

Kurpius, D. J., & Fuqua, D. R. (1993). Fundamental issues in defining consultation. *Journal of Counseling and Development, 71,* 598–600.

Lambert, N. M., Hylander, I., & Sandoval, J. (Eds.). (2003). *Consultee-centered consultation: Improving the quality of professional services in schools and community organizations.* Mahwah, NJ: Lawrence Erlbaum.

Maital, S. L. (1996). Integration of behavioral and mental health consultation as a means of overcoming resistance. *Journal of Educational and Psychological Consultation, 7,* 291–303.

Moe, J. L., & Perera-Diltz, D. M. (2009). An overview of systemic-organizational consultation for professional counselors. *Journal of Professional Counseling: Practice, Theory, and Research, 37,* 27–37.

Myrick, R. D. (1997). *Developmental guidance and counseling: A developmental approach.* Minneapolis, MN: Educational Media.

Neukrug, E. (2012). *The world of the counselor: An introduction to the counseling profession.* New York: Brooks/Cole.

Ohlsen, M. M. (1983). *Introduction to counseling.* Itasca, IL: F. E. Peacock.

Olivos, E. M., Gallagher, R. A., & Aguilar, J. (2010). Fostering collaboration of culturally and linguistically diverse families of children with moderate to severe disabilities. *Journal of Educational and Psychological Consultation, 20,* 28–40.

Remley, T. P. (1993). Consultation contracts. *Journal of Counseling and Development, 72,* 157–158.

Rockwood, G. F. (1993, July/August). Edgar Schein's process versus content consultation models. *Journal of Counseling and Development, 71,* 636–638.

Ryan, R. M., & Deci, E. L. (2000). Self-determination theory and the facilitation of intrinsic motivation, social development, and well-being. *American Psychologist, 55,* 68–78.

Schein, E. H. (1969). *Process consultation.* Reading, MA: Addison-Wesley.

Schein, E. H. (1990). Organizational culture. *American Psychologist, 45,* 109–119.

Schein, E. H. (1997). The concept of "client" from a process consultation perspective: A guide for change agents. *Journal of Organizational Change Management, 10,* 202–216.

Schmidt, J. J. (2003). *Counseling in schools: Essential services and comprehensive programs* (4th ed.). Boston: Allyn & Bacon.

Sears, R., Rudisill, J., & Mason-Sears, C. (2006). *Consultation skills for mental health professionals.* Hoboken, NJ: Wiley.

Seligman, M. E. P., & Csikszentmihalyi, M. (2000). Positive psychology: An introduction. *American Psychologist, 55,* 5–14.

Tindal, G., Parker, R., & Hasbrouck, J. E. (1992). The construct validity of stages and activities in the consultation process. *Journal of Educational and Psychological Consultation, 3,* 99–118.

Truscott, S. D., Kreskey, D., Bolling, M., Psimas, L., Graybill, E., Albritton, K., et al. (2012). Creating consultee change: A theory-based approach to learning and behavioral change processes in school-based consultation. *Consulting Psychology Journal: Practice and Research, 64,* 63–82.

CHAPTER 12

FINAL EVALUATIONS

This chapter is organized to help those involved in the practicum and internship to be formally evaluated. This process will help practicum students and interns determine their strengths and weaknesses. It also serves as a vehicle to help site personnel formally evaluate their training structures.

The Monthly Practicum Log (Form 3.7) permits the student to quantify the number of hours spent in particular counseling areas while in the practicum. The practicum student should detail the time spent in the various training activities. The student should have his/her supervisor sign the practicum log monthly in recognition of these activities.

The function of the remaining evaluation forms (Forms 12.1 through 12.6) is explained in the following information:

- The Weekly Internship Log (Form 12.1) parallels the function of the practicum log and is used by interns.
- The Summary Internship Log (Form 12.2) quantifies the total number of hours spent within the identified counseling activities during the internship. The site supervisor will sign these logs and submit them to the university field site coordinator or the university supervisor.
- The Evaluation of Intern's Practice in Site Activities (Form 12.3) complements the practicum and internship logs. The supervisor utilizes this form to evaluate the student's work in each relevant and appropriate category. This is to be used with Form 7.6 (Supervisor's Final Evaluation of Intern) to provide a comprehensive evaluation of the intern's counseling performance at the field site.
- The Client's Assessment of the Counseling Experience (Form 12.4) allows the practicum student's or intern's clients to address the satisfaction experienced during the counseling process. The student should have his/her client fill out the form when counseling has been terminated.
- The Supervisee Evaluation of Supervisor (Form 12.5) is completed by the practicum student or intern at the midpoint and conclusion of the supervisory contract. Both the student and his/her supervisor should sign the form.
- The Site Evaluation Form (Form 12.6) is to be used so that site personnel and university program faculty can assess the quality of their training sites.

These final evaluation forms are included because they are similar to those typically used in agencies and schools. The final assessment by the student, supervisor, and client at the culmination of the internship experience is an important component of the training process and provides an excellent opportunity for these individuals to evaluate the internship as a whole. It is only through a final assessment of the internship that the student is truly able to reflect on the material and skills learned. In the same way, feedback provided by the client and supervisor is instrumental in communicating to the student which skills have been used effectively and which need to be further refined. The student or supervisor might consider adapting these forms to address the specific and particular needs of the internship experience.

APPENDICES

THE SUPERVISEE PERFORMANCE ASSESSMENT INSTRUMENT[1]

The Supervisee Performance Assessment Instrument (SPAI) is a multifaceted tool that allows for self-assessment by the supervisee, collaboration between the supervisor and the supervisee, and/or supervisor assessment. The design of this instrument is to focus on the collaborative process between the supervisor and the supervisee through the option of choosing both the evaluation criteria and the performance scale items. In developing this instrument as a collaborative tool, we decided to depart from many other scales by introducing a large number of evaluation criteria and by using a nonhierarchical type of scaling. Our rationale behind these two ideas is to provide the user with as much flexibility as possible in creating an evaluation tool that meets the needs of both the supervisee and the supervisor.

The absence of a traditional evaluation scale is a foundational feature of this instrument. Traditional scales often succumb to response styles such as the halo effect. The evaluation criteria of the SPAI are arranged in five categories. These categories consist of skill development, case conceptualization, and personalization as defined by Bernard's (1979) discrimination model, with the addition of professional issues and supervision skills. We have attempted to include as many different criteria for assessment in each category as possible, and thus you will find there are far too many for any one situation. This allows the supervisor and supervisee to choose the specific criteria for evaluation and tailor these to specific individuals or groups. This instrument also has the flexibility of accommodating additional criteria to customize the evaluation for individuals or unique applications. The absence of a traditional evaluation scale is a foundational feature of this instrument. Traditional scales often succumb to response styles such as the halo effect, generosity, and central tendency. We are suggesting the use of some combination of the following instrument scale items.

A. I have not been trained in using this skill.
B. I seldom use this skill.
C. I use this skill often.
D. This is a skill that does not fit my model/style.
E. I am comfortable in using this skill.
F. I am uncomfortable in using this skill.
G. I would like additional information and training on this skill.

Supervisees may choose one or more of these scale items based on their own self-reflection. This type of scale is far less hierarchical and lends itself to more discussion and action. Although this scale is designed for supervisees, supervisors could adapt it to fit their needs by inserting more hierarchical words such as adequate/inadequate, sufficient/insufficient, satisfactory/unsatisfactory, or effective/ineffective.

We describe this as a collaborative instrument. The collaboration takes place between the supervisor and supervisee in developing specific criteria and scaling it to be used in each application. The following is a brief example of this assessment in action.

Example: The supervisor and supervisee collaborate and focus on each of the five categories, together choosing the criteria which best apply to the supervisee's situation. In this example, we have chosen the criterion "Helps clients build on their strengths." Once the criteria have been identified, the supervisee decides which scale items best describe his/her situation and goals. In this example, the supervisee might pick the following:

B, F, G Helps clients build on their strengths.

Note: B, F, and G represent instrument scale items above. B = I seldom use this skill; F = I am uncomfortable using this skill; and G = I would like additional information and training on this skill.

In discussion with the supervisor, the supervisee says that she is not using the skill often because it feels awkward, as though she is praising the client. This dialogue both identifies the area of weakness and provides sufficient information to begin forming a plan to increase the efficacy of the behavior.

The SPAI

Place the letter(s) of the instrument scale items chosen in the space preceding the criterion.

Intervention Skills

_____ Listens to verbal and nonverbal communications.

_____ Projects warmth, caring, and acceptance.

_____ Communicates empathy and genuineness with clients.

_____ Communicates effectively, using basic skills such as paraphrasing, reflections, questions, and summaries.

_____ Establishes effective therapeutic relationships.

_____ Observes in-session behavior (e.g., client language) and uses it to facilitate the client–counselor relationship.

_____ Uses silence as an effective intervention technique.

_____ Times interventions to maximize effectiveness.

_____ Attends to the relationship with clients.

_____ Demonstrates readiness to explore charged areas.

_____ Understands and uses resistance to assist clients.

_____ Demonstrates effectiveness in making formal assessments.

_____ Performs effective harm assessments.

_____ Assists clients in goal setting.

_____ Helps clients build on their strengths.

_____ Assists clients in assuming responsibility for their progress in therapy.

_____ Assists clients in normalizing their behavior.

_____ Understands how to help clients change their behavior.
_____ Understands how to assist clients who are in crisis.
_____ Demonstrates an ability to be concrete and specific.
_____ Assists clients in identifying and exploring presenting problems.
_____ Demonstrates the use of multiple approaches to treatment.
_____ Works effectively with immediacy.
_____ Exhibits control of the session.
_____ Models effectively for clients.
_____ Assists clients by partializing behavior.
_____ Effectively uses reinforcement.
_____ Rehearses new behaviors and skills with clients.
_____ Effectively uses contracts and homework assignments.
_____ Makes referrals when necessary.
_____ Is knowledgeable about planned breaks, interruptions, and unplanned endings.
_____ Is knowledgeable about termination.
_____ Reviewing the treatment process.
_____ Giving and receiving feedback.
_____ Saying goodbye.

Conceptualizing Skills

_____ Identifies relevant client themes and patterns.
_____ Assists clients in perceiving situations from different points of view.
_____ Assists clients in creating new perspectives.
_____ Uses client information to develop working hypotheses and hunches.
_____ Makes relevant observations about client behavior.
_____ Identifies and uses client discrepancies.
_____ Perceives underlying client issues.
_____ Uses clients' cultural background in assessment, diagnosis, and treatment.
_____ Encourages clients to hypothesize about their own behavior.
_____ Assists clients in developing relevant focus and direction.
_____ Evaluates the efficacy of interventions.
_____ Is knowledgeable about systems and their impact on client behavior.
_____ Accurately ascertains the reality of the client.
_____ Adapts theory and techniques to meet the client's reality.
_____ Grasps the complexity of issues involved with each client.
_____ Willing to reevaluate the conceptualization of the client.

Diagnosis and Treatment

_____ Identifies presenting symptoms and formulates _DSM_ diagnoses.
_____ Formulates hypotheses based on client information.
_____ Develops appropriate strategies and interventions based on established counseling theories and techniques.

Personalization Skills

_____ Recognizes personal assets and liabilities.

_____ Perceives self in relation with clients.

_____ Directly addresses the relationship process.

_____ Understands differences between client and self.

_____ Understands the dynamics of transference and countertransference.

_____ Perceives and addresses countertransference.

_____ Understands power and influence and their use in enhancing client development.

_____ Perceives and understands boundaries in the client–counselor relationship, e.g., limit setting, sexual involvement, time limits, gifts.

_____ Sets and maintains appropriate boundaries.

_____ Understands the advantages and disadvantages of self-disclosure.

_____ Responds effectively to personal questions.

_____ Is knowledgeable concerning out-of-office contacts.

_____ Works effectively with clients who are culturally different.

_____ Is aware of own cultural background and how it may influence the counselor–client relationship.

_____ Is aware of own feelings and uses them in assisting clients.

Professional Behavior

_____ Participates in continuing education activities such as supervision, consultation, personal counseling, courses, workshops, teaching, reading, and writing.

_____ Completes paperwork, such as intakes and case notes, in a concise and timely manner.

_____ Communicates written information clearly and effectively.

_____ Provides a thoughtful disclosure statement to clients.

_____ Communicates oral information clearly and effectively.

_____ Respects appointment times with clients and supervisors.

_____ Possesses working knowledge of relevant professional literature.

_____ Dresses appropriately.

_____ Is aware of and responsive to relevant ethical standards.

_____ Is knowledgeable about professional primary ethical issues.

_____ Effectively applies ethical standards to practice situations.

_____ Has begun to think ethically.

_____ Seeks consultation on complex ethical situations.

_____ Is aware of and responsive to relevant legal standards.

_____ Is knowledgeable concerning laws that pertain to counseling practice.

_____ Applies legal mandates to practice situations.

_____ Seeks consultation on complex legal matters.

_____ Makes a conscious effort to improve counseling knowledge and skill.

_____ Exhibits willingness to work on personal issues.

_____ Exhibits respectful behavior toward clients and peers.

_____ Demonstrates an awareness of personal influence and impact on clients.

Supervision Skills for the Supervisee

_____ Initiates dialogue with the supervisor.
_____ Arrives prepared at each supervision session.
_____ Identifies questions, concerns, and issues relevant to current cases.
_____ Creates professional development goals for supervision.
_____ Shows interest in learning.
_____ Understands and incorporates suggestions.
_____ Willing to take risks for learning and identifying troublesome situations.
_____ Seeks clarification of unfamiliar situations.
_____ Accepts encouragement and constructive criticism.
_____ Demonstrates concern for and commitment to clients.
_____ Actively participates in the supervisory process.
_____ Shows willingness to engage in and use role-plays effectively.

Note

1 From Fall, M., & Sutton, J.M., Jr. (2004). *Clinical supervision*, pp. 12–16. Upper Saddle River, NJ: Pearson. Reprinted with permission.

Reference

Bernard, J. M. (1979). Supervision training: A discrimination model. *Counselor Education and Supervision, 19*, 60–68.

APPENDIX II

PSYCHIATRIC MEDICATIONS

Traditionally, counselor training programs have not focused on psychopharmacology as a major content area of training. Philosophical as well as ethical issues regarding the use of medications are contributing factors in the lack of training in this area.

Unfortunately, today's counselors in both schools and agencies are confronted with the fact that a portion of their clientele may be taking medications or is in need of medications to function more effectively. It is therefore critical that counselors have at least a rudimentary understanding of the types of medications commonly prescribed and their uses in treating mental health issues. Counselors are expected to consult and cooperate with other mental health professionals in the treatment of clients. Familiarity with medications is especially helpful in understanding the pharmacological treatment regimens prescribed for clients by physicians and psychiatrists.

The following listing of medications, used in the treatment of mental health issues, is provided for the purposes of

- providing interns in schools and agencies with a listing of common psychotropic medications used in the treatment of mental disorders;
- familiarizing the intern with basic pharmacological terms, symbols, and definitions;
- providing interns with suggested readings to help in their understanding of psychopharmacological treatment; and
- encouraging interns to learn more about the use and abuse of medications.

The number and types of medications used for the treatment of mental health issues are vast. The following is a representative sampling of the more commonly used medications in the United States.

Antidepressant Medications

All antidepressants have similar effects, and most have different side effects. About 50 percent of patients will respond to the medications with some symptom reduction within the first several days to week of treatment. Remission of symptoms is harder to achieve and may take 8 to 12 weeks. Those patients who do not achieve remission of symptoms are more likely to relapse back into depression and are at an increased risk of suicide (Wegman, 2012).

There are six classes of antidepressant medications on the US drug market:

- cyclics,
- selective serotonin reuptake inhibitors (SSRIs),
- serotonin and norepinephrine reuptake inhibitors (SNRIs),
- norepinephrine reuptake inhibitors (NRIs),
- monoamine oxidase inhibitors (MAOIs), and
- atypical antidepressants.

Cyclics

Tricyclic antidepressants (TCAs): This includes tricyclics and tetracyclics, which have similar chemical structures. TCAs are 65% to 75% effective in relieving the somatic features associated with depression. The cyclics are effective treatments for depression and were used primarily from the 1950s through the 1990s. Unfortunately, they can have serious side effects. They can be dangerous in overdose and can increase the sedative effects of alcohol and cause life-threatening heart rhythm disturbances when taken in overdose (Smith, 2012).

Trade Name	Generic Name	Daily Dosage
Anafranil	clomipramine	150–200 mg
Desyrel	trazodone	150–400 mg
Elavil	amitriptyline	100–200 mg
Norpramin	desipramine	150–300 mg
Pamelor	desipramine	75–150 mg
Sinequan	doxepin	150–300 mg
Tofranil	imipramine	100–200 mg

Note: See Wegman, 2012.

Selective Serotonin Reuptake Inhibitors (SSRIs)

SSRIs, a second-generation antidepressant, have fewer side effects than TCAs and monoamine oxidase inhibitors (see below). Generally, SSRIs cause less weight gain and less sedation and hypotension than TCAs. In addition, SSRIs are less lethal when taken in overdose.

Trade Name	Generic Name	Daily Dosage
Celexa	citalopram	20–80 mg
Lexapro	escitalopram	10–40 mg
Luvox	fluvoxamine	100–400 mg

Trade Name	Generic Name	Daily Dosage
Paxil	paroxetine	20–50 mg
Prozac	fluoxetine	10–80 mg
Sarafem	fluoxetine	20–80 mg
Viibryd*	vilazodone	10–40 mg
Zoloft	sertraline	50–200 mg

*SSRI/atypical.

Serotonin and Norepinephrine Reuptake Inhibitors (SNRIs)

These are considered dual action antidepressants.

Trade Name	Generic Name	Daily Dosage
Cymbalta	duloxetine	20–80 mg
Effexor	venlafaxine	75–350 mg
Effexor XR	venlafaxineXR	75–350 mg
Pristiq	venlafaxine	75–350 mg

Norepinephrine Reuptake Inhibitors (NRIs)

NRIs are noted for providing an energy boost as well as for decreasing distractibility and improving the attention span. *Strattera* (atomoxetine) is pharmacologically considered an antidepressant but is approved by the Food and Drug Administration for the treatment of attention deficit–hyperactivity disorder. *Remeron* (mirtazapine) helps with the anxiety and sleep problems common to depression.

Monoamine Oxidase Inhibitors (MAOIs)

MAOIs were first developed in the 1950s and today are rarely used. MAOIs are indicated for some patients who are unresponsive to other antidepressants. Because of their side-effects profile and a potential for serious interactions with other drugs and food, MAOIs are no longer used as a first drug of choice when treating depression (Buelow, Hebert, & Buelow, 2000).

Trade Name	Generic Name	Daily Dosage
Emsam	selegiline	patch 6–12 mg
Nardil	phenelzine	10–30 mg
Parnate	tranylcypromine	10–30 mg

Atypical Antidepressants

Trade Name	Generic Name	Daily Dosage
Aplenzin	bupropion(Hbr)	174–522 mg
Remeron	mirtazapine	15–45 mg
Oleptro	trazodone ER	150–300 mg
Symbyax	olanzapine/fluoxetine	6 mg olanzapine/25 mg fluoxetine
Viibryd*	vilazodone	10–40 mg
WellbutrinSR	bupropionSR	150–300 mg
WellbutrinLA	bupropionLA	150–300 mg

Antianxiety Medications

Anxiolytics or Minor Tranquilizers

Benzodiazepines (BDZs): BDZs are a group of structurally related compounds that have sedative properties. Because of the greater safety margin of BDZs, their use has, for the most part, replaced the use of barbiturates, a more dangerous class of sedatives (Buelow, Hebert, & Buelow, 2000). BDZs are often the treatment of choice for anxiety. While BDZs are popular and widely used, the risk of dependence is significant. They can also be dangerous when used in overdose, particularly when combined with alcohol. Their use should be monitored. When discontinued, their dose should be reduced slowly, over days, weeks, or even months, to prevent withdrawal symptoms (Wegman, 2012). These medications are often used with SSRIs in the treatment of panic. Antianxiety medication is not indicated for obsessive-compulsive disorder, which is typically treated with higher doses of serotonin antidepressants (SSRIs) in combination with cognitive behavioral therapy.

Trade Name	Generic Name	Daily Dosage
Ativan	lorazepam	1–10 mg
Klonopin	clonazepam	0.25–1.5 mg
Librium	chlordiazepoxide	20–40 mg
Valium	diazepam	20–40 mg
Xanax	alprozolam	0.5–1.5 mg

Antianxiety Agents Other Than Benzodiazepines

Trade Name	Generic Name	Daily Dosage
Atarax	hydroxyzine	100–400 mg
Buspar	buspirone	15–30 mg
Vistaril	hydroxyzine pamoate	100–400 mg

Mood-Stabilizing Medications

These medications are used primarily for the treatment of bipolar disorder.

Lithium (Lithobid) is considered as a first-line agent in the treatment of acute mania and hypomania as well as for the maintenance treatment of bipolar I and II. It is safe and effective when closely monitored. Therapeutic doses can be close to toxic, and consequently blood levels must be carefully monitored. Other medications used in the treatment of bipolar disorders are the anticonvulsants and the atypical antipsychotics.

Anticonvulsant Medications Used in the Treatment of Bipolar Disorder

Trade Name	Generic Name	Daily Dosage
Depakote	divalproex	750–3000 mg
Lamictal	lamotrigine	100–200 mg
Tegretol	carbamazepine	600–1200 mg
Topamax	topiramate	200–400 mg

In addition to the mood stabilizers and the anticonvulsant medications, all second-generation antipsychotic medications have been approved for the treatment of bipolar mania. However, most are not effective in bipolar depression with the exception of Seroquel and Abilify. Traditional antidepressants have little, if any, advantage in the treatment of bipolar depression (Wegman, 2012).

Antipsychotic Medications

The modern era for the treatment of psychotic disorders began in the early 1950s when Thorazine was found to be an effective treatment for schizophrenia. All antipsychotic medications block dopamine receptors in the central nervous system. But because of their actions on the neurotransmitter systems, there can be many side effects. When the medications are effective the patient feels relaxed and less fearful, and thought distortion and mood may also improve (Wegman, 2012). These medications induce in schizophrenia a "neuroleptic state" that is characterized by decreased agitation, aggression, and impulsiveness, as well as a decrease in hallucinations and delusions and, generally, less concern with the external environment (Buelow, Hebert, & Buelow, 2000, p. 66). Antipsychotic medications fall into two main categories: the older conventional agents and the newer atypical agents.

Conventional Agents

The first antipsychotic medication on the US drug market was Thorazine in 1952. This was followed by several others. However, these first-generation medications are no longer considered agents of choice. These conventional agents fell out of favor because of the neurological side effects and because 20 percent of adult schizophrenics are unresponsive to these conventional medications (Wegman, 2012).

Trade Name	Generic Name	Daily Dosage
Haldol	haloperidol	1–40 mg
Mellaril	thioridazine	150–800 mg
Moban	molindone	20–225 mg
Navane	thiothixene	10–60 mg
Prolixin	fluphenazine	3–45 mg
Stelazine	trifluoperazine	2–40 mg
Thorazine	chlorpromazine	60–800 mg

Atypical Antipsychotic Agents

The atypicals are not a single homogeneous class of drugs. They carry a lower risk of neurological side effects and tardive dyskinesis. All of the atypicals are approved for use with bipolar mania, but effectiveness varies depending on symptomatic circumstances.

Trade Name	Generic Name	Initial Dosage
Abilify	aripiprazole	10–15 mg
Clorazil	clozapine	300–600 mg
Fanapt	iloperidone	12–24 mg
Geodon	ziprasidone	120–160 mg
Invega	paliperidone	3–12 mg
Risperdal	risperidone	2 mg/divided/bid
Saphris	asenapine	10–20 mg
Symbyax	olanzapine/fluoxetine	5–20 mg
Seroquel	quetiapine	100–150 mg
Zyprexa	olanzapine	5–20 mg

Special Populations: Psychopharmacological Treatments for Children and Adolescents

Disorder	Medications
Major depression	SSRIs
Bipolar disorder	Lithium, Depakote, Risperdal, Abilify
Schizophrenia	Risperdal, Abilify, Zyprexa, Seroquel
Obsessive-compulsive disorder	Luvox, Zoloft

Separation anxiety disorder	Buspar, Vistaril, SSRIs
Attention-deficit/hyperactivity disorder (ADHD)	RitalinLA, AdderallXR, Daytrana, Vyvanse, WellbutrinSR/LA, Intuniv
Psychotic disorder	Seroquel, Zyprexa

These lists of medications are offered to provide an overview of medications currently used in treatment and are not intended to be used prescriptively. The information reflects currently accepted practice, but any recommendations must be held up against individual circumstances at hand. These lists of medications were adapted from the following sources. Miller's (2009) book is particularly helpful to use with patients.

Buelow, G., Hebert, S., & Buelow, S. (2000). *Psychotherapists resource on psychiatric medications: Issues of treatment and referral*. Belmont, CA: Wadsworth.

Ingersoll, R. E., & Rak, C. F. (2006). *Psychopharmacology for helping professions*. Pacific Grove, CA: Thompson Brooks/Cole.

Miller, F. (2009). *My mental health medication workbook*. Eau Claire, WI: PESI.

PDR: Drug guide for mental health professionals. (2004). Montvale, NJ: Thomson PDR.

Smith, T. (2012). *Psychopharmacology: What you need to know about psychiatric medications*. Eau Claire, WI: CMI Education.

Wegman, J. (2012). *Straight talk on mental health medications*. Eau Claire, WI: Premier Publishing & Media.

FORMS

Form 2.1: Practicum Contract

This agreement is made on _____ by and between _____
(date)   (field site)

and _____. The agreement will be effective for a period
(university program)

from _____ to _____ for _____ per week for _____.
(starting date)   (ending date)   (number of hours)   (student name)

Purpose

The purpose of this agreement is to provide a qualified graduate student with a practicum experience in the field of counseling or psychology.

The University Program Agrees

1. to assign a university faculty liaison to facilitate communication between university and site;
2. to provide the site prior to placement of the student the following information:
   a. a profile of the student named above, and
   b. an academic calendar that shall include dates for periods during which student will be excused from field supervision;
3. to notify the student that he/she must adhere to the administrative policies, rules, standards, schedules, and practices of the site;
4. that the faculty liaison shall be available for consultation with both site supervisors and students and shall be immediately contacted should any problem or change in relation to student, site, or university occur; and
5. that the university supervisor is responsible for the assignment of a fieldwork grade.

The Practicum Site Agrees

1. to assign a practicum supervisor who has appropriate credentials, time, and interest for training the practicum student;
2. to provide opportunities for the student to engage in a variety of counseling activities under supervision and for evaluating the student's performance (suggested counseling experiences included in the "Practicum Activities" section);
3. to provide the student with adequate work space, telephone, office supplies, and staff to conduct professional activities;
4. to provide supervisory contact that involves some examination of student work using audio- or videotapes, observation, and/or live supervision; and
5. to provide written evaluation of student based on criteria established by the university program.

The Practicum Student Agrees

1. to obtain transportation to and from the site;
2. to schedule and attend weekly supervision sessions with on-site supervisor and attend weekly supervision sessions with faculty supervisors;
3. to adhere to the ethical guidelines of the American Counseling Association *Code of Ethics*; and
4. to adhere to the policies and procedures, rules, and standards of the placement site.

Within the specified time frame, _____ (site supervisor) will be the primary practicum site supervisor. The training activities (checked below) will be provided for the student in sufficient amounts to allow an adequate evaluation of the student's level of competence in each activity.

_____ (faculty liaison) will be the faculty liaison with whom the student and practicum site supervisor will communicate regarding progress, problems, and performance evaluations.

Practicum Activities

1. Individual counseling/psychotherapy
   Personal/social nature
   Occupational/educational nature

2. Group counseling/psychotherapy
   Coleading
   Leading

3. Intake interviewing
   Taking social history information

4. Testing
   Administration
   Analysis
   Interpretation of results

5. Report writing
   Record keeping
   Treatment plans
   Treatment

6. Consultation
   Referrals
   Professional team collaboration

7. Psychoeducational activities
   Parent conferences
   Outreach

8. Career counseling

9. Individual supervision

10. Group or peer supervision

11. Case conferences or staff meetings

12. Other (please list) _____
    _____
    _____
    _____

Practicum site supervisor _____ Date _____

Student _____ Date _____

Faculty liaison _____ Date _____

248

Form 2.2: Internship Contract

This agreement is made this _____ day of _____ , by and between

_____ (hereinafter referred to as the

AGENCY/INSTITUTION/SCHOOL) and _____

(hereinafter referred to as the UNIVERSITY). This agreement will be effective for a period from

_____ to _____ for student _____.

Purpose

The purpose of this agreement is to provide a qualified graduate student with an internship experience in the field of counseling/therapy.

The UNIVERSITY Shall Be Responsible for the Following:

1. Selecting a student who has successfully completed all of the prerequisite courses and the practicum experience.
2. Providing the AGENCY/INSTITUTION/SCHOOL with a course outline for the supervised internship counseling that clearly delineates the responsibilities of the UNIVERSITY and the AGENCY/INSTITUTION/SCHOOL.
3. Designating a qualified faculty member as the internship supervisor who will work with the AGENCY/INSTITUTION/SCHOOL in coordinating the internship experience.
4. Notifying the student that he/she must adhere to the administrative policies, rules, standards, schedules, and practices of the AGENCY/INSTITUTION/SCHOOL.
5. Advising the student that he/she should have adequate liability and accident insurance.

The AGENCY/INSTITUTION/SCHOOL Shall Be Responsible for the Following:

1. Providing the intern with an overall orientation to the agency's specific services necessary for the implementation of the internship experience.
2. Designating a qualified staff member to function as supervising counselor/therapist for the intern. The supervising counselor/therapist will be responsible, with the approval of the administration of the AGENCY/INSTITUTION/SCHOOL, for providing opportunities for the intern to engage in a variety of counseling activities under supervision and for evaluating the intern's performance. (Suggested counselor/therapist experiences are included in the course outline.)
3. Providing areas for conducting counseling sessions and for doing paperwork. Provisions will be made to ensure that students have the ability to meet course requirements for internship, especially regarding direct service hours with clients.

The STUDENT Shall Be Responsible for the Following:

1. Obtaining transportation to and from the site.
2. Scheduling and attending weekly supervision sessions with on-site supervisor and attending weekly supervision sessions with faculty supervisors.

3. Adhering to the ethical guidelines of the American Counseling Association's *Code of Ethics*.
4. Adhering to the policies and procedures, rules, and standards of the placement site.

Equal Opportunity

It is mutually agreed that neither party shall discriminate on the basis of race, color, nationality, ethnic origin, age, sex, or creed.

Financial Agreement

Financial stipulations, if any, may vary from one AGENCY/INSTITUTION/SCHOOL to another. If a financial stipulation is to be provided, the agreement is stipulated in a separate agreement and approved by the intern, the AGENCY/INSTITUTION/SCHOOL, and the UNIVERSITY.

Termination

It is understood and agreed by and between the parties hereto that the AGENCY/INSTITUTION/SCHOOL has the right to terminate the internship experience of the student whose health status is detrimental to the services provided to the patients or clients of the AGENCY/INSTITUTION/SCHOOL. Furthermore, it has the right to terminate the use of the AGENCY/INSTITUTION/SCHOOL by an intern if, in the opinion of the supervising counselor/therapist, such person's behavior is detrimental to the operation of the AGENCY/INSTITUTION/SCHOOL and/or to patient or client care. Such action will not be taken until the grievance against any intern has been discussed with the intern and with UNIVERSITY officials.

The names of the responsible individuals at the two institutions charged with the implementation of the contract are as follows:

_____   _____
Internship supervisor at the UNIVERSITY   Agency supervising counselor/therapist at
                                           the AGENCY/INSTITUTION/SCHOOL

   In witness whereof, the parties hereto have caused this contract to be signed the day and year first written above.

_____   _____
AGENCY/INSTITUTION/SCHOOL   Witness
(Administrator)

_____   _____
UNIVERSITY (Representative)   Witness

Form 2.3: Student Profile Sheet

Directions: The student counselor is to submit this form in duplicate to the field site.

Practicum Student Counselor/Psychologist

Name _____

Address _____

_____

Telephone: (home) _____

(office) _____

Date _____

I hold the degree of _____ from

_____ and have completed the following

courses as part of the _____ (degree)

program, with a major in _____

from _____.

Psychology of Human Development _____   Tests and Measurements _____

Diagnosis and Treatment _____   Personality Development _____

Counseling Skills _____   Career Development _____

Intro to Counseling _____   Legal and Ethical Issues _____

Theories of Counseling _____   Process and Techniques of
                                                Group Counseling _____

Multicultural Counseling _____

Other (please specify) _____

_____

_____

Professional and nonprofessional work experience _____

_____

_____

Form 2.4: Student Practicum/Internship Agreement

Directions: Student is to complete this form in duplicate and submit a copy of this agreement to the university practicum supervisor or internship coordinator.

1. I hereby attest that I have read and understood the American Psychological Association and/or the American Counseling Association *Code of Ethics* and will practice my counseling in accordance with these standards. Any breach of these ethics or any unethical behavior on my part will result in my removal from practicum/internship and a failing grade, and documentation of such behavior will become part of my permanent record.
2. I agree to adhere to the administrative policies, rules, standards, and practices of the practicum/internship site.
3. I understand that my responsibilities include keeping my practicum/internship supervisor(s) informed regarding my practicum/internship experiences.
4. I understand that I will not be issued a passing grade in practicum/internship unless I demonstrate the specified minimal level of counseling skill, knowledge, and competence and complete course requirements as required.
5. I understand I must obtain proper clearances (e.g., child abuse clearance, criminal background checks) or health tests (e.g., TB test) as required by the program and/or my site prior to the start of practicum and internship.
6. I understand that my placement site is subject to the approval of the program faculty.

Signature _____

Date _____

Form 3.1a: Parental Release Form: Secondary School Counseling

_____ school district offers short-term individual counseling and group counseling to students as the need arises. Parents/guardians or school staff may refer students for counseling, or students may request counseling. These counseling services are provided by _____ , the school counselor, or _____ , the counseling intern. Should it be determined that more extensive services are needed, it is the parent's responsibility, with the assistance of the counselor, to arrange outside counseling or psychiatric services.

School counseling services are short-term services aimed to enhance the education and socialization of students within the school community. Trust is a cornerstone of the relationship between the counselor and student. Information shared by the student will be kept confidential except in certain situations in which ethical responsibility limits confidentiality. You will be notified if:

1. The student reveals information about hurting himself/herself or someone else.
2. The student or someone else may be in physical danger.
3. A court order is received directing disclosure of information.

We encourage you to contact us whenever you have a question, input, or concern.

The counseling intern is an advanced-level master's degree student in the Department of Counseling and Psychology at _____University. The University requires that the counseling sessions conducted by the counseling intern be audio/video-recorded for confidential supervision purposes. Personal identifying details will be deleted, and the tape will be reviewed by the supervisor and peer members of the supervision group to review the counseling practice of the intern. The tape will be destroyed after the supervision review. Supervision requires that ethical standards regarding confidentiality be followed.

Student's name _____

By signing this form, I give permission for my child to receive counseling services during the 20___ school year. I understand that anything my child shares is confidential except in the above-mentioned cases.

Parent/guardian _____   Date _____

I do _____ do not _____ give permission for the taping of sessions for confidential supervision purposes.

Form 3.1b: Elementary School Counseling Permission Form

Short Form

We, the parents of _____ , acknowledge and approve of our child being seen by the elementary school counselor or counselor intern. The counselor may engage our child in any counseling services deemed appropriate in encouraging positive educational and social development.

We understand that that the intern is an advanced-level graduate student in the Department of Counseling and Psychology at _____ University and will audio/videotape counseling sessions for supervision purposes. The tape will be reviewed by the University supervisor and peer group members of the supervision seminar to evaluate the intern's counseling practice. The tape will be erased after supervision. Supervision requires following confidentiality standards established in the professional code of ethics.

_____

Parent signature

_____

Date

OR

We, the parents of _____ , acknowledge but do not give our permission for our child to be seen by the elementary school counselor or counseling intern to receive counseling services. We decline the offer of services at this time but reserve the opportunity to reconsider services at a later date.

_____

Parent signature

_____

Date

Form 3.2: Client Permission to Record Counseling Session for Supervision Purposes

    I, _____, give my permission for the counseling intern, _____ _____ to audio/videotape my counseling sessions _____ (fill in date or inclusive dates if over a period of time). [If client is under 18, change wording to "tape the counseling sessions with my child" and fill in child's name.] I understand that the counseling intern at _____ Agency is an advanced-level master's degree student in the Department of Counseling and Psychology at _____ University. The University requires that the counseling sessions conducted by the counseling intern be audio/video-recorded for confidential supervision purposes. Personal identifying details will be deleted, and the tape will be reviewed by the supervisor and peer members of the supervision group to review the counseling practice of the intern. The tape will be destroyed after the supervision review. Supervision requires that ethical standards regarding confidentiality be followed.

_____ Name of agency supervisor

_____ Name of university supervisor

_____   _____

Client's signature   Date

_____

Parent/guardian signature

Form 3.3: Initial Intake Form

Name _____ Date _____

Address _____ City _____ State _____ Zip _____

Telephone (home) _____ (work) _____ (cell) _____

Counselor's name _____ Date _____

Identifying Information

Age _____ Date of birth _____ / _____ / _____ Place _____

Sex: Male _____ Female _____ Height _____ ft. _____ in. Weight _____ lbs.

Race: White _____ Black _____ Asian _____ Hispanic _____ Other _____

Marital status: M _____ S _____ D _____ W _____ Sep _____

If married, spouse's name _____ Age _____

Occupation (client) _____ Employer _____

Occupation (spouse)_____ Employer _____

Referral source: Self_____ Other _____

Name of referral source _____

Address of referral source _____

Treatment History (General)

Are you currently taking medication? Yes _____ No _____

If yes, name(s) of the medication(s) _____

Dosage of medication(s) _____

Provider of medication(s) _____

Have you received previous psychiatric treatment? Yes _____ No _____

If yes, name provider _____

Dates of service _____ Location _____

Reason for termination of treatment _____

Presenting problem or condition (current) _____

Presenting factors (contributors) _____

Symptoms (describe) _____

_____

Acute _____ Chronic _____

Family History (General)

Father's name _____ Age _____ Living _____ Deceased _____

Occupation _____ Full-time _____ Part-time _____

Mother's name _____ Age _____ Living _____ Deceased _____

Occupation _____ Full-time _____ Part-time _____

Brother(s)/sister(s)

Name _____ Age _____ Living _____ Deceased _____

Name _____ Age _____ Living _____ Deceased _____

Name _____ Age _____ Living _____ Deceased _____

Educational History (General)

	Name of institution	*Location*	*Dates*	*Degree*
Secondary				
College				
Trade				
Graduate				

Employment History (General)

Title/description	*From when to when*	*Full- or part-time*

Form 3.4: Psychosocial History

Directions: Practicum/internship students should review/complete this form prior to the initiation of therapy and after completion of the Initial Intake Form.

I. Identifying Information

Name_____Age_____

Address _____ Date of birth _____

Phone _____ Cell phone _____ Marital status _____

II. Presenting Problem/Complaint

Nature of complaint? _____

_____

When did the problem begin? (date of onset) _____

How often does it occur? (be specific) _____

How does it affect your daily functioning? _____

_____

Are there events, situations, and person(s) that precipitate it? _____

_____

Symptoms:

Acute (describe) _____

_____

Chronic (describe) _____

_____

Previous treatment (list by whom, outcome, and reason(s) for termination of treatment) _____

_____

_____

_____

Medical:

Physician's name _____

Treatment dates from _____ to _____

Describe _____

_____

Psychiatric:

Therapist's name _____

Treatment dates from _____ to _____

Substance use _____

_____

III. Developmental History

Pregnancy _____

_____

Delivery _____

_____

Infancy (developmental milestones) _____

_____

Middle childhood (developmental milestones) _____

_____

Young adulthood (developmental milestones)

_____

IV. Family History

Where were you born and raised? _____

What culture/ethnic group do you identify with? _____

What is your primary language? _____

Parent (names, ages, occupations) _____

_____

Were your parents married?   Yes _____ No _____

Do they remain married?   Yes _____ No _____

If divorced, how were you affected by it? _____

_____

Who was primarily responsible for your upbringing? _____

Describe the relationship between your parents _____

_____

Describe your relationship with your parents _____

_____

Do you feel supported by your family? Explain _____

_____

Do you feel loved in your family? Explain _____

_____

Describe how love was expressed in your family _____

_____

Who was the disciplinarian in your family? _____

How was discipline handled? _____

_____

Were you physically, verbally, or emotionally abused in any way? _____

_____

Describe your best memory _____

_____

Describe your worst memory _____

_____

V. Educational/Occupational History

Education (highest grade achieved) _____

Describe your school performance _____

_____

Did you take any special classes? Explain _____

_____

Did you have any special needs? _____

_____

Do you have adequate reading skills?   Yes _____ No _____

Do you have adequate math skills?   Yes _____ No _____

Occupational

Have you served in the military?_____

When and where did you serve?_____

What was your rank? _____

Describe your duties _____

Usual occupation _____

Present status: Employed? _____ Unemployed? _____ Full time _____ Part time _____

Job satisfaction: Good _____ Fair _____ Poor _____

Estimate the number of jobs that you have held _____

Longest continued employments (dates) _____

Reason(s) for leaving? Explain _____

_____

What impact does your present concern have on your employment?

None _____ Terminated _____ Absenteeism _____ Tardiness _____ Laid off _____

Poor work performance _____ Conflict with fellow workers _____

Conflict with employer _____

VI. Health History

Childhood diseases (list) _____

_____

Surgeries? _____

_____

Current health (describe) _____

_____

_____

Family health (grandparents, parents, children) _____

_____

_____

Current medications (prescribed and over the counter). List _____

_____

_____

Do you have any chronic medical problems? _____

_____

Do you have any bio-medical problems requiring medical monitoring? _____

_____

VII. Relationship History

Single _____ Married _____ Separated _____ Divorced _____ Widowed _____

Common law _____ Years married? _____

Number of children (names and ages) _____

_____

_____

Problems, stressors in the relationship? Explain _____

_____

_____

Your perception of sexual relationship (attitudes/behavior) _____

_____

_____

Have you ever been physically or emotionally abused in the relationship?

_____

_____

VIII. Additional Information

Information that has not been covered that you feel is an important consideration in your treatment (explain, be specific) _____

_____

_____

Form 3.5: Case Notes

These case notes are confidential and must be kept in a secure place under the control of the counselor.

Counselor's name _____   Agency/school _____

CLIENT IDENTIFYING DATA

Client's ID _____ Age _____ Sex _____

Date of session _____ Session number _____

Taping: Audio _____ Video _____

Presenting/current concern

_____

_____

_____

Key issues addressed

_____

_____

_____

Summary of the session

_____

_____

_____

Diagnostic impression(s) and interventions

_____

_____

_____

Client progress/setbacks (current internal/external dynamics that support or inhibit change)

_____

_____

_____

Plan

_____

_____

Counselor's comments

_____

_____

_____

Supervisor's comments

_____

_____

_____

Date _____   Counselor's signature _____

Date _____   Supervisor's signature _____

Form 3.6: Weekly Schedule/Practicum Log

Day of week	Location	Time	Practicum activity	Comment

Student counselor name _____

Week beginning _____ Ending _____

Total hours of direct service _____ Indirect service _____

Site supervisor signature _____ Date _____

Form 3.7: Monthly Practicum Log

Directions:

1. Record the dates of each week at the site where indicated.
2. Record the total number of hours per week for each activity under the appropriate column.
3. Total the number of hours for the week at the bottom of the week's column.
4. At the end of the month, total the hours spent in each activity by adding the hours across each activity; indicate the total in the monthly totals column.
5. Get the supervisor's signature. Keep this in your file to be submitted to the university internship coordinator at the completion of the internship.

Activities	Week 1 From: To:	Week 2 From: To:	Week 3 From: To:	Week 4 From: To:	Monthly Totals
Intake interview*					
Individual counseling*					
Group counseling*					
Family counseling*					
Consulting/intervention*					
Psychoeducation/guidance*					
Community work					
Career counseling*					
Report writing					
Case conference					
Program planning					
Testing/assessment					
Individual supervision					
Other					
Weekly totals					
Total direct contact*					

*Indicates direct contact

Intern's name _____

Supervisor's signature and date _____

Form 4.1: Elementary School Counseling Referral Form

Please complete and return this confidential referral form to me. The form should be closed in a sealed envelope and placed in my office mailbox. Do not duplicate.

To: _____ School Counselor _____ Date _____

Priority

Low (schedule when available); High (as soon as possible); Emergency (see now)

Student's name and grade _____

Referred by _____

Please check any behaviors of concern that you have observed:

☐ aggression   ☐ academics

☐ dramatic change in behavior   ☐ homework completion

☐ bullying—victim   ☐ study skills

☐ bullying—bully   ☐ organizational skills

☐ daydreams/fantasizes   ☐ impulsive

☐ poor peer relationships   ☐ always tired

☐ poor social skills   ☐ inattentive

☐ family concerns (illness, divorce) ☐ disruptive

☐ suspected abuse   ☐ worried/anxious

☐ cries easily/often for age   ☐ scared

☐ self-image/self-confidence   ☐ sadness

☐ personal hygiene   ☐ withdrawn/shy

☐ lying   ☐ depressed

☐ stealing   ☐ defiant

☐ grief and loss   ☐ difficulty making friends

☐ other

Explanation: _____

_____

_____

_____

_____

Best time to pull child from class: 1st choice _____   2nd choice _____

I recommend this child for individual counseling _____; small group counseling _____.

Thank you for taking the time to share this information with me.

Form 4.2: Secondary School Counseling Referral Form

Please complete this confidential counseling referral form, place it in a sealed envelope, and place it in the mailbox of the counselor to whom you are making the referral. Do not duplicate.

Date referral received _____

Counselor's name _____

Student's name and grade _____

Referred by _____

Priority:

Low (schedule when available)   High (as soon as possible)   Emergency (see now)

Have you had a discussion with the child's parent(s) regarding this referral? Yes or no

Student's Present Functioning (as you perceive it)

	Excellent	*Above average*	*Average*	*Below average*	*Poor*
Self-directed learner					
Attention span					
Quality of writing					
Self-image					
Attitude toward authority					
Peer relationships					
Works well with others					
Completes assignments					
Follows classroom rules					

Please check any behaviors of concern that you have observed or have knowledge of:

☐ academic

☐ absences

☐ anger/aggression

☐ truancy

☐ suicidal thoughts

☐ tardiness

☐ depression

☐ family issues (illness, divorce)

☐ stress/anxiety

☐ health/hygiene

☐ peer relationships   ☐ student/teacher issues

☐ boyfriend/girlfriend issues   ☐ student/parent issues

☐ dramatic change in behavior   ☐ hurts/cuts self

☐ sexuality issues   ☐ child neglect/abuse

☐ dropout risk   ☐ work habits/organization

☐ grief/loss   ☐ withdrawn

☐ bullying—victim   ☐ substance abuse

☐ bullying—bully   ☐ other

Special skills, talents, or competencies this student has _____
_____

Reason for referral (based on your observations) _____
_____

Signature _____   Date _____

Position _____

Form 4.3: Mental Status Checklist

Appearance and Behavior

	Check if applies	*Circle*	*Therapist's Comments*
1. Posture	Normal _____	Limp, rigid, ill at ease	_____
2. Gestures	Normal _____	Agitated, tics, twitches	_____
3. Grooming	Neat _____	Well groomed,	_____
		disheveled,	_____
		meticulous	_____
		Dirty, careless,	_____
4. Dress	Casual _____	inappropriate,	_____
	Formal _____	seductive	_____
5. Facial expression	Appropriate _____	Poor eye contact, dazed, staring	_____
6. Speech			_____
a. Pace	Normal _____	Retarded, pressured,	_____
		blocking	_____
b. Volume	Normal _____	Soft, very loud,	_____
		monotone	_____
c. Form	Logical _____	Illogical, rambling,	_____
	Rational _____	incoherent, coherent	_____
d. Clarity	Normal _____	Garbled, slurred	_____
e. Content	Normal _____	Loose, associations, rhyming, obscene	_____

Attention/Affect/Mood

	Check if applies	*Circle*	*Therapist's Comments*
1. Attention	Normal _____	Short span, hyper,	_____
	Alert _____	alert, distractible	_____
2. Mood	Normal _____	Elated, euphoric,	_____
		agitated, fearful,	_____
		hostile, sad	_____
3. Affect	Appropriate _____	Inappropriate,	_____
		shallow, flat,	_____
		intense	_____

Perception and Thought Content

	Check if applies	*Description*
1. Hallucination	_____	_____
a. Auditory	_____	_____
b. Visual	_____	_____
c. Tactile	_____	_____
d. Gustatory	_____	_____
e. Olfactory	_____	_____

2. Delusion

a. Paranoid	_____	b. Persecutor	_____
c. Grandiose	_____	d. Reference	_____
e. Control	_____	f. Thought	_____
g. Broadcasting	_____	h. Insertion	_____
i. Thought withdrawal	_____		

3. Illusions

a. Visual _____

b. Auditory _____

Describe _____

_____

4. Other derealization

a. Phobias	_____	b. Obsessions	_____
c. Compulsions	_____	d. Ruminations	_____

Describe _____
_____

5. Suicide/homicide

   Ideation _____ Plans _____

   Describe _____
   _____

Orientation   Oriented × 3   Yes _____ No _____

Disoriented to: Time _____ Place _____ Person _____

Judgment   Intact _____   Impaired _____

Describe _____
_____

Concentration/Memory

1. Memory   Intact _____   Impaired _____
2. Immediate recall Good _____   Poor _____
3. Reversals   Good _____   Poor _____
4. Concentration   Good _____   Poor _____

Abstract Ability

1. Similarities   Good   _____   Poor   _____   Bizarre   _____
2. Absurdities   Recognized   _____   Not recognized   _____
3. Proverbs   Appropriate _____   Literal   _____   Concrete _____ Bizarre _____
Insight   Good   _____   Fair   _____   Poor   _____ Absent   _____

Form 4.4: Therapeutic Progress Report

Date _____

Therapist's name _____

Therapist's phone _____

Client's name/ID _____

Client's age _____ Sex _____

Sessions to date with client _____
                                              (dates from/to and total number)

Client's presenting complaint

_____

_____

_____

Therapeutic summary

_____

_____

_____

Methods of treatment

_____

_____

_____

Duration of treatment

_____

_____

_____

Current status

_____

_____

_____

Treatment recommendations

_____

_____

_____

_____   _____
Therapist's signature   Supervisor's signature

Form 5.1: Counseling Techniques List

Directions

1. First, examine the techniques listed in the first column. Then, technique by technique, decide the extent to which you use or would be competent to use each. Indicate the extent of use or competency by circling the appropriate letter in the second column. If you do not know the technique, then mark an "X" through the "N" to indicate that the technique is unknown. Space is available at the end of the techniques list in the first column to add other techniques.
2. Second, after examining the list and indicating your extent of use or competency, go through the techniques list again and circle in the third column the theory or theories with which each technique is appropriate. The third column, of course, can be marked only for those techniques with which you are familiar.
3. The third task is to become more knowledgeable about the techniques that you do not know—the ones marked with an "X." As you gain knowledge relating to each technique, you can decide whether you will use it and, if so, with which kinds of clients and under what conditions.
4. The final task is to review the second and third columns and determine whether techniques in which you have competencies are within one or two specific theories. If so, are these theories the ones that best reflect your self-concept? Do those techniques marked reflect those most appropriate, as revealed in the literature, for the clients with whom you want to work?

Extent of Use Key

N = None	M = Minimal	A = Average	E = Extensive

Theory for Technique Key

Ad = Adlerian (Adler, Dreikurs)	Ge = Gestalt (Perls)
Be = Behavioral (Skinner, Bandura, Lazarus)	PC = Person Centered (Rogers)
CBT = Cognitive behavioral (Beck, Ellis, Meichenbaum)	Ps = Psychodynamic (Freud, Erikson)
Ex = Existential (May, Frankl)	Re = Reality (Glasser, Wubbolding)
FS = Family systems (Bowen, Satir, Minuchin)	SF = Solution focused (Berg, deShazur)

Technique	Extent of Use	Theory for Technique
ABC Model	N M A E	Ad Be CBT Ex FS Ge PC Ps Re SF
Acceptance	N M A E	Ad Be CBT Ex FS Ge PC Ps Re SF
Accurate empathic understanding	N M A E	Ad Be CBT Ex FS Ge PC Ps Re SF
Analysis of resistance	N M A E	Ad Be CBT Ex FS Ge PC Ps Re SF
Analysis of transference	N M A E	Ad Be CBT Ex FS Ge PC Ps Re SF
Analyze cognitive triad	N M A E	Ad Be CBT Ex FS Ge PC Ps Re SF
Analyze defense mechanisms	N M A E	Ad Be CBT Ex FS Ge PC Ps Re SF
Analyzing cognitive distortions	N M A E	Ad Be CBT Ex FS Ge PC Ps Re SF
Assertiveness training	N M A E	Ad Be CBT Ex FS Ge PC Ps Re SF
Assignment of tasks	N M A E	Ad Be CBT Ex FS Ge PC Ps Re SF
Avoid focus on symptoms	N M A E	Ad Be CBT Ex FS Ge PC Ps Re SF

Technique	Extent of Use	Theory for Technique
Behavioral tasks	N M A E	Ad Be CBT Ex FS Ge PC Ps Re SF
Bibliotherapy	N M A E	Ad Be CBT Ex FS Ge PC Ps Re SF
Birth order	N M A E	Ad Be CBT Ex FS Ge PC Ps Re SF
Boundary setting	N M A E	Ad Be CBT Ex FS Ge PC Ps Re SF
Bridging compliments to tasks	N M A E	Ad Be CBT Ex FS Ge PC Ps Re SF
Change faulty motivation	N M A E	Ad Be CBT Ex FS Ge PC Ps Re SF
Change focused questions	N M A E	Ad Be CBT Ex FS Ge PC Ps Re SF
Change maladaptive beliefs	N M A E	Ad Be CBT Ex FS Ge PC Ps Re SF
Changing language	N M A E	Ad Be CBT Ex FS Ge PC Ps Re SF
Clarify personal views on life and living	N M A E	Ad Be CBT Ex FS Ge PC Ps Re SF
Classical conditioning	N M A E	Ad Be CBT Ex FS Ge PC Ps Re SF
Cognitive homework	N M A E	Ad Be CBT Ex FS Ge PC Ps Re SF
Cognitive restructuring	N M A E	Ad Be CBT Ex FS Ge PC Ps Re SF
Commitment to change	N M A E	Ad Be CBT Ex FS Ge PC Ps Re SF
Communication analysis	N M A E	Ad Be CBT Ex FS Ge PC Ps Re SF
Communication training	N M A E	Ad Be CBT Ex FS Ge PC Ps Re SF
Compliments	N M A E	Ad Be CBT Ex FS Ge PC Ps Re SF
Confrontation	N M A E	Ad Be CBT Ex FS Ge PC Ps Re SF
Co-therapy	N M A E	Ad Be CBT Ex FS Ge PC Ps Re SF
Detriangulation	N M A E	Ad Be CBT Ex FS Ge PC Ps Re SF
Disputing irrational beliefs	N M A E	Ad Be CBT Ex FS Ge PC Ps Re SF
Dramatization	N M A E	Ad Be CBT Ex FS Ge PC Ps Re SF
Dream analysis	N M A E	Ad Be CBT Ex FS Ge PC Ps Re SF
Dreamwork	N M A E	Ad Be CBT Ex FS Ge PC Ps Re SF
Early recollections	N M A E	Ad Be CBT Ex FS Ge PC Ps Re SF
Empty chair	N M A E	Ad Be CBT Ex FS Ge PC Ps Re SF
Enactments	N M A E	Ad Be CBT Ex FS Ge PC Ps Re SF
Encouragement	N M A E	Ad Be CBT Ex FS Ge PC Ps Re SF
Exaggeration exercise	N M A E	Ad Be CBT Ex FS Ge PC Ps Re SF
Examine source of present value system	N M A E	Ad Be CBT Ex FS Ge PC Ps Re SF
Examining automatic thoughts	N M A E	Ad Be CBT Ex FS Ge PC Ps Re SF
Exception questions	N M A E	Ad Be CBT Ex FS Ge PC Ps Re SF
Experiential learning	N M A E	Ad Be CBT Ex FS Ge PC Ps Re SF
Experiments	N M A E	Ad Be CBT Ex FS Ge PC Ps Re SF
Explore quality world	N M A E	Ad Be CBT Ex FS Ge PC Ps Re SF
Explore subjective reality	N M A E	Ad Be CBT Ex FS Ge PC Ps Re SF
Exposing faulty thinking	N M A E	Ad Be CBT Ex FS Ge PC Ps Re SF
Family constellation	N M A E	Ad Be CBT Ex FS Ge PC Ps Re SF
Family-life chronology	N M A E	Ad Be CBT Ex FS Ge PC Ps Re SF
Finding alternative interpretations	N M A E	Ad Be CBT Ex FS Ge PC Ps Re SF
Flooding	N M A E	Ad Be CBT Ex FS Ge PC Ps Re SF
Focus on choice	N M A E	Ad Be CBT Ex FS Ge PC Ps Re SF

Technique	Extent of Use	Theory for Technique
Focus on personal responsibility	N M A E	Ad Be CBT Ex FS Ge PC Ps Re SF
Focus on present problems	N M A E	Ad Be CBT Ex FS Ge PC Ps Re SF
Focus on what client can control	N M A E	Ad Be CBT Ex FS Ge PC Ps Re SF
Formulate first-session task	N M A E	Ad Be CBT Ex FS Ge PC Ps Re SF
Foster social interest	N M A E	Ad Be CBT Ex FS Ge PC Ps Re SF
Free association	N M A E	Ad Be CBT Ex FS Ge PC Ps Re SF
Genogram	N M A E	Ad Be CBT Ex FS Ge PC Ps Re SF
Genuineness	N M A E	Ad Be CBT Ex FS Ge PC Ps Re SF
Guided imagery	N M A E	Ad Be CBT Ex FS Ge PC Ps Re SF
Hypothesizing systemic roots of problems	N M A E	Ad Be CBT Ex FS Ge PC Ps Re SF
Identify and define wants and needs	N M A E	Ad Be CBT Ex FS Ge PC Ps Re SF
Identify basic mistakes	N M A E	Ad Be CBT Ex FS Ge PC Ps Re SF
Immediacy	N M A E	Ad Be CBT Ex FS Ge PC Ps Re SF
Internal dialogue	N M A E	Ad Be CBT Ex FS Ge PC Ps Re SF
Interpersonal empathy	N M A E	Ad Be CBT Ex FS Ge PC Ps Re SF
Interpretation	N M A E	Ad Be CBT Ex FS Ge PC Ps Re SF
In vivo exposure	N M A E	Ad Be CBT Ex FS Ge PC Ps Re SF
Keep therapy in the present	N M A E	Ad Be CBT Ex FS Ge PC Ps Re SF
Lifestyle assessment	N M A E	Ad Be CBT Ex FS Ge PC Ps Re SF
Logotherapy	N M A E	Ad Be CBT Ex FS Ge PC Ps Re SF
Maintain analytic framework	N M A E	Ad Be CBT Ex FS Ge PC Ps Re SF
Making the rounds	N M A E	Ad Be CBT Ex FS Ge PC Ps Re SF
Miracle question	N M A E	Ad Be CBT Ex FS Ge PC Ps Re SF
Natural consequences	N M A E	Ad Be CBT Ex FS Ge PC Ps Re SF
Negative reinforcement	N M A E	Ad Be CBT Ex FS Ge PC Ps Re SF
Objective empathy	N M A E	Ad Be CBT Ex FS Ge PC Ps Re SF
Objective interview	N M A E	Ad Be CBT Ex FS Ge PC Ps Re SF
Observational tasks	N M A E	Ad Be CBT Ex FS Ge PC Ps Re SF
Operant conditioning	N M A E	Ad Be CBT Ex FS Ge PC Ps Re SF
Plan for acting	N M A E	Ad Be CBT Ex FS Ge PC Ps Re SF
Positive reinforcement	N M A E	Ad Be CBT Ex FS Ge PC Ps Re SF
Progressive muscle relaxation	N M A E	Ad Be CBT Ex FS Ge PC Ps Re SF
Psychoeducation	N M A E	Ad Be CBT Ex FS Ge PC Ps Re SF
Recognizing and changing unrealistic negative thoughts	N M A E	Ad Be CBT Ex FS Ge PC Ps Re SF
Reflection of feeling	N M A E	Ad Be CBT Ex FS Ge PC Ps Re SF
Reframing	N M A E	Ad Be CBT Ex FS Ge PC Ps Re SF
Rehearsal exercise	N M A E	Ad Be CBT Ex FS Ge PC Ps Re SF
Reject transference	N M A E	Ad Be CBT Ex FS Ge PC Ps Re SF
Reorientation	N M A E	Ad Be CBT Ex FS Ge PC Ps Re SF
Reversal exercise	N M A E	Ad Be CBT Ex FS Ge PC Ps Re SF
Scaling questions	N M A E	Ad Be CBT Ex FS Ge PC Ps Re SF

Technique	Extent of Use	Theory for Technique
Sculpting	N M A E	Ad Be CBT Ex FS Ge PC Ps Re SF
Self-evaluation	N M A E	Ad Be CBT Ex FS Ge PC Ps Re SF
Self-monitoring	N M A E	Ad Be CBT Ex FS Ge PC Ps Re SF
Shame-attacking exercises	N M A E	Ad Be CBT Ex FS Ge PC Ps Re SF
Social skills training	N M A E	Ad Be CBT Ex FS Ge PC Ps Re SF
Staying with the feeling	N M A E	Ad Be CBT Ex FS Ge PC Ps Re SF
Stress inoculation training	N M A E	Ad Be CBT Ex FS Ge PC Ps Re SF
Subjective empathy	N M A E	Ad Be CBT Ex FS Ge PC Ps Re SF
Subjective interview	N M A E	Ad Be CBT Ex FS Ge PC Ps Re SF
Systematic desensitization	N M A E	Ad Be CBT Ex FS Ge PC Ps Re SF
Unbalancing	N M A E	Ad Be CBT Ex FS Ge PC Ps Re SF
Unconditional positive regard	N M A E	Ad Be CBT Ex FS Ge PC Ps Re SF

*Adapted from Hollis, Joseph W. (1980). Techniques used in counseling and psychotherapy. In K. M. Dimick and F. H. Krause (Eds.), *Practicum manual in counseling and psychotherapy* (4th ed., pp. 77–80). Muncie, IN: Accelerated Development. Reprinted with permission. The Counseling Techniques List format was used. Theories and techniques listed have been updated and drawn from Corey, G. (2013). *Theory and practice of counseling and psychotherapy* (9th ed.). Belmont, CA: Brooks/Cole.

Form 6.1: Self-Assessment of Counseling Performance Skills

Purposes: To provide the trainee with an opportunity to review levels of competency in the performance skill areas of basic helping skills and professional procedural skills.

To provide the trainee with a basis for identifying areas of focus for supervision.

Directions: Circle a number next to each item to indicate your perceived level of competence.

Basic and Advanced Helping Skills	Poor		Average		Good
1. Ability to demonstrate active attending behavior	1	2	3	④	5
2. Ability to listen to and understand nonverbal behavior	1	2	3	④	5
3. Ability to listen to what client says verbally, noticing mix of experiences, behaviors, and feelings	1	2	3	④	5
4. Ability to understand accurately the client's point of view	1	2	3	④	5
5. Ability to identify themes in client's story	1	2	3	④	5
6. Ability to identify inconsistencies between client's story and reality	1	2	3	④	5
7. Ability to respond with accurate empathy	1	2	3	④	5
8. Ability to ask open-ended questions	1	2	3	4	⑤
9. Ability to help clients clarify and focus	1	2	3	④	5
10. Ability to balance empathic response, clarification, and probing	1	2	3	④	5
11. Ability to assess accurately severity of client's problems	1	2	③	4	5
12. Ability to establish a collaborative working relationship with client	1	2	3	④	5
13. Ability to assess and activate client's strengths and resources in problem solving	1	2	3	④	5
14. Ability to identify and challenge unhealthy or distorted thinking or behaving	1	2	3	④	5
15. Ability to use advanced empathy to deepen client's understanding of problems and solutions	1	2	③	4	5
16. Ability to explore the counselor–client relationship	1	2	3	④	5
17. Ability to share constructively some of own experiences, behaviors, and feelings with client	1	2	3	④	5
18. Ability to summarize	1	2	③	4	5
19. Ability to share information appropriately	1	2	3	④	5
20. Ability to understand and facilitate decision making	1	2	3	④	5
21. Ability to help clients set goals and move toward action in problem solving	1	2	3	④	5
22. Ability to recognize and manage client reluctance and resistance	1	2	3	④	5
23. Ability to help clients explore consequences of the goals they set	1	2	3	④	5
24. Ability to help clients sustain actions in direction of goals	1	2	③	4	5
25. Ability to help clients review and revise or recommit to goals based on new experiences	1	2	3	④	5

Procedural and Professional Skills	Poor		Average		Good
26. Ability to open the session smoothly	1	2	3	(4)	5
27. Ability to collaborate with client to identify important concerns for the session	1	2	3	(4)	5
28. Ability to establish continuity from session to session	1	2	(3)	4	5
29. Knowledge of policy and procedures of educational or agency setting regarding harm to self and others, substance abuse, and child abuse	1	2	(3)	4	5
30. Ability to keep appropriate records related to counseling process	1	2	3	4	(5)
31. Ability to end the session smoothly	1	2	(3)	4	5
32. Ability to recognize and address ethical issues	1	2	(3)	4	5
33. Ability to integrate privacy practices and informed consent into initial session	1	2	(3)	4	5

Trainee's signature _____

Supervisor's signature _____

Date _____

Form 6.2: Self-Awareness/Multicultural Awareness Rating Scale

KEY   1 = low—lack competence in this practice

2 = low average—some competence in this practice but need to improve

3 = average—adequate competence in this practice

4 = high average—competence level is more than adequate in this practice

5 = high—perform extremely well in this practice

Directions: Read each of the statements below and indicate the extent to which this applies to your counseling practice using the 1 through 5 key above.

____ 1. I explore how my personal attitudes can impact my clients.

____ 2. I understand how my family background impacts my activities and relationships.

____ 3. I understand how my early family experiences may trigger a reaction to my client's concerns.

____ 4. I am aware of and can avoid imposing my own needs on clients.

____ 5. I reflect on my own dynamics following a counseling session, particularly when I have strong emotional reactions or am uncomfortable with my client's emotional reactions.

____ 6. I reflect on my own dynamics following a counseling session, particularly when I have a strong negative judgment about my client's thoughts, feelings, and behaviors.

____ 7. I understand countertransference and am aware of how my unresolved personal issues and conflicts can be projected onto my clients.

____ 8. I am aware of my own biases and prejudices. This includes issues of gender, sexual orientation, poverty, privilege, and authority relationships.

____ 9. I pay attention to the worldview of my client and how it may be different from mine.

____10. I understand and am aware of how my own culture may impact my counseling relationships.

____11. I understand how my religious values, political values, and family values impact my counseling relationships.

____12. I can broach cultural issues with my client and discuss issues of diversity.

____13. I am involved with cultures of people different from me.

____14. I help clients make decisions that are congruent with their own worldview.

____15. I help clients define goals that are consistent with their life experiences and cultural values.

Review your ratings on the above items. Pay particular attention to items rated 1 or 2 as they may indicate areas of focus needed in this skill area.

Form 6.3: Directed Reflection Exercise on Supervision

Respond to the following questions or directives using one or two sentences.

1. Describe your anxiety level about being supervised.
2. What are your concerns about being evaluated?
3. What is your internal dialogue about your counseling practice (i.e., I'm really bad at this; I need a lot of back-up; I'll never be good enough; I'm very self-conscious)?
4. Describe your current level of confidence as a counselor.
5. What kind of structure and support do you hope for in supervision (a great deal, a moderate amount, a back-up)?
6. Describe the extent to which you feel dependent on your supervisor.
7. Describe what you need from your supervisor in the teacher role? The counselor role? The consultant role?
8. What areas of your counseling practice may need the most focus initially?
9. What is your comfort level for self-disclosing personal history as it relates to your work with clients?
10. How difficult would it be for you to give feedback to your supervisor about the supervisor–supervisee relationship?

Review your answers to the question and directives. You may want to discuss some of these questions with your peers in group supervision. Perhaps your peers could add additional questions to the list? Reviewing your answers can help you clarify your goals related to your developmental level in the supervision process.

Form 6.4: Supervisee Goal Statement

Directions: The student should complete this and provide a copy for your individual and/or group supervisor at the beginning of supervision. This will assist you in forming the supervision contract with your supervisor. The goal statements can be updated as appropriate when current goals are met and your contract is revised.

Student name _____

Supervisor name _____

Date submitted _____

Counseling Performance Skills

_____

_____

_____

_____

Cognitive Counseling Skills

_____

_____

_____

_____

Self-Awareness/Multicultural Awareness

_____

_____

_____

_____

Developmental Level

_____

_____

_____

_____

Form 6.5: Tape Critique Form

Student counselor's name _____

Client ID _____ No. of session _____

Brief summary of session content:

_____

_____

_____

Intended goals:

_____

_____

_____

Comment on positive counseling behaviors:

_____

_____

_____

Comments on areas of counseling practice needing improvement:

_____

_____

_____

Concerns, observations, or comments regarding client dynamics:

_____

_____

_____

Plans for further counseling with this client:

_____

_____

_____

Tape submitted to _____

Date _____

Form 6.6: Peer Rating Form

Purposes

1. To provide the trainee with additional sources of feedback regarding skill development.
2. To provide the rater with the opportunity to increase knowledge and recognition of positive skill behavior.

Directions

1. The trainee submits this sheet to be completed by peers who review the trainee's tapes in the group supervision class. The particular skills the counselor is working on are identified by the counselor trainee. All ethical guidelines regarding confidentiality must be followed for this tape review process, and the tape should be erased after the supervision session.
2. The peer writes remarks on all tapes reviewed, rating performance on the targeted skill behavior.
3. The information is cumulative to aid in review of progress.

Counselor's name _____

Targeted skills (to be identified by counselor) _____

_____

_____

_____

Remarks (based on all tapes reviewed during the week) _____

_____

_____

_____

Signature of rater _____

Date _____

Form 6.7: Interviewer Rating Form

Rating of a Counseling Session Conducted by a Student Counselor*

Client's identification _____

Student counselor's name _____

Check one:

___ Audiotape ___ Videotape ___ Observation ___ Other (specify) _____

Signature of supervisor or observer _____

Date of interview _____

Directions: Supervisor or peer of the student counselor circles a rating for each item and as much as possible provides remarks that will help the student counselor in his/her development.

Specific Criteria

Rating
(best to least)

Remarks

1. Opening: Was opening unstructured, friendly, and pleasant? Any role definition needed? Any introduction necessary?   5 4 3 2 1

2. Rapport: Did student counselor establish good rapport with client? Was the stage set for a productive interview?   5 4 3 2 1

3. Interview responsibility: If not assumed by the client, did student counselor assume appropriate level of responsibility for interview conduct? Did student counselor or client take initiative?   5 4 3 2 1

4. Interaction: Were the client and student counselor really communicating in a meaningful manner?   5 4 3 2 1

5. Acceptance/permissiveness: Was the student counselor accepting and permissive of client's emotions, feelings, and expressed thoughts?   5 4 3 2 1

6. Reflections of feelings: Did student counselor reflect and react to feelings, or did interview remain on an intellectual level?   5 4 3 2 1

7. Student counselor responses: Were student counselor responses appropriate in view of what the client was expressing, or were responses concerned with trivia and minutia? Meaningful questions?   5 4 3 2 1

8. Value management: How did the student counselor cope with values? Were attempts made to impose counselor values during the interview?   5 4 3 2 1

9. Counseling relationship: Were student counselor–client relationships conducive to productive counseling? Was a counseling relationship established?   5 4 3 2 1

10. Closing: Was closing initiated by student counselor or client? Was it abrupt or brusque? Any follow-up or further interview scheduling accomplished?   5 4 3 2 1

11. General techniques: How well did the student counselor conduct the mechanics of the interview?   5 4 3 2 1

A. Duration of interview: Was the interview too long or too short? Should interview have been terminated sooner or later?
B. Vocabulary level: Was student counselor vocabulary appropriate for the client?
C. Mannerisms: Did the student counselor display any mannerisms that might have adversely affected the interview or portions thereof?
D. Verbosity: Did the student counselor dominate the interview, interrupt, override, or become too wordy?
E. Silences: Were silences broken to meet student counselor needs, or were they dealt with in an effectual manner?

Comments for student counselor assistance: Additional comments that might assist the student counselor in areas not covered by the preceding suggestions.

Form 7.1: Supervision Contract

Purpose: The purpose of the supervision is to monitor client services provided by the supervisee and to facilitate the professional development of the supervisee. This ensures the safety and well-being of our clients and satisfies the clinical supervision requirements of _____ University and _____ school/agency.

Supervisor's Responsibilities:
- The supervisor agrees to provide face-to-face supervision to the supervisee for 1 hour per week at a regularly scheduled time for the fall/spring practicum/internship semester as required by _____ University.
- The supervisor will complete forms required by the University concerning hours, completion, verification, and evaluation of the supervisee's practicum/internship and make appropriate contact with University liaison concerning supervisee's progress.
- The supervisor will make a recommendation as to the student's grade, but responsibility for the final grade rests with the University.
- The supervisor will review audiotapes, case notes, and other written documents; do live observations; and co-lead groups as part of the supervision format.
- The supervision sessions will focus on professional development, teaching, mentoring, and the personal development of the supervisee.
- Skill areas will include counseling performance skills and professional practices, cognitive counseling skills, self-awareness/multicultural awareness, and developmental level in supervision.
- The supervisor will provide weekly formative evaluation, document supervision sessions, and provide summative evaluations based on mutually agreed-on supervision goals. Evaluation will be offered within the skill categories listed above and use evaluation instruments recommended by the University program.
- The supervisor will practice consistent with accepted ethical standards.

Supervisee's Responsibilities:
- Uphold the American Counseling Association/Canadian Counseling and Psychotherapy Association *Code of Ethics*.
- Prepare for weekly supervisions by reviewing audiotapes and framing concerns for focus of the supervision session.
- Be prepared to discuss and justify the case conceptualization made and approach and techniques used.
- Reflect on your own personal dynamics and any multicultural issues which may surface in your sessions.
- Review any ethical dimensions which may be important in your sessions.
- Contact supervisor immediately in any crisis situations involving harm to self or others or abuse of a child, vulnerable adult, or elder.
- Keep notes regarding the supervision sessions.
- Provide the supervisor with audio/videotapes to be reviewed prior to the supervision session.

GOAL 1: _____

     Objective 1: _____

     Objective 2: _____

     Objective 3: _____

GOAL 2: _____

     Objective 1: _____

     Objective 2: _____

     Objective 3: _____

GOAL 3: _____

     Objective 1: _____

     Objective 2: _____

     Objective 3: _____

GOAL 4: _____

     Objective 1: _____

     Objective 2: _____

     Objective 3: _____

Supervisor signature and date _____

Supervisee signature and date _____

Form 7.2: Supervisor Notes

Supervisor name _____

Supervisee name _____

_____

Session #

Supervisee concerns _____

Date _____

Supervision intervention/strategies/recommendations _____

_____

_____

_____

Supervisor observation of counselor's skill level _____

_____

Session #

Supervisee concerns _____

Date _____

Supervision intervention/strategies/recommendations _____

_____

_____

_____

Supervisor observation of counselor's skill level _____

_____

_____

Supervisor signature and date _____

Form 7.3: Supervisee Notes on Individual Supervision

The supervisee should keep brief notes summarizing the weekly supervision session.

For supervision from _____ to _____.

_____

Session Insights and/or comments _____

(Dates) _____

_____

_____

_____

Session Insights and/or comments _____

(Dates) _____

_____

_____

_____

Session Insights and/or comments _____

(Dates) _____

_____

_____

_____

Session Insights and/or comments _____

(Dates) _____

_____

_____

_____

Session Insights and/or comments _____

(Dates) _____

_____

_____

_____

_____

_____   _____
Supervisee's signature and date   Supervisor's signature and date

Form 7.4: Supervisor's Formative Evaluation of Supervisee's Counseling Practice

Name of student counselor _____

Identifying code of client _____

Date of supervision _____ or period covered by the evaluation _____

Directions: The supervisor, following each counseling session that has been supervised or after several supervisions covering a period of time, circles a number that best evaluates the student counselor on each performance at that point in time.

General Supervision Comments	Poor		Adequate		Good	
1. Demonstrates a personal commitment in developing professional competencies	1	2	3	4	5	6
2. Invests time and energy in becoming a counselor	1	2	3	4	5	6
3. Accepts and uses constructive criticism to enhance self-development and counseling skills	1	2	3	4	5	6
4. Engages in open, comfortable, and clear communication with peers and supervisors	1	2	3	4	5	6
5. Recognizes own competencies and skills and shares these with peers and supervisors	1	2	3	4	5	6
6. Recognizes own deficiencies and actively works to overcome them with peers and supervisors	1	2	3	4	5	6
7. Completes case reports and records punctually and conscientiously	1	2	3	4	5	6

The Counseling Process	Poor		Adequate		Good	
8. Researches the referral prior to the first interview	1	2	3	4	5	6
9. Keeps appointments on time	1	2	3	4	5	6
10. Begins the interview smoothly	1	2	3	4	5	6
11. Explains the nature and objectives of counseling when appropriate	1	2	3	4	5	6
12. Is relaxed and comfortable in the interview	1	2	3	4	5	6
13. Communicates interest in and acceptance of the client	1	2	3	4	5	6
14. Facilitates client expression of concerns and feelings	1	2	3	4	5	6
15. Focuses on the content of the client's problem	1	2	3	4	5	6
16. Recognizes and resists manipulation by the client	1	2	3	4	5	6
17. Recognizes and deals with positive affect of the client	1	2	3	4	5	6
18. Recognizes and deals with negative affect of the client	1	2	3	4	5	6
19. Is spontaneous in the interview	1	2	3	4	5	6
20. Uses silence effectively in the interview	1	2	3	4	5	6
21. Is aware of own feelings in the counseling session	1	2	3	4	5	6
22. Communicates own feelings to the client when appropriate	1	2	3	4	5	6
23. Recognizes and skillfully interprets the client's covert messages	1	2	3	4	5	6
24. Facilitates realistic goal setting with the client	1	2	3	4	5	6

25. Encourages appropriate action-step planning with the client	1	2	3	4	5	6
26. Employs judgment in the timing and use of different techniques	1	2	3	4	5	6
27. Initiates periodic evaluation of goals, action-steps, and process during counseling	1	2	3	4	5	6
28. Explains, administers, and interprets tests correctly	1	2	3	4	5	6
29. Terminates the interview smoothly	1	2	3	4	5	6

The Conceptualization Process	*Poor*		*Adequate*		*Good*	
30. Focuses on specific behaviors and their consequences, implications, and contingencies	1	2	3	4	5	6
31. Recognizes and pursues discrepancies and meaning of inconsistent information	1	2	3	4	5	6
32. Uses relevant case data in planning both immediate and long-range goals	1	2	3	4	5	6
33. Uses relevant case data in considering various strategies and their implications	1	2	3	4	5	6
34. Bases decisions on a theoretically sound and consistent rationale of human behavior	1	2	3	4	5	6
35. Is perceptive in evaluating the effects of own counseling techniques	1	2	3	4	5	6
36. Demonstrates ethical behavior in the counseling activity and case management	1	2	3	4	5	6

Additional comments and/or suggestions: _____
_____
_____
_____

Date _____ Signature of supervisor _____

or peer _____

My signature indicates that I have read the above report and have discussed the content with my site supervisor. It does not necessarily indicate that I agree with the report in part or in whole.

Date _____ Signature of student counselor _____

Form 7.5: Supervisor's Final Evaluation of Practicum Student

Supervisor name and signature _____

Supervisee name and signature _____

Date _____

Directions: The supervisor will indicate the degree to which the supervisee has demonstrated competency in each of the following areas by indicating 3 for exceeds expectations; 2 for meets expectations; or 1 for does not meet expectations. This completed form will be given to the faculty group supervisor to be considered as part of the final practicum grade.

_____ Consistently demonstrates the use of basic and advanced helping skills

_____ Has the ability to appropriately use additional theory-based techniques consistent with at least one theoretical framework

_____ Demonstrates skill in opening and closing sessions and managing continuity between sessions

_____ Demonstrates knowledge and integration of ethical standards into practice

_____ Has cognitive skills of awareness, observation, and recognition of relevant data to explain some client dynamics

_____ Writes accurate case notes, intake summaries, and case conceptualizations

_____ Recognizes how several of his/her personal dynamics may impact a client and the counseling session and demonstrates sensitivity to cultural differences

_____ Demonstrates moderate to low levels of anxiety and moderate to low levels of dependency on supervisor direction during supervision sessions

Additional comments and suggestions:

_____

_____

_____

_____

Form 7.6: Supervisor's Final Evaluation of Intern

Please indicate your evaluation of the intern on the following competencies using the following rating scale:

1 = low (lacks competency)

2 = low average (possesses competency but needs improvement)

3 = average (possesses adequate competency)

4 = high average (performance level more than adequate)

5 = high (performs extremely well)

Counseling Performance Skills

_____ 1. Uses basic and advanced counseling techniques.

_____ 2. Opens and closes sessions smoothly, incorporates privacy and informed consent information, and manages transitions between sessions.

_____ 3. Develops a therapeutic relationship with a wide variety of clients.

_____ 4. Appropriately uses theory-based techniques consistent with personal guiding theory.

_____ 5. Responds and intervenes appropriately in crisis situations.

_____ 6. Recognizes ethical dilemmas and follows a consistent ethical decision-making process.

_____ 7. Practices in a manner consistent with the American Counseling Association's *Code of Ethics* standards.

Cognitive Counseling Skills

1. Demonstrates competencies in

   _____ Assessment

   _____ Case conceptualization

   _____ Goal setting

   _____ Treatment planning

   _____ Record keeping and case notes

_____ 2. Practices using a personal guiding theory of counseling.

_____ 3. Conceptualizes cases accurately.

_____ 4. Develops appropriate goals as a result of conceptualization.

_____ 5. Identifies key themes relevant to the client.

_____ 6. Identifies key factors maintaining client problems.

_____ 7. Moves clients toward achieving mutually formed goals.

Self-Awareness/Multicultural Awareness

_____ 1. Examines transference/countertransference issues as related to clients.

_____ 2. Examines personal values as related to work with clients.

_____ 3. Recognizes how elements of culture impact the client's view of the counseling process.

_____ 4. Demonstrates the qualities of openness, flexibility, and emotional stability.

_____ 5. Communicates an understanding of each client's worldview as perceived by the client and develops goals consistent with client's worldview.

_____ 6. Identifies and examines multicultural elements related to assessment, goal setting, and intervention strategies.

Developmental Level in Supervision

_____ 1. Comes to supervision prepared and open to receiving feedback.

_____ 2. Identifies appropriate priorities for the work in supervision.

_____ 3. Functions with appropriate autonomy and knows when to consult.

_____ 4. Demonstrates self-confidence in the role of counselor.

_____ 5. Comfortably integrates all elements of practice when receiving supervision.

_____ 6. Demonstrates reflective thinking when reviewing a case.

In comparison with other counselors at this stage in their development, how would you rate this person?

1	2	3	4	5	6	7	8	9
Clearly deficient				Like others			Clearly excellent	

Comments _____

_____

_____

_____   _____

Supervisor   Supervisee

Date _____

Form 10.1: Suicide Consultation Form

Directions: Student will complete this form when working with a potentially suicidal client. The student will take this information to his/her supervisor for consultation, collaborate on a treatment plan, and place in client's file.

Part I

Name of institution _____

Intern's name _____ Supervisor's name _____

Supervisor's professional degree _____

Supervisor is licensed in _____ Supervisor is certified in _____

Client's name _____ Client's age _____

If the client is a minor, has the parent signed a consent form? _____

When was the counseling initiated? Month _____ Day _____ Year _____

Where was counseling initiated? _____

Number of times you have seen this client _____

Part II

Check the presenting symptoms often associated with a suicidal client.

Client is between the ages of 14 and 19. Yes _____ No _____

Client is depressed. Yes _____ No _____

If yes, include a description of the client's depressive behavior:

_____

_____

Has a previous attempt of suicide occurred? Yes _____ No _____

If yes, how long ago was the attempt? _____

Is the client abusing alcohol? Yes _____ No _____

If yes, how much does he/she drink? _____

_____

Is the client abusing some other substance? Yes _____ No _____

If yes, what other substance? _____

_____

Is rational thinking lost? Yes _____ No _____

If yes, explain how this behavior is manifested: _____

_____

_____

_____

Does the client have little social support? Yes _____ No _____

How does the client spend his/her time? _____

_____

_____

_____

Does the client have an organized suicide plan? Yes _____ No _____

If yes, what is the plan? _____

_____

_____

_____

If there is a plan, does it seem irreversible, for example, gunshot?

Yes _____ No _____

Is the client divorced, widowed, or separated? Yes _____ No _____

Is the client physically sick? Yes _____ No _____

If yes, describe the symptoms: _____

_____

_____

Does the client have sleep disruption? Yes _____ No _____

If yes, describe the disruption: _____

_____

_____

_____

_____

Has the client given his/her possessions away? Yes _____ No _____

Does the client have a history of previous psychiatric treatment or hospitalization?

Yes _____ No _____

If yes, describe for what the client was hospitalized: _____

_____

_____

_____

Does the client have anyone near him/her to intervene? Yes _____ No _____

Does the client seem agitated? Yes _____ No _____

If yes, describe the client's behavior: _____

_____

_____

Part III

Describe and summarize your interactions with the client. What are his/her basic problems? What is your goal with the client? What techniques are you using?

_____

_____

_____

_____

Describe your supervisor's reaction to the problem:

_____

_____

_____

_____

                                                    _____
                                                          Supervisor's signature

What are your plans for the client? _____

_____

_____

_____

Form 10.2: Harm to Others Form

Directions: Student completes the form prior to supervisory sessions and records supervisor's comments and reactions; student and supervisor then sign the completed form. The student should keep the form in his/her confidential records.

1. Student's name _____

    Client's name _____

2. Number of times the client has been seen _____

3. Dates client has been seen _____

    _____

    Client's presenting problem _____

    _____

    _____

Risk Assessment[1]

Does the client have any of the following characteristics, traits, or current life circumstances? (Check yes for all that apply.)

	Yes	No
History of previous violence toward others (e.g., hitting, slapping, punching, stabbing, etc.)		
History of violence at a young age		
Relationship instability		
Employment instability or problems		
Substance use history		
Current use of substances		
Mental illness diagnosis		
Presence of psychopathology		
Maladjustment early in life (e.g., problems in school, problems with peers)		
Diagnosis of a personality disorder		
Lacking in insight into the mental disorder		
Active symptoms of the mental disorder		
Negative perceptions toward authority or those trying to intervene to help		
History of impulsive behaviors		
Access to means of lethality (e.g., weapons, guns, knives, etc.)		
History of being unresponsive to treatment		
Presence of current life stressors		
Lack of support		

---

[1] Items for the checklist are adapted from C. D. Webster, K. S. Douglas, D. Eaves, & S. D. Hart (1997), HCR-20 risk assessment for violence (Version 2). Burnaby, Canada: Mental Health, Law, and Policy Institute, Simon Fraser Institute.

Additional Clinical Assessment Areas for Risk

4. What did the client do or say to make the counselor concerned that he/she could represent a "harm to others"? _____

_____

_____

_____

5. Describe the client's history of violence or criminal behavior _____

_____

_____

_____

6. Have you consulted the client's case notes/treatment records for such a history? _____

_____

7. Does the client have a history of child abuse and maltreatment? If yes, briefly describe:

_____

_____

_____

8. Does the client have a history of substance abuse? Describe the client's history and current use of substances? _____

_____

_____

_____

_____

9. Is the client experiencing hallucinations (auditory or visual), and does the client perceive that his/her life is being threatened? Describe: _____

_____

_____

_____

_____

10. What is the client's history of dealing with stress? Describe his/her level of impulse control, reactivity to stressful situations, and history of acting without thinking: _____

_____

_____

_____

_____

_____

11. What stressors is the client currently facing, and does he/she have any support in dealing with them? (Stressors can be relational, related to work, finances, housing, etc.) _____

_____

_____

_____

_____

_____

12. Was a specific victim(s) named? _____

_____

13. If the victim was not named, what was the relationship of the client to the victim? _____

_____

14. If the victim was not named, did the counselor suspect who the person was? _____

_____

15. Was a clear threat made? If yes, what threat? _____

16. Is serious danger present? For example, does the client have access to victims and to weapons and the setting in which to commit violence? _____

_____

_____

17. Is the danger believed to be imminent? _____

    If so, why? _____

_____

_____

    If not, why not? _____

_____

_____

18. Supervisor's reaction/advice? _____

_____

_____

19. What plan of action is to be taken? _____

_____

_____

_____

Student's signature

_____

Supervisor's signature

_____

Date of conference

Form 10.3: Child Abuse Reporting Form

Counselor trainee and position _____

Date and time _____

Alleged perpetrator _____ DOB _____

Address _____

Alleged victim _____ DOB _____

Address _____

Information obtained from _____ DOB _____

Address _____

Relationship to alleged perpetrator _____

Relationship to alleged victim _____

Brief description of incident or concern _____

_____

_____

Incident(s) ongoing? _____ Or specific date _____

Reported to immediate supervisor on _____

Supervisor's name and position _____

Reported to children and youth services on _____ Time _____

Children and youth worker's name _____

Alleged perpetrator aware of report?   Yes _____ No _____

Alleged victim aware of report?   Yes _____ No _____

Alleged perpetrator in counseling?   Yes _____ No _____

If so, where? _____

Alleged victim in counseling?   Yes_____ No_____

If so, where? _____

Results _____

_____

Counselor trainee's signature _____

Field supervisor's signature _____

cc: Client's file, Agency file

Form 10.4: Substance Abuse Assessment Form

Directions: Student asks the client the specific questions addressed on the form as a way to make a clinical assessment of the level of severity of use and abuse of substances in the client's life.

The completed form is kept in the student's confidential file.

1. What substances do you or have you used? _____
_____
_____
_____

2. How long have you used (beginning with experimentation)? _____
_____
_____
_____

3. How often are you high in a week? _____
_____
_____
_____

4. How many of your friends use? _____
_____
_____

5. Are you on medication? _____
_____

6. Do you have money for chemicals? How much? _____
_____

7. How much do you spend for drugs or alcohol in a month? _____
_____

8. Who provides if you are broke? _____
_____
_____

9. Have you ever been busted (police, school, home, DWIs)? _____
_____

10. Have you lost a job because of your use? _____
_____
_____

11. What time of day do you use? _____
_____
_____

12. Do you use on the job or in school? _____
_____
_____

13. Does it take more, less, or about the same amount of the substance to get you high? _____

_____

_____

14. Have you ever shot up? What substance? Where on your body? _____

_____

_____

15. Do you sneak using? How do you do it? _____

_____

_____

_____

16. Do you hide things? _____

_____

17. Do you have rules for using? What are they? How did they come about? _____

_____

_____

_____

18. Do you use alone? _____

_____

19. Have you ever tried to quit? How often have you tried to quit and not been able to? _____

_____

_____

20. Have you had any withdrawal symptoms? _____

_____

_____

_____

21. Have you lost your "good time highs"? _____

_____

_____

22. Have you ever thought about suicide? _____

_____

_____

23. Do you mix your chemicals when using? _____

_____

_____

24. Do you ever shift from one chemical to another? Yes _____ No _____

What happened that made you decide to shift? _____

_____

_____

_____

25. Do you avoid people who don't use? _____
_____
_____

26. Do you avoid talking about your drug or alcohol use? _____
_____
_____

27. Have you done things when using that you are ashamed of? Yes _____ No _____
What happened? _____
_____
_____
_____

28. Who is the most important person in your life, including yourself? _____
_____
_____

29. How are you taking care of him/her? _____
_____
_____

30. On a scale of 1 (*low*) to 10, how is your life going? _____
Explain _____
_____

31. Are there any harmful consequences you are aware of in your chemical use other than those
touched upon? _____
_____
_____
_____

32. Do you think your chemical is harmful to you? Yes _____ No _____
Do you think you have a chemical problem? Yes _____ No _____
Explain _____
_____
_____

_____

Student's signature

_____

Client's signature

_____

Supervisor's signature

_____

Date

Form 12.1: Weekly Internship Log

Directions: Fill in the number of hours spent in each activity for each day at your internship site. Activities with an * are those activities which are counted as direct contact hours.

Week of: From _____ to _____

Activity	Monday	Tuesday	Wednesday	Thursday	Friday	Total
Individual counseling*						
Group counseling*						
Family/couple counseling*						
Career counseling*						
Intake interview*						
Consulting with professionals or parents*						
Crisis intervention/referral*						
Psychoeducation/guidance*						
Testing/assessment						
Documentation						
Program/case planning						
Case conference						
Professional development						
Other/please list						
Individual supervision/site						
Group supervision						
Total direct contact hours*						
Total indirect contact hours						
Total hours						

_____   _____
Student signature and date   Supervisor signature and date

Form 12.2: Summary Internship Log

Directions: Fill in the dates of each week of internship where indicated. Fill in the total number of hours spent in each activity for the week indicated. Indicate the total number of hours spent in direct contact with clients (activity indicated by *). Total the hours spent in indirect contact. Then indicate the total of all hours where indicated at the bottom of the form. Hours in supervision are not included in total hours.

Activity Week> Dates>	1	2	3	4	5	6	7	8	Total
Individual counseling*									
Group counseling*									
Couple/family counseling*									
Career counseling*									
Intake interview*									
Consulting with professionals/parents*									
Testing/assessment									
Crisis intervention/ referrals*									
Psychoeducation/guidance*									
Documentation/report writing/grant preparation									
Program/case planning									
Case conference									
Professional development									
Other/please list									
Individual supervision/site									
Group supervision									
Total direct contact hours									
Total indirect contact hours									
Total hours									

_____   _____

Student signature and date   Supervisor signature and date

Form 12.3: Evaluation of Intern's Practice in Site Activities

Directions: The site supervisor is to complete this form in duplicate. One copy is to go to the student; the other copy is sent to the faculty liaison. The areas listed below serve as a general guide for the activities typically engaged in during counselor training. Please rate the student on the activities in which he/she has engaged using the following scale:

A = Functions extremely well and/or independently

B = Functions adequately and/or requires occasional supervision

C = Requires close supervision in this area

NA = Not applicable to this training experience

Training Activities

_____ 1. Intake interviewing

_____ 2. Individual counseling/psychotherapy

_____ 3. Group counseling/psychotherapy

_____ 4. Testing: Administration and interpretation

_____ 5. Report writing/documentation

_____ 6. Consultation with other professionals or parents/family

_____ 7. Psychoeducational activities

_____ 8. Career counseling

_____ 9. Family/couple counseling

_____ 10. Case conference or staff presentation

_____ 11. Other

Additional Comments

Please use the additional space for any comments that would help us evaluate the student's progress. Student may comment on exceptions to ratings, if any.

_____

_____

_____

_____

_____   _____

Student name   Supervisor signature

_____   _____

Site   Date

Form 12.4: Client's Assessment of the Counseling Experience

Counselor's name _____

Date _____

Directions: Please read the following statements and place a check next to the ones that accurately describe your counseling experience with this counselor.

_____ I got the help that I needed with my concerns.

_____ I was satisfied with the relationship I had with my counselor.

_____ I received help with concerns that were in addition to my original concerns.

_____ I feel much better now compared to how I was feeling when I started counseling.

_____ The counseling helped me understand myself better.

_____ I would gladly return to this counselor if I wanted help with another concern.

_____ I would recommend this counselor to a friend.

_____ My counselor was competent and skilled.

_____ My counselor put me at ease right away.

_____ My counselor understood and was sensitive to my feelings and my situation.

_____ I didn't feel free to talk about all my concerns with my counselor.

_____ Counseling helped me see a number of things I could do to change and improve my situation.

_____ The counselor asked questions and made comments that made it easy for me to talk about my concerns.

_____ I felt I could not get my story across and that I couldn't get the counselor to understand me.

_____ I felt I could be honest and talk about my feelings and thoughts and behaviors openly.

_____ I would prefer to work with a counselor who has a different approach to counseling.

Thank you for completing this form. Your feedback will be very helpful.

Form 12.5: Supervisee Evaluation of Supervisor**

Directions: The student counselor is to evaluate the supervision received. Circle the number that best represents how you, the student counselor, feel about the supervision received. After the form is completed, the supervisor may suggest a meeting to discuss the supervision desired.

Name of practicum/internship supervisor _____

Period covered: From _____ to _____

	Poor		*Adequate*		*Good*	
1. Gives time and energy in observations, tape processing, and case conferences.	1	2	3	4	5	6
2. Accepts and respects me as a person.	1	2	3	4	5	6
3. Recognizes and encourages further development of my strengths and capabilities.	1	2	3	4	5	6
4. Gives me useful feedback when I do something well.	1	2	3	4	5	6
5. Provides me the freedom to develop flexible and effective counseling styles.	1	2	3	4	5	6
6. Encourages and listens to my ideas and suggestions for developing my counseling skills.	1	2	3	4	5	6
7. Provides suggestions for developing my counseling skills.	1	2	3	4	5	6
8. Helps me understand the implications and dynamics of the counseling approaches I use.	1	2	3	4	5	6
9. Encourages me to use new and different techniques when appropriate.	1	2	3	4	5	6
10. Is spontaneous and flexible in the supervisory sessions.	1	2	3	4	5	6
11. Helps me define and achieve specific concrete goals for myself during the practicum experience.	1	2	3	4	5	6
12. Gives me useful feedback when I do something wrong.	1	2	3	4	5	6
13. Allows me to discuss problems I encounter in my practicum/internship setting.	1	2	3	4	5	6
14. Pays appropriate amount of attention to both my clients and me.	1	2	3	4	5	6
15. Focuses on both verbal and nonverbal behavior in me and in my clients.	1	2	3	4	5	6
16. Helps me define and maintain ethical behavior in counseling and case management.	1	2	3	4	5	6

---

* This form was designed by two Purdue graduate students based on material drawn from *Counseling Strategies and Objectives*, by H. Hackney and S. Nye (1973). Englewood Cliffs, NJ: Prentice Hall. Printed by permission from Harold Hackney, Ph.D.

* This form originally was printed in chapter 10 of the *Practicum Manual for Counseling and Psychotherapy*, by K. Dimick and F. Krause (Eds.) (1980). Muncie, IN: Accelerated Development.

17. Encourages me to engage in professional behavior.	1	2	3	4	5	6
18. Maintains confidentiality in material discussed in supervisory sessions.	1	2	3	4	5	6
19. Deals with both content and affect when supervising.	1	2	3	4	5	6
20. Focuses on the implications, consequences, and contingencies of specific behaviors in counseling and supervision.	1	2	3	4	5	6
21. Helps me organize relevant case data in planning goals and strategies with my client.	1	2	3	4	5	6
22. Helps me to formulate a theoretically sound rationale of human behavior.	1	2	3	4	5	6
23. Offers resource information when I request or need it.	1	2	3	4	5	6
24. Helps me develop increased skill in critiquing and gaining insight from my counseling tapes.	1	2	3	4	5	6
25. Allows and encourages me to evaluate myself.	1	2	3	4	5	6
26. Explains his/her criteria for evaluation clearly and in behavioral terms.	1	2	3	4	5	6
27. Applies his/her criteria fairly in evaluating my counseling performance.	1	2	3	4	5	6

Additional Comments and/or Suggestions

_____

_____

_____

My signature indicates that I have read the above report and have discussed the content with my supervisee. It does not necessarily indicate that I agree with the report in part or in whole.

_____

Supervisee's signature and date

310

Form 12.6: Site Evaluation Form

Directions: The student completes this form at the end of the practicum and/or internship. This should be turned in to the university supervisor or internship coordinator as indicated by the university program.

Name_____Site_____

Dates of placement _____ Site supervisor _____

Faculty liaison _____

Rate the following questions about your site and experiences with the following scale:

A. *Very satisfactory*   B. *Moderately satisfactory*   C. *Moderately unsatisfactory*   D. *Very unsatisfactory*

1. _____   Amount of on-site supervision

2. _____   Quality and usefulness of on-site supervision

3. _____   Usefulness and helpfulness of faculty liaison

4. _____   Relevance of experience to career goals

5. _____   Exposure to and communication of school/agency goals

6. _____   Exposure to and communication of school/agency procedures

7. _____   Exposure to professional roles and functions within the school/agency

8. _____   Exposure to information about community resources

9. _____   Rate all applicable experiences that you had at your site:

   _____   Report writing

   _____   Intake interviewing

   _____   Administration and interpretation of tests

   _____   Staff presentation/case conferences

   _____   Individual counseling

   _____   Group counseling

   _____   Family/couple counseling

   _____   Psychoeducational activities

   _____   Consultation

   _____   Career counseling

   _____   Other

10. _____   Overall evaluation of the site

Comments: Include any suggestions for improvements in the experiences you have rated *moderately unsatisfactory* (C) or *very unsatisfactory* (D)._____

_____

_____

_____

INDEX

AAPC (American Association of Pastoral Counselors) 4, 7, 136
ABC model of crisis intervention 166–7
abstaining behaviors 199–200
abused clients 189–96
ACA (American Counseling Association) 4, 137; *Code of Ethics* 30–1, 111, 119, 138, 140; *Practitioner's Guide to Ethical Decision-Making, A* 142
acceptance 85
Acceptance and Commitment Therapy (ACT) 86
accounting requests 30
accreditation standards 4–7
ACES (Association for Counselor Education and Supervision): *Best Practices in Clinical Supervision* 119
ACT (Acceptance and Commitment Therapy) 86
action, taking 68
addictions, clients with 196–201
addictions counseling 47
Addictions Counselor 9
Adler, A. 73
administration site 17
administrative consultation 208, 209
administrative supervision 112
advanced helping skills 36–7
affiliations of the site 16–17
agreement form 21
Aguilar, J. 213
Alcohol Use Disorders Identification Test (AUDIT) 57
Allport, G. 74
amendment requests 30
American Academy of Experts in Traumatic Stress 171–2
American Association for Marriage and Family Therapy 4, 9, 136
American Association of Pastoral Counselors (AAPC) 4, 7, 136
American Association of Suicidology 181
American Counseling Association (ACA) 4, 136–7; *Code of Ethics* 30–1, 111, 119, 138, 140; *Practitioner's Guide to Ethical Decision-Making, A* 142
American Mental Health Counselors Association 136; *Code of Ethics* 144
American Psychiatric Association 56; *Diagnostic and Statistical Manual of Mental Disorders* 196

American Psychological Association (APA) 136–8
American Psychological Association Commission on Accreditation (APA-CoA) 7
American School Counselors Association 136, 215; *Ethical Standards for School Counselors* 43
American Society for Suicide Prevention: Risk Factors for Suicide 174–5
Anastasi, A. 57
Anderson, S. K. 137–8, 140–1
APA (American Psychological Association) 136–8
APA-CoA (American Psychological Association Commission on Accreditation) 4, 7
apologizing 26–7
Appelbaum, P. S. 186, 188
assessing: client progress 57–60; danger in clients 186–8; suicide risk 176–9
assessment and case conceptualization 47–65; of client progress 57–60; diagnostic use of 52–6; goals 50; information gathering 48–50, 57; information sharing 56–7; initial assessment 48–50; of mental status of client 52
assessment tools 178–9, 186
Association for Counselor Education and Supervision (ACES): *Best Practices in Clinical Supervision* 119
Association for Multicultural Counseling and Development 136
attending behaviors 37
AUDIT (Alcohol Use Disorders Identification Test) 57
Authoritative Interventions 116
authorization forms 34
autonomy, respect for 138
awareness 84–5

BAI (Beck Anxiety Inventory) 57
Baker, S. B. 214–15, 220
Bandura, A. 73
Barnett, J. E. 189
Baruth, L. G. 135
basic and advanced counseling skills 93–4
basic helping skills 36–7
BDI-II (Beck Depression Inventory II) 57
Beauchamp, T. L. 173–4
Beck, A. T. 83
Beck, J. C. 186
Beck Anxiety Inventory (BAI) 57
Beck Depression Inventory II (BDI-II) 56, 57

behavioral assessments 58
behaviors, abstaining 199–200
Behring, S. T. 212
beneficence 138
Benshoff, J. M. 71
Bergan, J. R. 220
Bergner, R. 61–2
Berliner, L. 193
Bernard, J. M. 107, 111, 115, 118
Best Practices in Clinical Supervision (ACES) 119
Beton, E. J. 61
Beutler, L. E. 52, 58
Binder, J. L. 61
Boes, S. R. 121
Borders, L. D. 104, 107, 112–13
Bordin, E. S. 113
boundaries, setting 37
Brainer, C. J. 194
Brandse, E. 194
Braun, S.: "Managed Mental Healthcare: Intentional Misdiagnosis of Mental Disorders" 160
breaching confidentiality 156–9
breach notification rule 29
Brief Family Therapy Center 82
brief therapy 80–2
Brown, D. 221
Bryce, G. K. 159
buffers against suicide 177

CACREP (Council for the Accreditation of Counseling and Related Educational Programs) 4–7, 20, 47, 93, 105–6, 117, 129
Callahan, C. J. 170–1
Cameron, S. *42*
Canada, confidentiality law in 159
Canadian Certified Counsellor (CCC): CCPA 8
Canadian Counselling and Psychotherapy Association (CCPA) 4, 8, 129, 136, 137, 138; *Code of Ethics* 138
Canadian Counselling and Psychotherapy Association's Council on Accreditation of Counselling Education Programs (CACEP) 20, 108
Canadian Professional Counsellors Association 8–9
Canadian Psychological Association 136, 137
Canadian regulation standards for counselling and school counselling 9
capacity to commit suicide 176–7
Caplan, G. 208–10; *Theory and Practice of Mental Health Consultation, The* 208
Captain, C. 174
Carlson, J. 195
case conceptualization 57–63
case consultation 208
case laws 150
case notes 42–3
Case Notes (Form 3.5) 43
Cattell, R. 74
CCC (Canadian Certified Counsellor) 8
CCPA (Canadian Counselling and Psychotherapy Association) 4, 8, 129, 138; *Code of Ethics* 138
Certified Rehabilitation Counselor (CRC) 8
Cerundolo, P. 186
change in the organization 223–4
change model 67–8
child abuse 158, 189–96

Child Abuse Prevention and Treatment Act (US Department of Health and Human Services) 192
Child Abuse Reporting Form (Form 10.3) 192
childhood suicide 173–4
children, interviewing sexually abused 193–4
children, post-crisis responses of 172
civil law 150
classification system 54–5
class requirements 26
Clawson, Thomas W. 4
clearances, pre-placement 16
Clemens, E. 216–17
client: assessment discussions with 56–7; developing rapport with 31, 34; emotions 58–9; forming relationship with 34–5; goals 69; initial session with 28–9, 35–9; problems 47, 51–2, 57; progress 57–60
client autonomy 160
client-centered case consultation 208
client-centered therapy 34
Client Permission to Record Counseling Session for Supervision Purposes (Form 3.2) 34
client population and site selection 18–19
client records 161–2
clients: abused 189–96; with addictions 196–201; cultural needs of 71; high-risk 184–9
Clinical Mental Health Counselor or Licensed Professional Counselor 9
clinical supervision 112, 119–26
COAMFTE (Commission on Accreditation for Marriage and Family Therapy Education) 4
Cobia, D. C. 121
Cochran, F. R. 173
Code of Ethics (ACA) 30–1, 111, 119, 138, 140
Code of Ethics (American Mental Health Counselors Association) 144
Code of Ethics (CCPA) 138
Code of Professional Ethics for Rehabilitation Counselors 136
codes, ethical 135–7
coding system 54–5
Cogdal, P. 165
cognitive: behavioral methods of counseling 194; counseling skills 94, 106; restructuring brief therapy 83
collaboration to change 113
collaborative consultation 211
collaborator role 213–14
Collins, D. R. 4, 103
Commission on Accreditation for Marriage and Family Therapy Education (COAMFTE) 4
commitment procedures laws 180
commitments to treatment 179
communication 153
competence 30, 106, 153, 160
concepts in group supervision 97–9
Conceptual Interventions 116
Concrete style 216–17
confidential communication channel requests 30
confidentiality 41, 154–9, 160
constitutional laws 149
consultant entry into system 219
consultation 28, 207–26; guidelines 218–21; impact of 221–2; intervention 220–1; peer 102–4; resistance to 221–3; school 213–18

consultee-centered administrative consultation 208, 209
consultee-centered case consultation 208
contact person 19
contemplation 68
continuous assessments 58
contracts 20, 152, 179, 223–4
Cook, L. 211
coping skills brief therapy 83–4
CORE (Council on Rehabilitation Education) 4, 6
Corey, G. 80, 94, 139
Cormier, S. 6–7, 35, 40, 48, 49, 50, 58, 68–9, 71, 95
Council for Accreditation of Counseling and Related Educational Programs (CACREP) 4–7, 47, 93, 105–6, 117
Council on Accreditation of Counsellor Education Programs (CACEP) 4
Council on Rehabilitation Education (CORE) 4, 6
counseling: clients with addictions 199–200; definition 3; goal setting in 67–9; overview 71–5; Overview of Theories of 72–5; personal theory of 71–5; person-centered approach 194; preferences 75–80; sexually abused persons 194–6; skills necessary for 93–7; suicidal clients 179–80; theoretical approach to 71
counseling performance skills 36–7
counseling psychology 7
Counseling Techniques List (Table 5.2) 76–80
counselor-in-training 20
counselors: beginning 24–8; certification 7–9; personal theory development by 72; professional 4; state licensure for 9–10; techniques 80–4
Course Objectives and Assignments (syllabus sample) 101–2
course of action, selecting 188
course requirements 26
cover letter 19
Cowell Memorial Hospital 184
Cox, J. 160; "Managed Mental Healthcare: Intentional Misdiagnosis of Mental Disorders" 160
CRC (Certified Rehabilitation Counselor) 8
crimes, reporting 188–9
criminal law 150
crisis 165–72
criteria 16–18
Crothers, L. M. 213
Crucianni, M. 45, 102
Culbreth, J. R. 107
culture 63, 107, 212–13

dangerous clients 157–8, 186–8
DAP (data, assessment, and plan) 41
data, assessment, and plan (DAP) 41
data, relevant 58–9
data-gathering 57
DBT (Dialectical Behavioral Therapy) 84, 86–7
DCT (developmental counseling and therapy) 216
decision-making self-tests 142
defamation 43, 152
defendant 151
demographic factors 186
dependence–reinforcing cognitions of substance abuse 199
descriptive metaphor 107
de Shazer, S. 80–2

desire to die 176
development 12
developmental counseling 215
developmental counseling and therapy (DCT) 216
developmental crises 165
developmental level 95
DHHS (US Department of Health and Human Services) 158; Child Abuse Prevention and Treatment Act 192; Children's Bureau 189
diagnosis in counseling 53–6
Diagnostic and Statistical Manual of Mental: Disorders (DSM) (American Psychiatric Association) 47, 159, 196
diagnostic classifications 47
Dialectical Behavioral Therapy (DBT) 84, 86–7
Dialectic/Systemic 217
dilemmas, ethical 139
Dimick, K 80
direct observation 52–3
disclosure restriction requests 29
disclosure statements 31
discovery process 151
discrimination model 116–17
Doctor-Patient Model 212
documentation 40–5, 153
"do no harm" 27
Douglas, K. S. 186
Draucker, C. B. 194
dress codes 21
DSM (Diagnostic and Statistical Manual of Mental Disorders) 47, 159, 196
DSM-5 196–7; codes and classification 56; "Emerging Measures and Models" 54–5
DSM-IV-TR 54
due process 151
duty and the law 156–8
Dye, A. 111
dysfunctional behaviors 103–4

Eaves, D. 186
eclectic selection model 52
Edwards, N. 194
Eels, T. D. 61
Egan, G. 36, 67, 214
Egan model 36, 93–4
elder abuse 159
electronic mail 143
Electronic PHI 29
Ellis, A. 73, 83
"Emerging Measures and Models" (*DSM-5*) 56
emotions: client 58–9; and substance abuse 199
Engels, E. W. 128
EPL (Exceptional Professional Learning) 218–19
Erikson, E. 73
ethical codes for counselors 135–7
ethical decision making 137–40
ethical guidelines 30
ethical issues 129–47
ethical mandates relating to danger to self 180–1
ethical responsibility 57, 139–40
Ethical Standards for School Counselors (American School Counselors Association) 43
ethics defined 135–6
evaluating suicide risk 178

evaluation: in group supervision 104–5, 108–9; in individual supervision 126–8
evidence-based treatment approaches 58
Exceptional Professional Learning (EPL). 217–18
existential crises 165
Existentialists 75
expert role 213
external consultation 210

Facilitative Interventions 116
faculty liaison 21, *42*
failure to warn 185
Fall, M. 124, 127
False Claims Act 160
Family Education Rights and Privacy Act 41–3
family history data 49
federal guidelines 29
feedback 108, 112
felony, misprision of a 188–9
fidelity 138
field site choice 25
final evaluation 227–8
focused observations 104
forces of change 223–4
Formal-Operational style 216–17
formative evaluation 104–5, 126
Fouad, N. 128
Fowers, B. J. 135
Fowler, J. C. 179
Freud, S. 72
Friend, M. 211
Fromm, E. 74
Fujimura, L. E. 173
Fulton, P. R. 84
functioning, level of 51
Fuqua, D. R. 213–15, 218–19, 223

Galassi, J. P. 58
Gallagher, R. A. 213
gambling addiction 196
Gehart, D. R. 70–1
Germer, C. K. 84
Geroski, A. M. 54
Gilliland, B. E. 165–8
Glosoff, H. L. 155
goals: assessment 50; brief therapy 82; of consultation 214–15; evaluation of 128; statement 121; for substance-abusing clients 200; types of 68–9
goal setting, treatment planning, and treatment modalities 67–89
Gold, Dr. Stuart 184
Gonzales, J. E. 223
good supervision 112
Goodyear, R. K. 107, 111, 115, 118
Gould, M. S. 181
Granello, D. H. 178
Gravois, T. A. 215
Greenberg, T. 181
Greene, D. B. 173
Greenstone, J. L. 171
group supervision: activities in 102–4; concepts in 97–9; in internship 105–9; models 107–8; in practicum 99–102
Gutkin, T. B. 223

Hackney, H. 35, 40, 48, 49, 68–9, 95, 153
Hanson, S. 34, 43
harm to others 184–6
harm to self 173–84
Harrison, R. 194–5
Hart, S. D. 186
Harwood, T. M. 52, 58
Hasbrouck, J. E. 218
Hatcher, R. L. 106
HCR-20 assessment tool 186
Health Insurance Portability and Accountability Act (HIPAA) 29–30, 40, 54
help, seeking 27, 108
helping skills 36–7
Henderson, Donna A. 4
Herlihy, B. 31, 47, 51, 54, 93, 154, 157
"Highlights of Changes From DSM-IV-TR to DSM-5" 56
high-risk clients 184–9
high-risk situations, avoiding 200
Hill, N. R. 118
HIPAA (Health Insurance Portability and Accountability Act) 29–30, 40, 54
history of violence 186
Hohenshil, T. H. 54
Horney, K. 74
hours, documenting 129
Howatt, W. A. 50
Huber, C. H. 135
hypothesis-testing 57

ICD (International Classification of Disorders) 47
ICD-9-CM codes 54, 56
ICD-10-CM codes 54, 56
implanted false memories 194
incompetence 152
individual supervision, approaches to 113–17
Individual supervision in practicum and internship 111–31
influencing skills 37
information gathering 35, 50
informed consent 29, 30–4, 119–21, 160; document (sample) 31–4; elements of 30–1
Ingraham, C. L. 212
initial assessment 48–50
Initial Intake Form (Form 3.3) 39–40, 48, 50
initial session with client 28–9, 35–9
insurance 16, 53, 153, 154
intake: information 39–40, 56; interview 48–9; session 35, 38–9; summary 40
integrated developmental model 115–16
Integrative Model 61–2
intent to commit suicide 177
internal consultation 210
International Classification of Disorders (ICD) 47
internship: group supervision in 105–9; hours 129; summative evaluations in 128; transitioning into 105
interpersonal influence 37
interpersonal skills 47
intervention: consultation 220–1
interventions: range of 69; in schools 169–72
interview questions 19–20
interviews, structured and unstructured 35–7

interviews, third parties during 194
Inverted Pyramid Model 61–3
involuntary commitment 180
"is evidenced by" phrase 41
issue-specific skills 37, 94
Ivey, A. E. 36–7, 67, 94, 216
Ivey, M. B. 216

James, R. K. 165–8
James and Gilliland model of crisis intervention 167–8
Joiner, T. E. 173, 176, 177
Jongsma, A. E. 70
Juhnke, G. A. 57–60
Jung, C. 72
justice 138

Kahn, B. B. 215, 217
Kaiser, T. L. 113
Kanel, K. 166–9
Kanel model of crisis intervention 166–7
Kanfer, F. H. 59–60
Kelly, G. 73
Kelly, K. 152
Kendjelic, E. M. 61
Kilburg, R. R. 222
Kitchener, K. S. 137–8, 140–1
Kitchener, R. F. 138
Kleist, D. M. 118
Knapp, S. 153, 185
Knotek, S. E. 209
Kratochwill, T. R. 220
Krause, F. 80
Kurpius, D. J. 213–15, 218–19, 223

Lambie, G. 194
Lassiter, K. D. 106, 107
law, the 136, 149–50
lawsuits 150–2
learning process, development in the 12
legal issues in child abuse reporting 192
legal issues in counseling 149–64
legal mandates relating to danger to self 180–1
Leib, R. 193
Leviton, S. C. 171
liability and suicide 181
liability insurance 154
libel 152
license to practice 7
licensure for counselors and psychologists 9–10
Life Span Model 116
lifestyle behaviors 200
linchpin model 61–2
locus of control in substance abuse 199
Loganbill, Hardy, and Delworth model 116
"Lousy" supervision 113–14
Lucas, C. P. 61

McDaniel, J. 169–70
McKaskill, Kristi 4
McNeill, B. W. 116
Magnuson, S. 113–14; "Profile of Lousy Supervision: Experienced Counselors' Perspectives, A" 113–14
Mahaffy, A. 159

maintenance 68
Maital, S. L. 223
malpractice 151–2
malpractice insurance 16
managed care 159–61
"Managed Mental Healthcare: Intentional Misdiagnosis of Mental Disorders " (Braun and Cox) 160
mandatory reporting 156, 158–9
Marlyere, K. 189
Marriage, Couple, and Family Therapist 9
Martsolf, D. S. 194
Maslow, A. 74
MAST (Michigan Alcohol Screening Test) 57
MBCT (Mindfulness-based Cognitive Therapy) 85–6
MBSR (Mindfulness-based Stress Reduction) 85
MBT (Mindfulness-based Therapy) 84–5
mediator role 214
medical record access 29
Meichenbaum, D. 173, 179
Meisel, M. A. 188
memories, implanted false 194
mental disorders, definitions of 54–5
mental events 85
mental health 51; consultation 209–11; counseling 47; law 150
Mental Research Institute 82
Mental Status Checklist (Form 4.3) 52
mental status examination 52–3
Merlone, L. 41–4
Michigan Alcohol Screening Test (MAST) 57
microskills training model 36–7
Midpoint Narrative Evaluation of a Practicum Student (sample) 126–7
Mindfulness-based Cognitive Therapy (MBCT) 84, 85
Mindfulness-based Stress Reduction (MBSR) 85
Mindfulness-based Therapy (MBT) 84–5
Minnesota Coalition Against Sexual Assault 195–6
misdiagnosis 160
misprision of a felony 188–9
models 60–3
monitoring 58–9, 188
Monthly Practicum Log (Form 3.7) 43, 45, 127
moods 85–6
Moore, L. 184
morality defined 136
multiaxial assessment system 55
multicultural awareness skills 94–5
multicultural consultation 213
multicultural-intensive observer 107
Murdock, N. 75
Murray, H. 74
Muse-Burke, J. 102
Myer, R. A. 165, 168–9
Myers, J. E. 216
myths about suicide 173–4

NAADAC—The Association for Addiction Professionals 136
Napolitano, L. 107
National Board of Certified Counselors (NBCC) 7, 8, 136; *Policy Regarding the Provision of Distance Professional Services* 144

National Career Development Association 9, 136
National Certified Counselor (NCC) 7–8
National Counselors Exam (NCE) 7–8
National Institute on Drug Abuse (NIDA) 198
NBCC (National Board of Certified Counselors) 7, 8;
    *Policy Regarding the Provision of Distance Professional
    Services* 144
NCC (National Certified Counselor) 7–8
NCE (National Counselors Exam) 8
neglect, child 189
negotiating placement 19–20
Nelson, J. R. 223
Nelson, M. L. 52
Ng, K. M. 107
NIDA (National Institute on Drug Abuse) 198
nonaxial documentation of diagnoses 55
nonmaleficence 138
Norcross, J. C. 67, 68
Norem, K. 113–14; "Profile of Lousy Supervision:
    Experienced Counselors' Perspectives, A" 113–14
Notice of Privacy Practices (NPP) 29–30
NPP (Notice of Privacy Practices) 29–30
Nurius, P. S. 50, 58, 71

Olivos, E. M. 213
orientation 17, 20–1, 219–20
Osborne, C. J. 58, 71
others, information from 50
other specified designation 55–6
Otto, R. 186
outcome goals 68–9
outcome oriented review 58
overdocumentation 153
Overview of Theories of Counseling and
    Psychotherapy (Table 5.1) *72–5*

Parental Release Form (Forms 3.1a and 3.1b) 34
Parker, R. 218
Partlett, D. F. 152
pastoral counseling, standards for 7
Pastoral Counselor 9
Patterson, T. 56, 58
peer consultation 102–4
performance skills 93–4
Perot, A. P. 58
personal files of counselor 42–3
personal history data 49
Personal Information Protection and Electronics
    Documents Act (Office of the Privacy
    Commissioner of Canada, May, 2014) 30
personality change, conditions for 34
personal theory of counseling 71–5
person-centered approach to counseling 194
Peterson, M. 70
phases of practicum and internship 11–12
PHI (Protected Health Information) 29
Piaget, J. 216
placement, negotiating 19–20
plaintiff 151
plea for help 108
Poddar, Prosenjit 184
*Policy Regarding the Provision of Distance Professional
    Services* (NBCC) 144
Pope, K. S. 138, 142, 143

post-crisis responses of children 172
practicum: competencies in professional psychology
    106; experience 24–8; final evaluation in
    105; group supervision in 99–102; hours 45;
    summative evaluation in 126
Practitioner's Guide to Ethical Decision-Making, A
    (ACA) 142
precontemplation 67
preentry 218–19
preferences, theory and technique 72–80
preparation 68
prepracticum 3–22, 10
prescriptive role 213
present moment 85
pretherapy intake information 39–40
pretrial hearings 151
Prevent Child Abuse America: Recognizing Child
    Abuse 189–91
prevention consultants 170
preventive approaches to care 208
principle-based ethics 137–8
privacy 28–30, 154–6
privacy rule, the 29
privileged communication 154–6
problem identification 220
problems, client: assessing 50–2; highest-priority
    82–3; hypotheses and 47
procedural skills 37, 94
Process Consultation 212
process goals 68–9
Prochaska, J. O. 67, 68
professional: codes of ethics 137; functioning 116;
    obligation 184; practices 16–17; skills 94
professional counselor 3–4
professionalization 3
"Profile of Lousy Supervision: Experienced
    Counselors' Perspectives, A" (Magnuson,
    Wilcoxon, and Norem) 113–14
profile sheet guides 21
program-centered administrative consultation 208
program structure 11–12
progress, assessing client 57–60
progress notes 40, 59–60
Prosser, W. I. 152
Protected Health Information (PHI) 29
psychodynamic supervision 115
psychological inflexibility 86
Psychologist licensure 9
psychologists, state licensure for 9–10
Psychosocial History form (Form 3.4) 39–40, 48, 50
psychotherapy supervisors 111
Purchase-of-Expertise Model 211

qualitative assessments 58
questions: to determine potential violence 187; and
    information gathering 47; for site selection 16–18
Quick, E. 82

rapport, developing 31
rational emotive brief therapy 83
RCP (Registered Professional Counsellor): Canadian
    Professional Counsellors Association 8–9
Recognizing Child Abuse (Prevent Child Abuse
    America) 189–91

record keeping 40–5, 153
recovery, stages of 198
recycling 68
Reflective Model 116
Registered Professional Counsellor (RPC): Canadian
    Professional Counsellors Association 8–9
regulations 149
Rehabilitation Counselors 9
relapse 68, 200–1
relationship dynamics 35
relationships, supervisor–supervisee 112–13
release of information 156
relevant data 58–9
Remley, T. P. 31, 47, 51, 54, 93, 154, 157, 223–4
reporting therapeutic progress 60
resistance to consultation 222–3
response teams 170
responsibility, ethical 139
restorying 37
résumé preparation 19
Reyna, C. F. 194
Riley, P. L. 169–70
risk assessment: for dangerous clients 186–8; for
    suicide 176–9
Risk Factors for Suicide (American Foundation for
    Suicide Prevention) 174–5
risk management 153–4
Rockwood, G. F. 211
Rodgers, K. A. 54
Rogers, C. 34, 75
role taking 104

SAFE-T (Suicide Assessment Five Step Evaluation and
    Triage) 178
safety guidelines 171
Sandoval, J. 209
scheduling 26
Schefft, B. K. 59–60
Schein, E. H. 211
Schmidt, J. J. 213
school counseling services 34
school counselors 41–4, 169–72, 210, 213–18
schools: crisis intervention in 169–72; suicide
    prevention programs in 181–2; suicide risk
    assessment and prevention in 181–4
Schwartz, V. E. 152
Schweiger, Wendi K., 4
Schwitzer, A. M. 62
Scott, J. 113
secondary relationships 137
Secondary School Counseling Referral Form (Form
    4.2) 50
security rule, the 29
self-assessment instruments 96
Self-Assessment of Counseling Performance Skills
    (Form 6.1) 104
self-assessment skills 96–7
self-awareness skills 94–5
self-care 154
self-determination 216
self-tests after ethical decision-making 142
Seligman, L. 69, 135
seminars 106–7
semi-structured interview 35–6

Sensorimotor style 216
sessions timing 37
sexually abused children, interviewing 193–4
sexual misconduct 152
sexual relationships 137
SGS (Structured Group Supervision Model) 108
shadowing 21
Shaffer, D. 181
sharing assessment information with client 56–7
Shwery, C. 223
Siegel, R. D., 84
site selection 15–22; criteria for 16–19; guidelines for
    choosing 15–16; negotiating 19–20; orientation at
    20–1; questions before 10; student role at 21
situational crises 165
skills: case formulation 61; counseling 93–7; helping
    36–7; interpersonal 47; for transitioning into
    internship 105
Skinner, B. F., 73
slander 152
Slavik, S. 195
SOAP (subjective, objective, assessment, and plan)
    41
SOAP definitions and examples (Table 3.1) 42
Social media 144–5
solution-focused therapy 36–7, 69, 80–3, 215–17
Sommers-Flanagan, J. 37
Sommers-Flanagan, R. 37
SPAI (Supervisee Performance Assessment
    Instrument) 127
specifiers 55
Sperry, L. 195
SPGS (Structured Peer Group Supervision Model)
    104, 107–8
Spice, C. G. 117
split-focus form 118
Spruill, D. A. 71
staff, professional and site selection 16
standardization 47
standards, accreditation 5–7
state licensure 9–10
statutory laws 149–50
Steenbarger, B. N. 83
Stetson University School of Law Center for
    Excellence in Elder Law 159
Stinchfield, T. A. 118
Stoltenberg, C. D. 116
Stone, A. A. 185
Structured Group Supervision (SGS) Model 108
structured interview 35–6
Structured Peer Group Supervision Model (SPGS)
    104
structuring the initial session 38–9
student counselor 21, 27–8
Student Practicum/Internship Agreement (Form 2.4)
    21
Student Profile Sheet (Form 2.3) 21
students and suicide 181–4
students in crisis, assessing 171–2
subjective, objective, assessment, and plan (SOAP)
    41
subpoenas 151
Substance Abuse and Mental Health Services
    Administration 178

Substance Abuse Assessment Form (Form 10.4) 200
substance-related disorders 195–6
subtypes 55
suicidal client 156–7
suicide 152, 173–84; intervention 179–80; mandates relating to 180–1; myths about 173–5; risk assessment for 176–9; risk factors for 174–5; and students 181–4
Suicide Assessment Five Step Evaluation and Triage (SAFE-T) 178
Suicide Consultation Form (Form 10.1) 180
suicide contracts 179
suicide intervention policy 184
suicide prevention programs in schools 181–2
suicide risk assessment for students 183–4
summative evaluations 126–8
Supervisee Goal Statement (sample) 96–7
Supervisee Performance Assessment Instrument (SPAI) 96, 105, 127
supervision 153; administrative 112; group 105–9; ineffective 113–14; in internship 105–9; in practicum and internship 93–131; psychodynamic 115; session format 123–4
Supervision Continuum 97
Supervision Contract (sample) 122–3
Supervisor Informed Consent and Disclosure Statement (sample) 119–21
supervisors 12, 16, 111–12
Supervisor's Formative Evaluation of Supervisee's Counseling Practice (Form 7.4) 126
supervisor–supervisee relationship 112–13
Sutton, J. M., Jr. 124, 127
Swanson, C. D. 42–3
Sweeney, T. J. 216
Swenson, L. C. 149
systemic crises 165

Tape Critique Form sample (Form 6.5) 100
taping counseling sessions 99–100
Tarasoff, T. 184
Tarasoff Case 157–8, 184–6
techniques: appropriate 27; theory-based 80–4; and theory preferences 72–80
technology-assisted distance counseling 143–4
technology in counseling 142–6
telephones 142–3
termination of counseling services 160
testing 57, 142
theory: based techniques 80–4, 94; and technique preferences 72–80
Theory and Practice of Mental Health Consultation, The (Caplan) 208
therapeutic alliance 28, 34–5
therapeutic confrontation 200
therapeutic progress 60
therapies, third-wave 84–7
therapist, definition of 185
therapy, solution-focused 69
therapy and informed consent 30
third-wave therapies 84–7
threat against self or others 37
time boundaries 37
timing 26, 37, 45
Tindal, G., 218

tort 151
training: for crisis response 170–2; and supervision values 17
transitioning Into internship 105
trauma, understanding 165–9
treatment for substance-related disorders 197–8
treatment planning 69–71, 160
treatment procedures 30
triadic consultation relationship 213
triadic model of supervision 117–18
trial phase 151
triggering events 199
Truscott, S. D. 216
Turtle-Song, I. 42

underdocumentation 153
University of California, Berkeley 184
University of Pittsburgh Counselor Education Program 117
university supervisors 111
unspecified disorder designation 55–6
unstructured interview 35–6
US Department of Health and Human Services: Child Abuse Prevention and Treatment Act 192
US Department of Health and Human Services (DHHS) 158, 189

values of supervisors and site selection 17
VandeCreek, L. 153, 185
Vasquez, M. J. T. 138, 142, 143
virtue-based ethics 140–2
vulnerable adults 159

Wade, J. W. 152
Walcott, D. M. 186
Walfish, S. 189
warning signs for suicide 175–6
Web-based professional discussion groups 145
Web counseling 143–4
websites for ethical codes 136
websites for state licensure 9–10
Webster, C. D. 186
Weekly Schedule (Form 3.6) 45
Weekly Schedule Form (Figure 3.1) 44
Weekly Schedule/Practicum Log (Form 3.6) 43, 127
Weis, D. M. 173
Welfel, E. 56, 154
wellness model of mental health 51
Whiston, S. C. 35–6
WHODAS (World Health Organization Disability Assessment Schedule) 55
WHODAS 2.0, 56
Wiger, D. E. 41
Wigmore, J. H. 155
Wilcoxon, S. A., 113–14; "Profile of Lousy Supervision: Experienced Counselors' Perspectives, A" 113–14
work performance review 128
World Health Organization Disability Assessment Schedule (WHODAS) 55

Zielke, R. 189
Zung Self-Rating Anxiety Scale 57